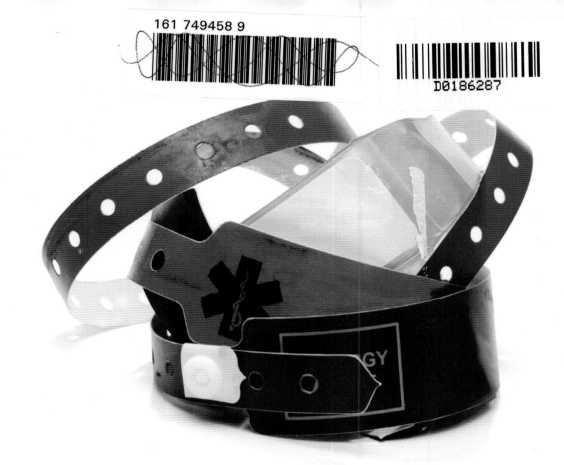

Psychology
for Medicine

'Really good. Interesting, enjoyable, succinct, robust in all areas ... THIS is what will get medical students to start thinking about the importance of psychology'

'Very good! Easy to read and interesting subject matter covered.'

'... flows well when reading and is easy to follow from one section to the next ... unlike many textbooks, it is really easy to read and follow.'

'I liked the use of examples and the non-intimidating style. It doesn't assume knowledge of the subject but at the same time manages not to be patronising!'

'The summaries at the end of each section were useful, as they helped break a large amount of information into sizeable chunks. The life orientation test is great, as it encourages you to think actively about what you have just read.'

'Excellent ... The factual tone will appeal to medical students and the inclusion of slightly quirky studies such as those looking at cardiovascular stress and football matches make it a very engaging read.'

'... succinct in style, highlighting relevant research that illustrates important psychological aspects of medicine. Nicely broken up by boxes, case studies and key research ... the textbook's final design could make it ideal for the intended 'dipping in and out'.

'I really liked reading the case studies on narratives of illness. For me, reading about actual people makes everything more interesting.'

'Really interesting and relevant ... incredibly useful for the first two years of medical school and also as a reference point if problems arise with communication in the future.'

'Overall I found it very easy to follow what was being said and I would definitely consider using this book to supplement a lecture and for reference.'

'Written at a good level, very understandable with good use of examples and references to popular culture. Interesting to read even not as an academic text.'

'Presented in a simple, yet engaging manner and suitable for a wide range of readers, from laypeople, to students and qualified professionals.'

'The inclusion of one of Churchill's most amusing quotes made me smile. This was both funny and still remained relevant.'

'I liked the critical analysis of the research that was presented and the clinical application of the research which was discussed.'

'I liked the part about how people's perception of asthma affected their management of their condition and felt this would be useful to future doctors in any area, who look after people with long-term health problems.'

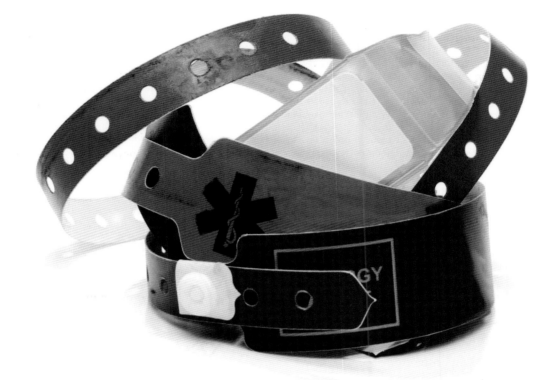

Psychology
for Medicine

Susan Ayers and Richard de Visser

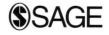

Los Angeles | London | New Delhi
Singapore | Washington DC

First published 2011

SAGE Publications Ltd
1 Oliver's Yard
55 City Road
London EC1Y 1SP

SAGE Publications Inc.
2455 Teller Road
Thousand Oaks, California 91320

SAGE Publications India Pvt Ltd
B 1/I 1 Mohan Cooperative Industrial Area
Mathura Road
New Delhi 110 044

SAGE Publications Asia-Pacific Pte Ltd
33 Pekin Street #02-01
Far East Square
Singapore 048763

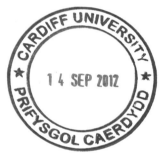

Library of Congress Control Number: 2010924821

British Library Cataloguing in Publication data

A catalogue record for this book is available from the British Library

ISBN 978-1-4129-4690-2
ISBN 978-1-4129-4691-9 (pbk)

Typeset by C&M Digitals (P) Ltd, Chennai, India
Printed in India at Replika Press Pvt Ltd
Printed on paper from sustainable resources

CONTENTS

ACKNOWLEDGEMENTS

There is more to writing a book than assembling its contents, and the story behind this one would make a good read in itself. The journey started because we were frustrated at the lack of a good comprehensive textbook on psychology for medical students. We happened to mention this in passing to the people at SAGE who harnessed all their enthusiasm and considerable expertise into helping us. SAGE started the ball rolling and supported us along the way so we are grateful for their impetus and help – particularly Matthew Waters and Anthony Haynes.

In the two years it has taken us to write this book it has been through many life events, including a new baby, moving house, building work, and travelling around the world. It has been transported by camper van to France and on long haul journeys to Japan, Africa, and Mexico. Unfortunately, close to our deadline one of us left it in a hotel safe in Mexico so we had a major panic in trying to get it back. In the end we enlisted the help of a fellow traveller to bring it back to England (thank you, Mike), who ironically turned out to be travelling with *the* medical director of the NHS! So from inauspicious beginnings this book has already been a big adventure.

Its real story, however, has been produced by the students who have been so important in making it happen. It was only really when students got involved that the book took on a life of its own. We are truly indebted to the many amazing people who have been an integral part of it. First there was our wonderful team of psychology students who gave up their summer vacation to work on the administrative side. Louise Fernay, Lizzie Shine, Gemima Fitzgerald, Amalia Houlton, and Michele McKenner spent many hours researching literature, sourcing copyright permissions, and arranging illustrations with the requisite amount of enthusiasm and unbelievable organisational skills to make sure this book was completed – and with plenty of good humour. We all laughed a lot along the way!

Sandra Popescu is a photography graduate from the University of Brighton who gave up weeks of her time to take many of the photographs that illustrate the book (and can be found in one of them). In fact, most of the models in this book are staff and students from Brighton and Sussex Universities (including we authors – see if you can guess who we are!). At this point we should say that many of the case studies are fictional and the photographs used are of volunteer models. Where real stories have been included this is usually made clear from the text and we have acknowledged each person in the case study.

The input from students didn't stop there. Simon Hall is a great artist who happened to be studying medicine whilst we were putting this book together. He spent much of his time between hospital shifts drawing the cartoons for this book so we are deeply indebted to him. We were also lucky in having excellent medical consultants advise us on chapters throughout the book.

In addition we must thank the medical students who read, re-read, and commented on every chapter through various drafts. They gave us their honest opinions and helped make this book what it is. When we asked for volunteers we never dreamt so many students would get involved. Students told us what they liked and didn't like; where we had the tone wrong; what features were missing. We were humbled by their enthusiasm, the amount of time they put in, and the expertise they brought to this book. Every review had something of importance and we learnt that some of our students had had previous careers as editors, journalists, lawyers, and other illustrious professions. The student reviews were single-handedly responsible for clinical notes being added to chapters. We have been inspired by many of these people and are very grateful for their input. We have listed all of these below in order to recognise their contribution to this book. We would also welcome any further feedback from you and can be contacted at psychologyformedicine@gmail.com.

By the time it went to press this book had already been a great experience and a witness to the combined efforts of many people who gave their considerable time and energy to get it there. This must clearly include our respective families who put up with two years of us being total book-bores and still supported us at every step. SA – love and thanks to my partner Andrew, children Hannah and Callum, and close family who support me in so many ways and remind me of the truly important things in life. RdV - thanks to Susan for asking me to be part of this book-writing process. Much love and many thanks to my partner Liz and children Thom, Felix, and Iris for giving me lots of 'book time' and for making the 'non-book time' so enjoyable.

RESEARCH AND ADMINISTRATIVE SUPPORT

Amalia Houlton, Clinical Psychology Department, University of Leicester
Gemima Fitzgerald, School of Psychology, University of Sussex
Lizzie Shine, School of Psychology, University of Sussex
Louise Fernay, School of Psychology, University of Sussex

COPYRIGHT PERMISSIONS

Michele McKenner, School of Psychology, University of Sussex

CARTOONS

Simon Hall, Brighton & Sussex Medical School

CHAPTER REVIEWS

Alice Hart-George, Brighton & Sussex Medical School
Alifa Isaacs Itua, Brighton & Sussex Medical School
Alison Burridge, Brighton & Sussex Medical School
Alison Pike, School of Psychology, University of Sussex
Amina Buba, Brighton & Sussex Medical School
Andrew Eagle, Central & North West London NHS Trust
Andy McGovern, Brighton & Sussex Medical School
Anna Crown, Brighton & Sussex University Hospitals
Ben Carter, Brighton & Sussex Medical School
Camilla Davis, Brighton & Sussex Medical School
Camilla Tooley, Brighton & Sussex Medical School
Charlotte Marks, Brighton & Sussex Medical School
Eleanor de Sausmarez, Brighton & Sussex Medical School
Georgie Kirby, Brighton & Sussex Medical School
Imogen Bone, Brighton & Sussex Medical School
Joseph Norris, Brighton & Sussex Medical School
Julia Montgomery, Brighton & Sussex University Hospitals
Julian Birch, Brighton & Sussex Medical School
Julie Appleton, Brighton & Sussex Medical School
Karen Walker-Bone, Brighton & Sussex Medical School
Katie Bishop, Brighton & Sussex Medical School
Leon Campbell, Brighton & Sussex Medical School
Lewys Morgan, Brighton & Sussex Medical School
Liam Mahoney, Brighton & Sussex Medical School
Lizzie Jackson, Brighton & Sussex Medical School
Meher Lad, Brighton & Sussex Medical School
Natalie Farmer, Brighton & Sussex Medical School
Patrick Harrington, Brighton & Sussex Medical School
Pollie Harrison, Brighton & Sussex Medical School
Rakshita Roplekar, Brighton & Sussex Medical School
Reshad Malik, Brighton & Sussex Medical School
Ruth Arnold, Brighton & Sussex Medical School
Sarah King, School of Psychology, University of Sussex
Sophie Binks, Brighton & Sussex Medical School

PHOTOGRAPH MODELS

Abeer Faisal Al Amin, University of Brighton
Alice Campion, Brighton & Sussex Medical School
Alison Burridge, Brighton & Sussex Medical School
Amy Tostevin, University of Sussex

Bobbie Farsides, Brighton & Sussex Medical School
Bradley Tully, University of Sussex
Callum Smith, University of Sussex
Cat Tighe, University of Brighton
Chris Boyson, Brighton & Sussex Medical School
Claire Brooks, Brighton & Sussex Medical School
Daisy Ryan, Brighton & Sussex Medical School
David Smalley, University of Sussex
Emma Brennan, Brighton & Sussex Medical School
Erica Strang, University of Brighton Postgraduate Medical School
Farrah Shah, Brighton & Sussex Medical School
Francesca Flohr, Brighton & Sussex Medical School
Gemima Fitzgerald, University of Sussex, and her daughter Emily Mason
Jim Price, University of Brighton Postgraduate Medical School
Joe Hinds, University of Sussex
Katie Stillwell, University of Brighton
Kuljinder Danjhal, University of Sussex
Liz Ford, University of Sussex, and her baby Eva Ford
Liz McDonnell, University of Brighton, and her children Thom, Felix, and Iris de Visser
Louise Fernay, University of Sussex, and her family Lindsay, Keith, and Zoe Fernay
Luke Holland, Brighton & Sussex Medical School
Mehreen Rizvi, Brighton & Sussex Medical School
Melanie Martin, University of Brighton
Natalie Farmer, Brighton & Sussex Medical School
Nathan Gardner, University of Sussex
Patrick Saintas, University of Brighton
Robert Miller, University of Brighton
Rose Meades, School of Psychology, University of Sussex
Sandra Popescu, graduate of University of Brighton
Sara Balouch, University of Sussex
Sara Smith, University of Brighton
Sarah Wade, University of Brighton
Warran Woodruff, University of Brighton
Wesely Scott-Smith, University of Brighton Postgraduate
    Medical School
Will Butterworth, Brighton & Sussex Medical School
Zonunmawia Zonunmtwit, University of Brighton

GUIDED TOUR

Chapter Contents Every chapter has a clear, numbered list of the contents of the chapter including major sections, subheadings, case studies, research boxes and other features.

LEARNING OBJECTIVES

This chapter is designed to enable you to:

- Describe motivation and discuss how it affects health.
- Outline the different components of emotion.
- Appreciate the role of positive and negative emotions in health.
- Consider whether expressing emotion is good or bad for health.

Motivation, emotion, and the way we respond to stress shape our lives in many ways. Emotions are powerful motivators that can even make us risk our lives in extreme cases, such as when parents risk their lives trying to save their children. In medicine, more than in any other profession, we are surrounded by stressful and emotional events as people face illness and death, either their own or others. How people respond to these situations varies hugely and there are many examples in medicine of people behaving in ways we might not understand. For example, the woman in Case Study 2.1 was prepared to risk her own and her unborn baby's life rather than have a Caesarean section.

The media are full of similar examples: parents refusing life-saving treatment for their child on religious grounds; a man with liver cirrhosis who continues to drink alcohol even though he knows it will kill him; a pregnant woman with cancer who refuses chemotherapy and then dies just after her daughter is born; a teenage girl who cuts her arms with a razor blade to blunt her feelings. These are real cases that illustrate the importance of beliefs, motivation, and emotion in how people respond to day-to-day stress and extreme situations. They also illustrate the complex interaction between motivation and emotion. In this chapter we shall look at motivation and emotion in turn, examining what these are, and how they are relevant to health.

Learning Objectives Learning objectives are given at the beginning of each chapter. These state the most important things we hope you will learn from each chapter.

decision making (see Chapter 17). Some motives are biological – for example, the desire to eat, drink, or reproduce. Others are more psychological and social – for example, the drive for achievement and status. Box 2.1 gives some examples of biological and social motives, although it is worth noting that the distinction between biological and social motives is not clear cut. For example, sexual motives can be both biological (the drive to reproduce) and social (e.g. affiliation and nurturance).

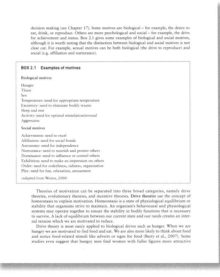

BOX 2.1 Examples of motives

Biological motives

Hunger
Thirst
Sex
Temperature: need for appropriate temperature
Excretory: need to eliminate bodily wastes
Sleep and rest
Activity: need for optimal stimulation/arousal
Aggression

Social motives

Achievement: need to excel
Affiliation: need for social bonds
Autonomy: need for independence
Nurturance: need to nourish and protect others
Dominance: need to influence or control others
Exhibition: need to make an impression on others
Order: need for orderliness, tidiness, organisation
Play: need for fun, relaxation, amusement

(adapted from Westen, 2004)

Theories of motivation can be separated into three broad categories, namely drive theories, evolutionary theories, and incentive theories. **Drive theories** use the concept of homeostasis to explain motivation. Homeostasis is a state of physiological equilibrium or stability that organisms strive to maintain. An organism's behavioural and physiological systems may operate together to ensure the stability in bodily functions that is necessary to survive. A lack of equilibrium between our current state and our needs creates an internal tension which we are motivated to reduce.

Drive theory is most easily applied to biological drives such as hunger. When we are hungry we are motivated to find food and eat. We are also more likely to think about food and notice food-related stimuli like adverts or signs for food (Berry et al., 2007). Some studies even suggest that hungry men find women with fuller figures more attractive

Boxes Boxes are used to illustrate key concepts described in the text. Some of these are lists of key points, some are descriptions of important issues, and others are diagrams or tables of information.

people could not consciously 'see' them. They found that even though people could not 'see' the words, they reported a more negative mood after being shown negative words. Other experiments have shown that if we 'see' something preconsciously we are more likely to prefer it or feel good if it is shown to us so we can consciously see it (Monahan et al., 2000).

Theories of emotion vary in focus. One way to conceptualise emotion is to divide it into positive and negative affect (Watson and Tellegen, 1985). Thus all emotions can be plotted according to whether they are positive (e.g. pleasurable) or negative (e.g. distressing), and on a second dimension according to intensity (high versus low) as shown in Figure 2.4. This has the advantage of simplifying emotions so it is easier to look at relationships between emotions, health, and illness. It also accounts for the *intensity* of emotion which may be important in the effect emotion can have on health. It is quite reasonable to assume that emotion at a low level of intensity (e.g. irritation) will have a different physiological effect and influence on health from a high intensity emotion (e.g. extreme anger).

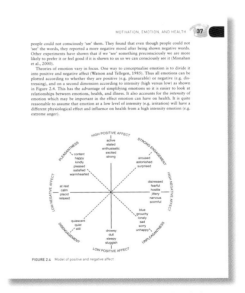

FIGURE 2.4 Model of positive and negative affect

Figures A variety of figures are used to help you understand the material described in the text. These include photographs, diagrams, flowcharts, and theoretical models.

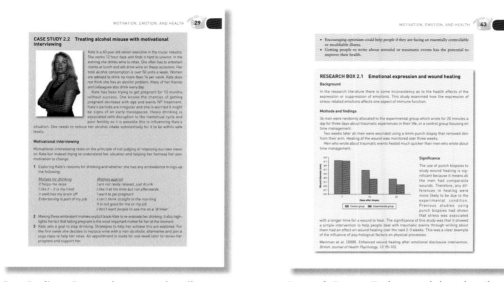

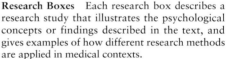

Case Studies   Case studies are used to illustrate patients' experiences of the issues described in the text. They also show how psychological theories and techniques can be used in clinical practice to help patients.

Research Boxes   Each research box describes a research study that illustrates the psychological concepts or findings described in the text, and gives examples of how different research methods are applied in medical contexts.

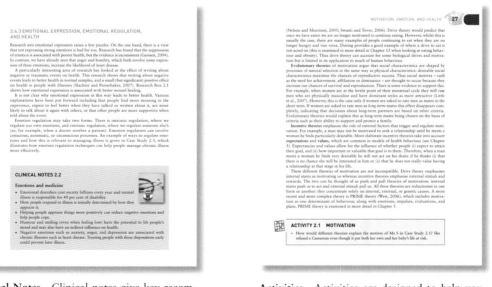

Clinical Notes   Clinical notes give key recommendations and tips for medical practice based on the psychological principles and techniques described in the text.

Activities   Activities are designed to help you stop and think about the information contained in the text and how it might apply to your own life.

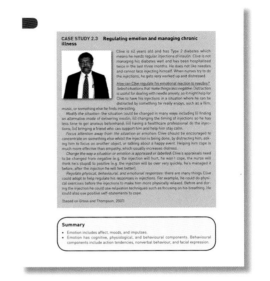

Cartoons Cartoons provide time out from the masses of words and provide a more humorous view of psychology and medicine!

Summaries Each section concludes with a bullet-point summary of the most important psychological theories and applications covered in that section. These summaries relate to the learning objectives and revision questions so will help you learn and revise.

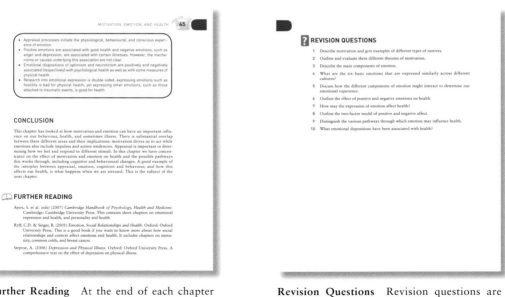

Further Reading At the end of each chapter there are suggestions for further reading, along with brief comments about each book to help you choose which ones to read.

Revision Questions Revision questions are included at the end of every chapter to help you learn and revise for exams.

1 PSYCHOLOGY AND MEDICINE

LEARNING OBJECTIVES

This chapter is designed to enable you to:

- Understand different definitions of health and discuss the implications of this for treatment.
- Describe the biomedical and biopsychosocial approaches to healthcare.
- Consider the role of psychological and social factors in healthcare.

1.1 PSYCHOLOGY AND MEDICINE

The importance of psychology for medicine is being increasingly recognised and psychological topics are now included in most medical curricula. In the UK, a report on *Tomorrow's Doctors* emphasised the need for a greater incorporation of psychological and social sciences in medical training (General Medical Council, 2009). This rests on a wealth of research evidence that psychological factors are important in many aspects of physical and mental health – as you will see throughout the course of this textbook.

Yet it has been our experience that there are a number of barriers to medical students learning about psychological topics. First, psychology is often seen as a 'soft' science in medicine. It is a bit like medical Marmite – students either love it or hate it! We will come back to this later on in the chapter but hope this book will encourage the sceptics among you to explore psychology more and use it in clinical practice. Second, psychology is a wide-ranging discipline that includes many specialisms. As a result, few students or doctors have the time to become familiar with the rich evidence base and psychological theory that are available. Box 1.1 shows the different psychological specialisms with examples of how these may be relevant to medicine. Psychology's breadth of scope makes it hard for healthcare professionals to work out which parts are most relevant to clinical practice. Third, being bombarded with psychobabble in the press makes it even more difficult to screen out evidence-based information from popular 'fact'. A further challenge is working out where medical care stops and psychological or social care begins.

A final difficulty is that, until now, there has been no integrated textbook that covered all the aspects of psychology that were relevant to medicine and highlighted the clinical relevance and application of this information. We hope this book solves this problem by providing a single, integrated overview of the psychology that is relevant to medicine and by considering how this can be used in medical practice. This is done in four sections. In this introductory chapter we examine fundamental conceptual issues of what we mean by health and illness, why psychology is important, and different approaches to medicine.

Section I focuses on psychology of health and covers theories and research relevant to most areas of medical practice, such as stress, symptoms, and chronic illness. Section II discusses knowledge from other areas of psychology that is relevant, such as brain and behaviour, development from infancy to old age, and the effects of social context on

BOX 1.1   Specialisms in psychology

Specialism	Focus	Relevance to medicine
Health	Psychological factors and health	Understanding health behaviour, effective health promotion and intervention, the link between psychosocial factors and health.
Clinical	Psychological disorders	Understanding emotions, emotional disorders (psychopathology), and developing effective interventions.
Developmental	Development and change over the lifespan	Understanding about normal and abnormal aspects of development across the lifespan.
Forensic	Criminal and judicial behaviour and systems	Understanding crime when relevant to medicine. Medico-legal investigations and testimony.
Social	Social and group processes	Understanding how social and group processes influence our own and patients' behaviour in medical settings.
Biological and Neuropsychological	Link between physiological and mental processes or behaviour	Understanding the interaction between psychological and physical systems.
Cognitive	Internal mental processes e.g. perception, memory	Understanding risk perception and decision making. How memory processes affect adherence to medication.
Occupational	Work, the workplace, and organisations	Understanding work performance and training requirements. How medical organisations function.
Educational	Learning and education	Improving education or training for healthcare professionals. Health education.

people's behaviour. Section III focuses on psychology that is relevant to different body systems, including cardiovascular, respiratory, gastrointestinal, immune, genitourinary, and reproductive systems. Finally, Section IV outlines psychology that is relevant to clinical practice, such as communication skills and psychological interventions.

Throughout the book you will find clinically relevant information and tips in the clinical notes boxes. Activity boxes will encourage you to apply psychology to your own experiences. Learning objectives and summary boxes also provide easy guides to the main learning points that may prove useful for exams. Revision questions are given at the end of every chapter to help you revise and test yourself.

1.2 WHAT IS HEALTH?

As healthcare professionals you will be embarking on careers that will commit you to helping people get better. But 'better', like 'health' is not the same for everyone. How then can we decide who to treat and who not to treat? Take a look at the examples in Case Study 1.1 and the definitions of health in Box 1.2.

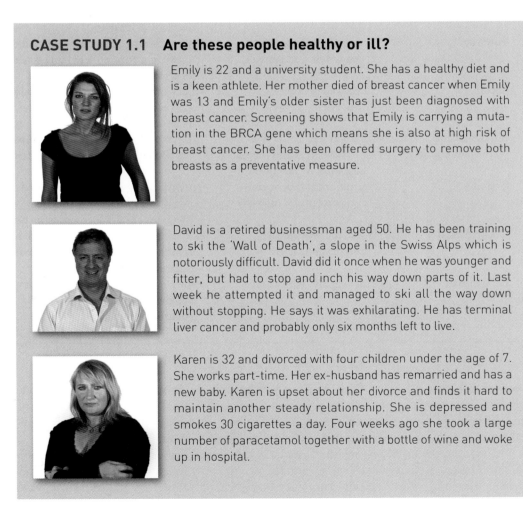

CASE STUDY 1.1   Are these people healthy or ill?

Emily is 22 and a university student. She has a healthy diet and is a keen athlete. Her mother died of breast cancer when Emily was 13 and Emily's older sister has just been diagnosed with breast cancer. Screening shows that Emily is carrying a mutation in the BRCA gene which means she is also at high risk of breast cancer. She has been offered surgery to remove both breasts as a preventative measure.

David is a retired businessman aged 50. He has been training to ski the 'Wall of Death', a slope in the Swiss Alps which is notoriously difficult. David did it once when he was younger and fitter, but had to stop and inch his way down parts of it. Last week he attempted it and managed to ski all the way down without stopping. He says it was exhilarating. He has terminal liver cancer and probably only six months left to live.

Karen is 32 and divorced with four children under the age of 7. She works part-time. Her ex-husband has remarried and has a new baby. Karen is upset about her divorce and finds it hard to maintain another steady relationship. She is depressed and smokes 30 cigarettes a day. Four weeks ago she took a large number of paracetamol together with a bottle of wine and woke up in hospital.

BOX 1.2   Definitions of health

Definition	Features of definition	Are they healthy or ill?		
		Emily	David	Karen
Physical	Absence of disease	Healthy	Ill	Healthy
	Not vulnerable to disease	Ill	Ill	Healthy
	Strong physical reserves	Healthy	Ill	Healthy
	Physically fit, has vitality	Healthy	Healthy	Ill
Subjective	No symptoms of physical illness	Healthy	Ill	Healthy
Behavioural	Living a healthy lifestyle	Healthy	Healthy	Ill
Functional	Able to function in day-to-day life	Healthy	Healthy	Ill
Psychosocial	Psychosocial wellbeing	Healthy	Healthy	Ill
Social	Able to contribute to society	Healthy	Healthy	Ill
Cultural	Matches cultural norm for health	Healthy	Ill	Ill

These cases illustrate that 'health' is not easy to define and is very individual. Research shows that people with a terminal illness generally have a reduced quality of life. Yet quality of life is not a single entity and although people may report worse physical symptoms, pain, and disability they may also report an increased appreciation of life and family and other positive benefits (as David's case illustrates). Karen may be particularly at risk, as research shows that young, divorced or widowed women are most likely to attempt suicide (although men are more likely to succeed at committing suicide). Being depressed is a critical risk factor – in Europe, 28 per cent of people with clinical depression will attempt suicide at some point during their lives (Bernal et al., 2007). Cases like Emily's will become more common as screening for genetic risk becomes more widespread. Women who have prophylactic mastectomies generally report a reduction in cancer-related distress afterwards, although there can be other negative impacts on their lives.

It should be clear that health issues are complex and require our consideration of the individual. We need to recognise that, for individuals, health and illness are subjective states of wellbeing. In other words, does the person *feel* or *think* they are healthy or ill? Do they have physical symptoms that they believe mean there is a problem with their health? We also need to take account of disease in the form of underlying pathology – although research shows that a physiological basis is not found for the majority of physical symptoms. In fact, an organic cause is usually only found for 10–15 per cent of symptoms reported by patients in primary care (Katon and Walker, 1998).

Health operates on many levels such as the physical, subjective, behavioural, functional, and social. One survey of around 9,000 people found that we generally think of health in six different ways (Blaxter, 1990):

1   Not having symptoms of illness.
2   Having physical or social reserves.
3   Having healthy lifestyles.
4   Being physically fit or vital.
5   Psychological wellbeing.
6   Being able to function.

Which of these definitions we use will have implications for who receives treatment. Box 1.2 applies these to the cases of David, Karen, and Emily. It shows, for each one, who would be considered healthy and who would be considered ill. Common sense would suggest that both David and Karen are ill and need treatment. David has terminal cancer and Karen has attempted suicide. Yet David would be classified as ill by physical definitions of health but not by behavioural, functional or psychosocial definitions. In contrast, Karen would be classified as ill by behavioural, function and psychosocial definitions but not by physical. In fact, the only definition of health that would classify both of them as ill is the cultural norm for health – in other words, they are both outside the norm within our society for what is regarded as healthy.

ACTIVITY 1.1   WHAT IS HEALTH?

- Rate your own health on a scale from 1 (very poor) to 10 (excellent).
- What factors were important in helping you decide where to rate your health?

We therefore need to think of health on many levels. The World Health Organisation (WHO) attempted this by defining **health** very broadly as *'a state of complete physical, mental, and social wellbeing and not merely the absence of disease or infirmity'* (WHO, 1992). The value of this definition is that it is inclusive and the emphasis on wellbeing accounts for individual differences in subjective perceptions of health. However, this definition has been criticised for being too broad to be useful and for referring to a Utopian 'perfect' state that few of us will reach, even when we feel healthy.

To quibble over definitions of health might seem pedantic but these have wide ranging implications for the treatments provided by health services. For example, if we aim for health as defined by the WHO it would put unrealistic pressures on countries to provide social circumstances and medical systems that mean everyone lives in a state of complete wellbeing. Others have pointed out that the conception of complete wellbeing confuses happiness with health (Saracci, 1997). This opens the door to limitless treatments if people view the pursuit of happiness as a legitimate medical goal. The rapid increase in cosmetic surgery to help people feel happier with their appearance is one example of this.

The way we define health therefore has implications for who can be seen as responsible for our health and for which treatments we offer. These implications are more than just medical and affect society's policies and laws. In the Western world, the dominant view is that individuals are responsible for their health by adopting healthy or unhealthy lifestyles. Policies have been implemented that attempt to improve our lifestyles and health, such as providing fruit for young school children and banning smoking in public places.

A striking example of the effect that our definition of health has on treatment is the increasing numbers of obese children being put into foster care by the authorities in an attempt to combat their obesity. The story of one such girl is given in Case Study 1.2. This course of action rests on a number of debateable assumptions, including the view that:

1 Obesity is an illness.
2 Obesity is controllable through diet.
3 Parental behaviour is the major cause of childhood obesity.
4 A child's physical health takes priority over the psychological impact of removing that child from their family.

Ultimately, the multidimensional nature of health makes finding an adequate definition difficult. Antonovsky (1987) therefore proposed that we think of **health as a continuum** from optimal wellness to death as shown in Figure 1.1. Health promotion techniques operate on the wellness side of the continuum to encourage people to choose a lifestyle that optimises their health. Medical treatment focuses on the illness side of the continuum when people show signs or symptoms of illness. The irony in the UK is that our medical system is called the National *Health* Service yet it deals predominantly with the illness end of the continuum!

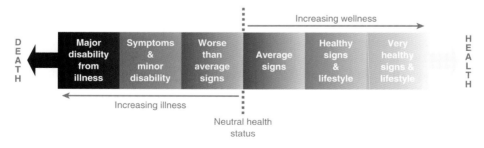

FIGURE 1.1 Illness–wellness continuum
Source: Antonovsky, 1987 – adapted from Sarafino, 2002

CASE STUDY 1.2   Anamarie Martinez-Regino

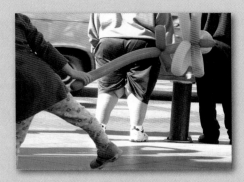

In August 2000, in a controversial case, New Mexico State took legal custody of 3 year old Anamarie Martinez-Regino because she was morbidly obese. She was removed from her parents and put in foster care for three months. A gagging order was put on her parents so they could not talk publicly about the case for five months.

Anamarie weighed three times more than a normal 3 year old and was 50 per cent taller. She had undergone numerous tests to determine what was causing her increased growth but doctors could not find a medical cause.

While in foster care, Anamarie was put on a strict diet, lost weight, and learned to walk unassisted. It is difficult to gauge the emotional impact of being taken from her parents (e.g. she stopped speaking Spanish, her father's language).

After three months of legal and political wrangling, Anamarie was returned to her parents, although the state kept legal custody of her for a while, monitoring her progress. Years later Anamarie lives at home with her parents on a strict diet and exercise programme. She is still obese and is growing much quicker than other children her age. At seven years of age she was 5 foot 1 inch and her condition continues to be a medical mystery. (Photograph reproduced courtesy of Malingering/www.flikr.com)

1.3 WHY IS PSYCHOLOGY IMPORTANT?

The importance of treating the person and not just the disease is widely recognised. Each person is a unique mix of thoughts, emotions, personality, behaviour patterns, and their own personal history and experiences. Understanding more about this will help us treat our patients better. Psychology, however, as we have said is a rather like medical Marmite – you either love it or hate it! Those who do not like it will often comment that 'It's just common sense', 'It's interesting but I can't see how it's useful', and 'I prefer to do real medicine'. Here we will consider each of these objections in turn.

'Psychology is just common sense'

Often statements from psychological research will indeed coincide with common sense. Examples of these include 'Stress is bad for you', 'A healthy lifestyle is important', and 'People with chronic illness have a worse quality of life'. If this was all we could take from psychology, then most of us would indeed dismiss the subject as mere common sense. The value of psychological research is that:

- It *tests* commonsense views empirically to confirm or disconfirm them.
- It goes *beyond* common sense.
- People don't always act according to common sense!

First, let's look at the empirical testing of commonsense views. Much common sense is in fact contradictory. For example, the proverbs 'Too many cooks spoil the broth' and 'Many hands make light work' contradict each other. In some cases psychological research has confirmed commonsense views, whilst for others it has rejected these. Some examples of commonsense views that have been tested by research are given in Box 1.3 – take a look at these statements and make up your own mind about whether these are facts or myths.

BOX 1.3   Common sense: fact or myth?

1 Getting old leads to depression and social withdrawal[1]
2 People are happier if they have a better standard of living[1]
3 Worried patients are reassured by negative test results[2]
4 Character is formed by parental discipline[1]
5 Being out in wet weather makes you more likely to catch a cold[3]
6 Taking vitamin C prevents colds[4]
7 Bed rest is a good adjunctive treatment for medical conditions[2]

Sources: 1 – McCrae & Costa (2003); 2 – Flaherty (2007); 3 – NIAID (2006); 4 – Hemilä et al. (2007)

In fact, all of the views given in Box 1.3 have not been supported by research. Research therefore not only challenges common sense but also examines the things that go beyond common knowledge, such as why depression puts people at a higher risk of heart disease, whether there are critical periods in development when babies are more sensitive to psycho-social or biological circumstances, and whether psychotherapy should try to change *what* people think or the *relationship* people have with their thoughts. There are many other examples of this that you will read about throughout the course of this book.

'Psychology is interesting but not useful'

Most people will find at least some parts of psychology interesting, but that does not necessarily mean it is useful. We need to ask what exactly it means in medicine for something to be useful. If the goal in medicine is to treat people effectively and restore them to health, what does this involve and how can psychology help? In order to treat people effectively we need to be able to (i) diagnose the problem accurately and (ii) treat that problem appropriately. Psychology can help in both these areas. Accurate diagnoses can be helped by understanding how people's beliefs shape their help-seeking behaviours, perceptions, and their reporting of symptoms (see Chapter 4). Negotiating an acceptable and effective treatment plan can be assisted by understanding decision making, what makes people more likely to adhere to treatment, and the influence of people's beliefs and emotions (see Chapter 17). In illnesses, such as HIV, where there is no medical cure behaviour change is crucial for limiting the spread of disease (see Chapter 15). Effective communication skills can facilitate this (see Chapter 18). Thus understanding psychological and social processes will help us both diagnose and treat people effectively.

Psychology can also help us to understand psychological *symptoms*, such as anxiety and depression, which can range from mild to severe, as well as *diagnostic disorders* such as panic disorder, major depressive disorder or schizophrenia. In the UK, psychological symptoms of anxiety and depression account for approximately 9 per cent of consultations in general practice (Office for National Statistics, 2000). However, the majority of patients with psychological symptoms will present with physical symptoms (Kroenke, 2003a). One study asked primary care physicians in the UK (GPs) to rate the content of 2,206 consultations and found that, in addition to consultations for psychological symptoms, 30 per cent of consultations were rated as involving some psychological content (Ashworth et al., 2003).

Evidently there is a strong link between physical health and psychological health and if we concentrate on only one side we risk missing important information and prescribing ineffective treatments. For example, chronic illness is associated with increased rates of psychological disorders (Cooke et al., 2007). People with psychological disorders are also at an increased risk of illness. A worldwide study of the link between medically unexplained symptoms and psychological disorders found that 69 per cent of patients with five or more unexplained symptoms had a psychological disorder, compared to 4 per cent of patients with no unexplained symptoms (Kisely et al., 1997). Psychological interventions, such as cognitive behaviour therapy (CBT), can be effective in managing or treating illnesses that have physical and psychological components, such as obesity, chronic pain, irritable bowel syndrome, and addiction (see Chapters 11 to 16). Psychological interventions can also be used to treat a range of psychological disorders, including bipolar disorder, personality disorder, and schizophrenia (see Chapters 16 and 19).

While psychological knowledge can help us be more effective medical practitioners, many students are put off psychology because of a sense that it is 'woolly' or 'interesting, but there's no right answer'. Psychology can appear abstract or ambiguous with many competing theories. The reasons for this are that when studying people we must deal with outcomes, such as behaviour, that are influenced by many factors. Explanatory theories are therefore tested by using a range of research methods and statistics to try to identify which factors are the most important. This means psychology will often present students with competing theories and supporting or conflicting evidence (and this book is no exception!). The ambiguity or uncertainty this involves may contrast directly with the large amount of physiological and anatomical facts students are required to learn in the first few years of their medical degree.

So psychology may require a different way of thinking, but there should be no doubt that this method of thinking is a useful skill in itself – and one that can prove essential in later medical practice. For example, patients will rarely present with a clearly defined textbook set of symptoms. In trying to diagnose and treat a patient, you will often have to form a hypothesis about what might be wrong, then find a way to test it, and then reformulate your hypothesis if the tests do not confirm it. There are still many medical conditions that do not have suitable tests to confirm them. Examples include chronic fatigue syndrome and irritable bowel syndrome (see Chapter 13). As with psychological learning, these conditions involve a tolerance of ambiguity and an openness to alternative explanations, particularly in the early stages of diagnosis and treatment.

'Psychology is not real medicine'

Most students will come to their medical studies keen to learn about the workings of the body, how it goes wrong, and how to fix it. Learning about the heart and how to resuscitate people is much closer to the common view of what it means to be a medical doctor than learning about such topics as health behaviour and stress. This implies a mechanical view of the body and medicine. Such a view is not new: it stems from a belief in dualism, according to which the mind and body are seen as independent. Dualism has its roots in classical philosophy and was reinforced by later thinkers, such as René Descartes (1637). Focusing on the mechanics of the body enabled rapid advances in medicine during the eighteenth and nineteenth century. Medical understanding grew exponentially as doctors and researchers focused on increasingly detailed physiological processes and identified the causes of pathology. Treatment also advanced: antibiotics and vaccines were developed and anaesthesia was introduced. The disadvantage of dualism is that it resulted in the **biomedical approach** or model, which dominated medicine for centuries. This approach, which is examined below, is based on a separation of body and mind that is unhelpful in many ways.

1.4 DIFFERENT APPROACHES TO MEDICINE

1.4.1 BIOMEDICAL APPROACH

The biomedical approach to medicine is summarised in Figure 1.2. This approach assumes that all disease can be explained in terms of physiological processes: therefore the treatment acts on the disease and not on the person. There is a linear progression of causality from the pathogen to the person and not the other way around. Psychological and social processes are separate and incidental. The person as a whole is therefore not considered by the biomedical approach.

Although this view has dominated medicine and led to great advances it has been criticised for many reasons, in particular that it does not consider the influence of (i) social or

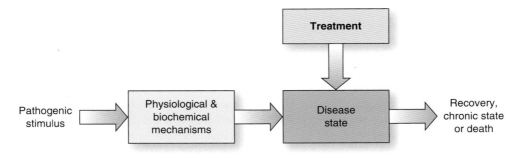

FIGURE 1.2 Biomedical approach to health (adapted from Lovallo, 2004)

(ii) psychological factors on health. Historically, the influence of social factors on population health is clear. Let us take the example of infectious diseases. Figure 1.3 shows the rapid decline in deaths from infectious diseases in the UK between 1859 and 1978 and also shows when vaccines were introduced. You can see that the largest decreases in deaths from infectious diseases occurred *before* most vaccines were introduced. Some of the reason for this can

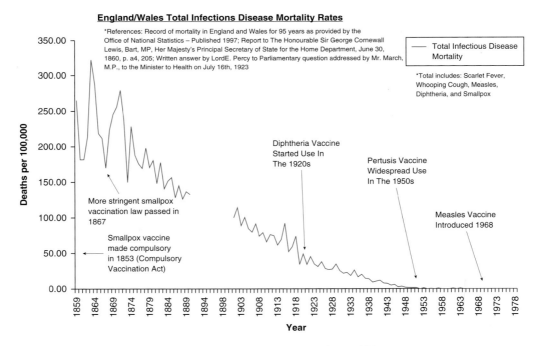

FIGURE 1.3 Decline in mortality from infectious diseases in the UK
Graph reproduced courtesy of Roman Bystrianyk (www.healthsentinel.com)

be explained by more effective treatments, but a lot was due to changes in people's understanding of illness and the effect of lifestyle. For example, in the mid-1800s a physician, John Snow, noticed that patterns of cholera outbreaks clustered around particular water supplies in London. This led to a better understanding of the cause and transmission of cholera; as well as social changes such as an improved water supply and sanitation. Here we can see that biomedical or public health knowledge provided the impetus for social change and that the reduction of cholera and many other diseases cannot be explained on a purely biomedical basis.

Social factors are just as important today. One of the most consistent findings from public health research is the influence of social class on health. People in lower social classes are at more risk of illness (**morbidity**) or death (**mortality**) from a variety of causes. This increased risk is partly due to differences in lifestyles. For example, people in lower social classes have a poorer diet, harder working and living conditions, and are more likely to smoke. However, studies that examine this indicate that even after these factors are taken into account people in lower social classes still remain at an increased risk of poor health (see Research Box 1.1).

RESEARCH BOX 1.1   Social class and morbidity

Background

In addition to being affected by health behaviours, morbidity and mortality rates are affected by socioeconomic status. This study was designed to determine the relative importance of social class and health behaviour.

Methods and findings

The Danish National Work Environment Cohort Study was a prospective study of 5,001 people aged 18 to 59 years-old and assessed over five years. Participants were interviewed in the first year and five years later. Measures were taken of self-rated health, social class, lifestyle factors, and work.

People in the lowest social class were over three times more likely to report poor health than people in the highest social class, and their health was more likely to deteriorate over the five years of the study. However, poor health was also associated with lifestyle (smoking, obesity) and work factors (repetitive, unskilled job, poor security, more exposure to weather, and physical risks). Lifestyle and work factors accounted for 66 per cent of the effect of social class on health, with work factors making the strongest contribution (see figure). However, while the influence of social class on health reduced it remained significant.

Significance

Although this study relied on a single self-reported rating of health, and did not examine other factors known to be important to health (e.g. social resources and

(Cont'd)

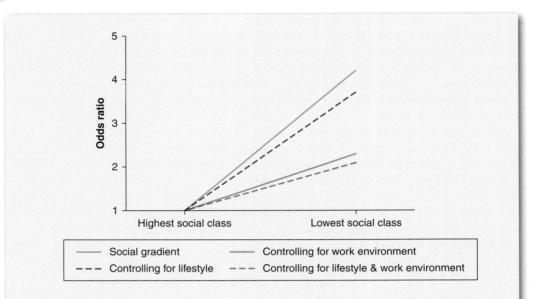

support), it showed that most of the effect of social class on health is due to work and lifestyle factors.

Borg, V. & Kristensen, T.S. (2000) Social class and self-rated health: Can the gradient be explained by differences in life style or work environment?, *Social Science & Medicine, 51*: 1019–1030.

The role of lifestyle in illness illustrates the importance of psychosocial factors, yet these are not considered by the biomedical model. Understanding and changing health behaviour would do more than anything else to reduce morbidity and mortality in our society (see Chapter 5). For example, one in four deaths from cancer in the UK are estimated to be due to unhealthy diets and obesity (Cancer Research UK, 2010). Increased alcohol use is directly related to increased rates of liver disorders and cancers of the GI tract (see Chapter 13). Smoking is directly related to lung cancer – the third highest cause of mortality in the UK (see Chapter 12).

It is not only lifestyle that is important. Individual factors such as personality, health behaviours, and beliefs also affect health. For example, individuals who are high on the personality trait of conscientiousness are less likely to engage in risky behaviours and more likely to engage in positive health behaviours. Perhaps unsurprisingly, they are therefore also more likely to live longer (Stone and McCrae, 2007). Stress and depression are strongly implicated in a range of illnesses, including cardiovascular disease where evidence suggests both these factors are associated with the onset of heart disease (see Chapter 12).

A good example of the effect of our beliefs on health and illness is the **placebo effect,** where people recover because they think they are going to recover, as opposed to recovering because of pharmacological or physical treatment. The placebo effect is typically tested by giving one group of patients a fake drug (placebo group), and comparing their recovery to another group of patients given an active drug (drug group) or no drug (control). The placebo effect is the recovery that occurs in the group given the fake drug, which is over and above any recovery observed in the control group. This effect is well established and there is evidence that beliefs are responsible for a large part of it. For example, a study of surgery for osteoarthritis compared two different types of procedure (arthroscopic debridement or lavage) with placebo surgery where the patients were anaesthetised and skin incisions made but the arthroscope was not inserted. Those who had placebo surgery showed the same level of improvements up to two years later (Moseley et al., 2002). The placebo effect is considered in more detail in Chapter 4.

The biomedical approach cannot account for any of these effects of social and psychological factors on health. Even when the biomedical approach dominated medicine most healthcare professionals realised that psychological and social factors were still important. However, working within the biomedical framework meant these factors were not made explicit or used to the advantage of medicine. They therefore remained part of the *art* of medicine rather than the *science* – although ironically the term 'medicine' comes from the Latin *medicīna* (*ars*) – the (art of) healing.

CLINICAL NOTES 1.1

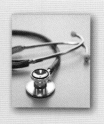

In primary care:

- Up to a third of the patients you see may have psychological disorders and many more will have psychological issues or symptoms.
- Physical causes are usually only found for around 15 per cent of people's symptoms.
- Psychological and physical symptoms are highly related. Many patients will only mention physical symptoms, so it is important to ask about psychological symptoms as well.
- In treatment, a lot of the effect of drugs can be due to patients believing they will recover rather than the drug itself.

1.4.2 BIOPSYCHOSOCIAL APPROACH

The **biopsychosocial approach,** proposed by Engel (1977), is a framework that does take into account the effect of biological, psychological, and social factors. This approach was later expanded to include such factors as ethnicity and culture (Kaplan, 1990; Matarazzo, 1980; Schwartz, 1982). A schematic diagram of the biopsychosocial approach is shown in Figure 1.4. which shows the personal and external factors that, according to this approach, impact on health.

The external factors include the sociocultural environment such as poverty, available support structures, access to healthcare and other facilities, and legislation that impacts on health. External factors also include pathogenic stimuli, which can range from, for example, being exposed to a virus, passive smoking, to living in an area high in radon gas. External factors also include any treatment that the individual receives which can act on the pathogenic stimuli or the person. All of these external factors both influence the person and are influenced by the person.

Internal factors include personal history, psychosocial processes, and physiological and biochemical mechanisms. Personal history involves multiple factors such as ethnicity, genetic make-up, learned behaviour, developmental processes, and previous illnesses. These inevitably influence psychosocial processes such as lifestyle, sociability, personality, mood, perception of symptoms, behaviour, adherence to treatment and so on, so that all in turn will influence, and be influenced by, physiological mechanisms.

Consider smoking, for example. Many people report that their first taste of a cigarette is fairly disgusting, so why do people persist in smoking until they are addicted? Most people will start smoking in adolescence when it is important to them to gain peer approval and fit in with group norms. The prevalence of smoking is highest in people from deprived backgrounds with a low socioeconomic status (West and Hardy, 2007). Thus a child

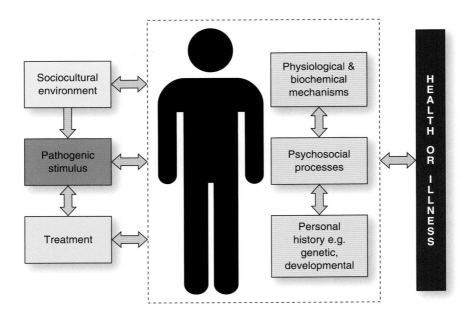

FIGURE 1.4   Biopsychosocial approach to health

growing up in a deprived area may be more exposed to others who smoke and more likely to start smoking which further reinforces the group norm. Without a motivation to quit smoking this child is also unlikely to seek help.

The pathogens in cigarettes mean that, with continued use, smokers are at increased risk of many illnesses including lung cancer, chronic obstructive pulmonary disease, heart disease, head and neck cancer, impotence, infertility, gum disease, back pain, and type II diabetes (West and Hardy, 2007). Whether an individual develops any of these illnesses will be determined by the other aspects in the biopsychosocial approach, such as their individual vulnerability, physiological processes, other lifestyle behaviours, and exposure to other pathogens. However, to return to our example, not all children in deprived circumstances will smoke. Therefore the sociocultural environment interacts with the characteristics of each child to determine exposure to the pathogen of cigarettes, the likelihood of seeking treatment, and the risk of disease.

The biopsychosocial approach provides a clear framework that sums up what many healthcare professionals already intuitively know. It is an improvement on the biomedical approach in that it makes the links between psychological and social factors and health explicit. Illness is seen to be caused by many factors at different levels, rather than purely by pathogens as posited by the biomedical model. Responsibility for health and illness therefore rests on individuals and society rather than on the medical profession alone. Similarly, treatment considers physical, psychological and social contributing factors as opposed to the physical in isolation. A further comparison of the key features of the biomedical and biopsychosocial approaches is given in Box 1.4.

BOX 1.4   Comparison of biomedical and biopsychosocial approaches

	Biomedical	Biopsychosocial
Mind-body relationship	Separate; independent (dualism)	Part of dynamic system; influence each other
Cause of disease	Pathogens	Multiple factors at different levels
Causality	Linear	Circular
Psychosocial factors	Irrelevant	Essential
Approach to illness and treatment	Reductionist	Holistic
Responsibility for health	Medical professionals – e.g. to combat disease	Individuals/society – e.g. healthy lifestyle
Focus of treatment	Eradication or containment of pathology	Physical, psychological, and social factors contributing to illness
Focus of health promotion	Avoidance of pathogens	Reduction of physical, psychological, and social risk factors

The biopsychosocial approach has implications for research, education, and clinical practice. It should lead to more comprehensive research that examines the multiple levels, systems, and factors involved in health. Moreover, in clinical practice the biopsychosocial approach should result in a more complete understanding of the many factors that can contribute to health or illness. This in turn should lead to a more **holistic approach** – that is, treatment of the whole person. The biopsychosocial approach has already resulted in a more patient-centred approach to medicine (Borrell-Carrio et al., 2004). It should also lead to better medical training, with the inclusion of education about psychological and social factors.

Thus the biopsychosocial approach is an improvement on the biomedical approach and should result in clear clinical benefits if used. It is therefore puzzling that, more than thirty years after it was proposed, the biopsychosocial approach still is not widely used or practised in medicine or psychology. Whilst the biopsychosocial approach is taught in most training courses for healthcare professionals, it tends to be taught more as a theoretical framework than applied to clinical work. As one medic observed 'The term was thrown around as often as possible in the first two years in the classroom and then disappeared entirely during the final two clinical years' (Myunclestu, 2005).

So we still have a long way to go to properly incorporate the biopsychosocial approach into medicine. There are many reasons why this might be. The biomedical approach has been dominant for centuries and modern medicine has developed within this framework. Although the biopsychosocial approach may appear simple, in fact the inclusion of all the different elements makes research and medicine more complicated to carry out in practice. In addition, the biopsychosocial approach suggests circular or nonlinear causality. In other words, that physical, psychological and social factors all influence, and are influenced by, each other. This means there is rarely a simple and linear cause-effect relationship between one factor and illness. This raises difficulties in clinical practice because we need to choose or prioritise one treatment. To do this, we have to think in terms of a hierarchy of causes (e.g. one cause is more important than others) and linearity of treatment (e.g. removing this cause will remove illness) (Borrell-Carrio et al., 2004).

Consider the case of Anne, a 50 year old woman with hypertension. This hypertension could be due to Anne's high cholesterol, obesity, smoking, demanding job, lack of support at home, or perfectionist tendencies and inflated beliefs about responsibility that mean she works long hours and is stressed. Which of these explanations we adopt will influence the treatment we offer. If we take the biological cause (high cholesterol) then we would treat Anne with cholesterol-reducing drugs. If we take the behavioural explanations (smoking and obesity), we might offer Anne support to stop smoking or lose weight. If we adopt the psychological explanation (stress and maladaptive beliefs) we might offer Anne stress-management or psychotherapy sessions. Finally, if we adopt the social explanations (work stress and a lack of support) we might refer her to a local support group, self-help groups, or an occupational health worker. In reality Anne's hypertension is probably affected by all these factors but we need to treat her in the most effective way. What would constitute 'effective' treatment here? To decide this, we would need to consider which treatment will provide the best outcome for Anne at the least cost and time for the health service.

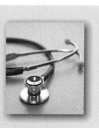

CLINICAL NOTES 1.2

In clinical practice:

- Promoting healthy lifestyles is an important aspect of medicine and has the potential to save thousands of lives.
- People respond differently to illness so it's important not to assume you know how they feel.
- Tolerance of ambiguity and the ability to test alternative explanations for symptoms are necessary clinical skills.
- The holistic approach means we should consider biomedical factors, lifestyle behaviour, psychological factors (e.g. beliefs, emotions, symptoms), and social factors.

ACTIVITY 1.2   DIFFERENT APPROACHES TO MEDICINE

- Reflect on the last time you saw a doctor.
- To what extent did they appear to be working with a biomedical framework and to what extent with a biopsychosocial one?
- How would their treatment have differed if they altered their framework(s)?

We can see that barriers to applying the biopsychosocial approach include the facts that (i) it is not possible to address all the factors that influence illness and (ii) in order to plan treatment we need to think in terms of linear causality rather than circular causality. However, this does not mean we should abandon it and return to the biomedical approach, which ignores psychosocial and environmental factors completely. There is, after all, a crucial difference between, on the one hand, recognising all potential determinants and then selectively treating an individual and, on the other, focusing only on biomedical factors because that's all we must look at. Psychologists also need to be reminded of this. Just as medics naturally err towards biological explanations, psychologists naturally err towards psychological explanations.

Therefore we all need to consciously remind ourselves to explore factors at each level of the biopsychosocial approach when assessing and treating patients. This will give us a more complete understanding of the illness, encourage an holistic treatment of the person, include a consideration of potential psychosocial barriers to treatment efficacy, and allow us to change or modify treatments accordingly if our first approach is not as effective as expected.

Summary

- It is difficult to define health. The choice of definition has implications for medical practice and society.
- No single definition of health is adequate and it is perhaps easier to think of health and illness on a continuum from complete wellness to death.
- The separation of psychology and medicine was initially founded on the mind-body divide (dualism).
- Medicine was dominated by the biomedical approach for many years.
- The more recent biopsychosocial approach has the capacity to unify disciplines in theory and practice, and encourage an holistic approach to medicine.

FURTHER READING

Frankel, R.M., Quill, T.E. & McDaniel, S.H. (eds) (2003) *The Biopsychosocial Approach: Past, Present, Future*. Rochester: University of Rochester Press. A comprehensive edited book on the biopsychosocial approach, clinical applications, patient-centred clinical methods, educational/administrative issues, and the future of this approach.

White, P. (ed.) (2005) *Biopsychosocial Medicine: An Integrated Approach to Understanding Illness*. Oxford: Oxford University Press. Edited book based on experts discussing the application of the biopsychosocial approach in medicine.

REVISION QUESTIONS

1   What are the various specialisms in psychology?

2   Describe two specialisms in psychology. How are they relevant to healthcare?

3   Outline four different definitions of health.

4   Compare and contrast two definitions of health. What are the implications of each definition for treatment?

5   What is dualism? How has it influenced medicine?

6   Describe the biomedical approach to medicine and outline the strengths and weaknesses of this approach.

7   Describe the biopsychosocial approach to medicine and outline the strengths and weaknesses of this approach.

8   Compare and contrast the biomedical and biopsychosocial approaches to medicine.

PSYCHOLOGY AND HEALTH

2 MOTIVATION, EMOTION, AND HEALTH

CHAPTER CONTENTS

(Cont'd)

LEARNING OBJECTIVES

This chapter is designed to enable you to:

- Describe motivation and discuss how it affects health.
- Outline the different components of emotion.
- Appreciate the role of positive and negative emotions in health.
- Consider whether expressing emotion is good or bad for health.

Motivation, emotion, and the way we respond to stress shape our lives in many ways. Emotions are powerful motivators that can even make us risk our lives in extreme cases, such as when parents risk their lives trying to save their children. In medicine, more than in any other profession, we are surrounded by stressful and emotional events as people face illnesses and death, either their own or others. How people respond to these situations varies hugely and there are many examples in medicine of people behaving in ways we might not understand. For example, the woman in Case Study 2.1 was prepared to risk her own and her unborn baby's life rather than have a Caesarean section.

The media are full of similar examples: parents refusing life-saving treatment for their child on religious grounds; a man with liver cirrhosis who continues to drink alcohol even though he knows it will kill him; a pregnant woman with cancer who refuses chemotherapy and then dies just after her daughter is born; a teenage girl who cuts her arms with a razor blade to blunt her feelings. These are real cases that illustrate the importance of beliefs, motivation, and emotion in how people respond to day-to-day stress and extreme situations. They also illustrate the complex interaction between motivation and emotion. In this chapter we shall look at motivation and emotion in turn, examining what these are, and how they are relevant to health.

CASE STUDY 2.1   Refusing life-saving treatment

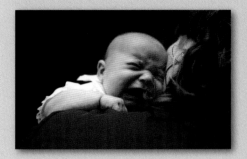

Ms S was a 29 year old single woman who did not see a doctor for the majority of her pregnancy. When she was 36 weeks pregnant she registered with a doctor who found she had severe pre-eclampsia – a life-threatening condition marked by high blood pressure, which can develop very quickly and lead to the death of the mother and baby.

Women with this condition are usually admitted to hospital immediately, and the baby is delivered by inducing labour or performing a Caesarean section.

However, Ms S repeatedly refused to be admitted to hospital despite two doctors recommending it. She insisted that she wanted to give birth naturally in a barn in the countryside. When told that she and the baby might die Ms S responded 'so be it'.

The doctors called in a social worker who concluded Ms S had 'little interest in her own survival and certainly none in the survival of her baby'. Ms S talked of punishing her ex-boyfriend and hoping he felt guilty if she died. The social worker and doctors therefore admitted Ms S to a psychiatric hospital against her will. Although a psychiatrist judged her mentally competent, Ms S was then quickly transferred to a nearby hospital and a court application was made to perform an emergency Caesarean section. The court granted the injunction and Ms S was forced to have a Caesarean section. Her daughter was born healthy.

Ms S took her case to the High Court. Her admission to hospital and Caesarean section were deemed unlawful and she was awarded financial compensation. The judge acknowledged that the social worker and doctors appeared to be well-motivated, but concluded that women have the right to refuse operations even if they risk their own life or that of their baby. Ms S argued that she did not want a hospital birth because she did not like medical procedures and was prepared to risk both her own and her daughter's life because she felt very strongly about it.

Photograph © Johanna Goodyear/Fotolia

2.1 MOTIVATION

2.1.1 WHAT IS MOTIVATION?

Motivation is essentially a drive to act. People are motivated to do (or, indeed, not do) things in their life by a wide range of factors. Because of this, theories from many areas of psychology and other disciplines are relevant. These include health behaviour (see Chapter 5) and decision making (see Chapter 17). Some motives are biological – for example, the desire to eat, drink, or reproduce. Others are more psychological and social – for example, the drive for achievement and status. Box 2.1 gives some examples of biological and social motives, although it is worth noting that the distinction between biological and social motives is not clear cut. For example, sexual motives can be both biological (the drive to reproduce) and social (e.g. affiliation and nurturance).

BOX 2.1   Examples of motives

Biological motives

Hunger
Thirst
Sex
Temperature: need for appropriate temperature
Excretory: need to eliminate bodily wastes
Sleep and rest
Activity: need for optimal stimulation/arousal
Aggression

Social motives

Achievement: need to excel
Affiliation: need for social bonds
Autonomy: need for independence
Nurturance: need to nourish and protect others
Dominance: need to influence or control others
Exhibition: need to make an impression on others
Order: need for orderliness, tidiness, organisation
Play: need for fun, relaxation, amusement

(adapted from Weiten, 2004)

Theories of motivation can be separated into three broad categories, namely drive theories, evolutionary theories, and incentive theories. **Drive theories** use the concept of homeostasis to explain motivation. Homeostasis is a state of physiological equilibrium or stability that organisms strive to maintain. An organism's behavioural and physiological systems may operate together to ensure the stability in bodily functions that is necessary to survive. A lack of equilibrium between our current state and our needs creates an internal tension which we are motivated to reduce.

Drive theory is most easily applied to biological drives such as hunger. When we are hungry we are motivated to find food and eat. We are also more likely to think about food and notice food-related stimuli like adverts or signs for food (Berry et al., 2007). Some studies even suggest that hungry men find women with fuller figures more attractive

(Nelson and Morrison, 2005; Swami and Tovee, 2006). Drive theory would predict that once we have eaten we are no longer motivated to continue eating. However, whilst this is usually the case, there are many examples of people continuing to eat when they are no longer hungry and vice versa. Dieting provides a good example of where a drive to eat is not acted on (this is examined in more detail in Chapter 13 when looking at eating behaviour and obesity). Thus drive theory can account for some biological drives and motivation but is limited in its application to much of human behaviour.

Evolutionary theories of motivation argue that social characteristics are shaped by processes of natural selection in the same way as physical characteristics: desirable social characteristics maximise the chances of reproductive success. Thus social motives – such as the need for achievement, affiliation or dominance – are thought to occur because they increase our chances of survival and reproduction. There is some evidence to support this. For example, when women are at the fertile point of their menstrual cycle they will rate men who are physically masculine and have dominant styles as more attractive (Little et al., 2007). However, this is the case only if women are asked to rate men as mates in the short term. If women are asked to rate men as *long-term* mates this effect disappears completely, indicating that decisions about long-term partners are based on other criteria. Evolutionary theories would explain this as long-term mates being chosen on the basis of criteria such as their ability to support and protect a family.

Incentive theories emphasise the role of external factors that trigger and regulate motivation. For example, a man may not be motivated to seek a relationship until he meets a woman he finds particularly desirable. More elaborate incentive theories take into account **expectations** and **values**, which are common in models of health behaviour (see Chapter 5). Expectancies and values allow for the influence of whether people (i) expect to attain their goal, and (ii) how important or valuable that goal is to them. Therefore, when a man meets a woman he finds very desirable he will not act on his desire if he thinks (i) that there is no chance she will be interested in him or (ii) that he does not really value having a relationship at that stage in his life.

These different theories of motivation are not incompatible. Drive theory emphasises internal states as motivating us whereas incentive theories emphasise external stimuli and rewards. The two can be thought of as push and pull theories of motivation: internal states push us to act and external stimuli pull us. All these theories are reductionist in one form or another: they concentrate solely on internal, external, or genetic causes. A more recent and more complex theory is PRIME theory (West, 2006), which includes motivation as one determinant of behaviour, along with emotions, impulses, evaluations, and plans. PRIME theory is examined in more detail in Chapter 5.

ACTIVITY 2.1   MOTIVATION

- How would different theories explain the motives of Ms S in Case Study 2.1? She refused a Caesarean even though it put both her own and her baby's life at risk.

2.2 MOTIVATION AND HEALTH

Clearly, motivation is relevant to health and healthcare professionals. Understanding biological motivations can help us treat abnormal extremes of biological drives, such as obesity, eating disorders, smoking, addiction, risky sexual behaviour, and insomnia. Understanding social motivations can help us comprehend our own behaviour and what motivates us to work as healthcare professionals. It can also help us deal with other people's behaviour that we might not understand. Knowing more about another person's motives means we can address the situation more constructively. Interventions such as motivational interviewing have been developed to treat disorders with a strong motivational component, such as addiction. This is also used to encourage behaviour changes such as smoking cessation, exercise, and diet (Treasure and Maissi, 2007) and is an effective adjunct to standard treatment (Hettama et al., 2005).

Motivation is relevant to many health topics. These include smoking, which is discussed in Chapter 5, and obesity, which we look at in Chapter 13. Here we focus on alcohol use because it is a good example of complex motives preventing behaviour change. Alcohol-related problems are high in developed countries. They account for 9.2 per cent of the disease burden (WHO, 2005). Alcohol-related disorders are five times more common in men than women, but alcohol consumption in the UK is currently increasing faster in women. In a survey of over 8,000 adults in the UK, 39 per cent of men and 42 per cent of women reported heavy drinking (Office for National Statistics, 2002a). Another survey of over 3,000 university students found that 61 per cent of men and 48 per cent of women drank over the recommended limits (Webb et al., 1996). Increased alcohol consumption inevitably impacts on morbidity and mortality. In the UK there has been a dramatic increase in deaths in the UK from liver cirrhosis and alcohol disorders over the last fifty years (though in the USA and Australia alcohol-related mortality remains stable or is decreasing) (WHO, 2005). There is more information on alcohol abuse in Chapter 13.

The motivation to drink alcohol involves both biological and social factors. As with many activities that become habitual, drinking alcohol is usually pleasurable. For many people the immediate feeling or reward they get from drinking alcohol outweighs the long-term risks, especially when those risks seem removed or unlikely. The common bias of **health optimism** means that most people will consistently underestimate their own risk of disease compared to others. This is especially the case in young adults (Madey and Gomez, 2003). Therefore the long-term negative consequences are minimised and outweighed by short-term pleasure or gain. Drinking alcohol is also included in many social rituals and norms. Changing a habitual behaviour such as alcohol consumption is difficult, particularly when it is longstanding and associated with social functioning. Case Study 2.2 provides an example of using motivational interviewing with a woman who has an alcohol problem and wants infertility treatment.

CASE STUDY 2.2 Treating alcohol misuse with motivational interviewing

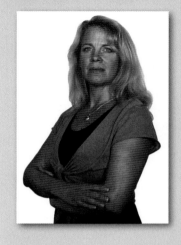

Kate is a 40 year old senior executive in the music industry. She works 12 hour days and finds it hard to unwind. In the evening she drinks wine to relax. She often has to entertain clients at lunch and will drink wine on these occasions. Her total alcohol consumption is over 50 units a week. Women are advised to drink no more than 14 per week. Kate does not think she has an alcohol problem. Many of her friends and colleagues also drink every day.

Kate has been trying to get pregnant for 10 months without success. She knows the chances of getting pregnant decrease with age and wants IVF treatment. Kate's periods are irregular and she is worried it might be signs of an early menopause. Heavy drinking is associated with disruption to the menstrual cycle and poor fertility so it is possible this is influencing Kate's situation. She needs to reduce her alcohol intake substantially for it to be within safe levels.

Motivational interviewing

Motivational interviewing rests on the principle of not judging or imposing our own views on Kate but instead trying to understand her situation and helping her harness her own motivation to change.

1 Exploring Kate's reasons for drinking and whether she has any ambivalence brings up the following:

Motives for drinking	*Motives against*
It helps me relax	*I am not really relaxed, just drunk*
I like it – it is my treat	*I like it at the time but not afterwards*
It switches my brain off	*I want to get pregnant*
Entertaining is part of my job	*I can't think straight in the morning*
	It is not good for me or my job
	I don't want people to see me as a 'drinker'

2 Making these ambivalent motives explicit leads Kate to re-evaluate her drinking. It also high-lights the fact that falling pregnant is the most important motive for her at the moment.

3 Kate sets a goal to stop drinking. Strategies to help her achieve this are explored. For the first week she decides to replace wine with a non-alcoholic alternative and join a yoga class to help her relax. An appointment is made for one week later to review her progress and support her.

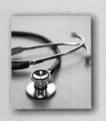

CLINICAL NOTES 2.1

Using motivation to encourage behaviour change

- Understanding motivation can help us treat abnormal extremes of biological drives such as obesity, eating disorders, smoking, addiction, risky sexual behaviour, and insomnia.
- If you ask people about perceived negative behaviours like smoking or alcohol intake they will often report them as less than they are.
- Educating people about the negative effects of these behaviours can trigger them to try to change.
- However, imposing our views and making people feel judged will not help them as much as assisting them to harness their own motivation.
- Try to understand why they behave in this way and empathise with their situation. Then support them to change their behaviour.
- Help them believe that they *can* change.

Summary

- Motivation is a drive to act for a range of reasons, including internal and external factors.
- Theories of motivation include drive theories, incentive theories, and evolutionary theories.
- Understanding motivational processes can be used to guide intervention for changing health-related behaviours, such as alcohol misuse.
- Theories of motivation have clinical applications.

2.3 EMOTION

Human life involves a wide range of emotions: indeed the English language has over 550 words referring to emotion. In psychology the term **affect** is used generally to include **emotions, moods,** and **impulses.** There is cross-cultural evidence of six basic common emotions that have their own distinct physiology. These are happiness, sadness, surprise, anger, fear, and disgust (Ekman, 1992) as shown in Figure 2.1. Additions to this list, including contempt, excitement, embarrassment, love, and jealousy, have also been proposed by some researchers (Ekman, 1999; Sabini and Silver, 2005).

Our emotions have a huge impact on the quality of our life. When feelings are negative, such as severe depression, this can motivate people to end their life. In healthcare settings

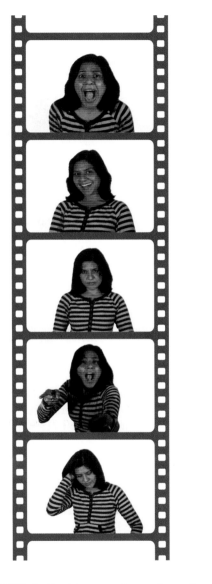
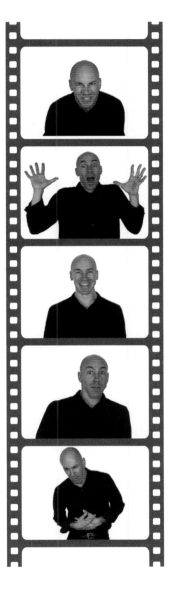

FIGURE 2.1 Facial expression and emotion

where patients face stress and personal difficulties, emotion has a huge impact on people's attitude, recovery and quality of life. For example, one person with terminal cancer may cope with humour and a renewed zest for life, while another person with curable cancer may feel devastated, depressed, and convinced they will die.

In the UK, emotional disorders cost £12 billion a year through loss of work, incapacity benefits, and absenteeism. Mental illness is also responsible for 40 per cent of physical and

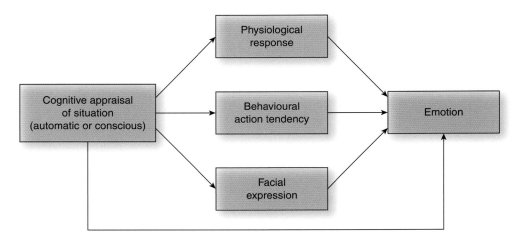

FIGURE 2.2   Components of emotions

mental disability (Layard, 2006). Much research and theory has therefore concentrated on negative emotions, such as anxiety and depression. The development of **positive psychology** over the last twenty years has encouraged the study of positive emotions, such as happiness, and the effect these can have on our wellbeing. There has also been research into normal emotions and their associated physiology: it is thought that they may provide a link between psychosocial factors – such as stress and social relationships – and health. Theories of emotion have therefore emerged from the study of both normal and abnormal emotional processes.

The range and complexity of emotional experiences make it difficult to define. Most theories of emotion start with the premise that emotion has three components: cognitive (thoughts), physiological, and behavioural. The **cognitive component** is the conscious experience of emotion including the meaning we attach to it. The **physiological component** of emotions is complex and involves the central nervous system, autonomic nervous system, and endocrine system. The **behavioural component** can be further separated into the nonverbal expression of emotions (facial expression, body posture, etc.) and behavioural responses. The interplay between these components is reflected in common phrases such as 'being frozen with fear' or 'blood boiling with anger'. Figure 2.2 shows how these different elements may interact to result in emotional experience.

ACTIVITY 2.2   REGULATING EMOTIONS

Think of the last time you were really upset or angry about something.

- What things did you do to calm yourself down?
- Did this involve cognitive factors, taking action, changing behaviour, social factors?

2.3.1 COGNITIVE COMPONENTS OF EMOTION

The *meaning* of a situation is critical to how a person responds to a situation emotionally. For example, if a woman finds a lump in her breast and interprets it as a harmless cyst she will not be hugely alarmed – whereas if she interprets the lump as cancer, she will be frightened and anxious. Strong negative emotions will usually motivate people to take action. Box 2.2 illustrates women's emotional responses to discovering a breast lump and how quickly they went to see their doctor (Meechan et al., 2003).

The first cognitive element of emotion is how people **appraise** a situation when it occurs, or what immediate meaning they make of it (for example, whether it is dangerous, threatening, or harmless). A second element is how people **label** their emotional state when it occurs. The physiological arousal experienced with many emotions is very similar. For example, sympathetic nervous system arousal occurs when we are anxious and excited, so how we label our emotional state will determine our emotional experience. On a roller-coaster some people will label their experience exciting or thrilling but some (including the authors) would label it terrifying and aversive! This leads us to a third important cognitive element, which is whether we **evaluate** our response as positive or negative. Those people who evaluate their experience on the roller-coaster as positive will enjoy it and want to do it again.

This process of appraisal, labelling, and evaluation therefore shapes our future emotional responses as well. Panic disorder is a good example of this. Between 3–9 per cent of people experience panic at some point in their lives (Grant et al., 2006). Panic is associated with extreme physiological arousal, which is part of the 'fight-flight' mechanism (see Chapter 3). Although panic is very unpleasant it is not life-threatening or uncommon. Long-term panic disorder is most likely to develop in people who interpret their initial experiences of panic in a catastrophic way, such as 'I'm going mad' or 'I'm going to die', and who label and evaluate the panic attack as extremely negative (Clark, 1986). Under these circumstances, people will worry about having another panic attack. This increases their anxiety levels and physiological arousal, thereby also increasing the likelihood they will experience panic again. In addition, if

---

BOX 2.2   Responses to discovering a breast lump

Visited doctor <4 days after discovering lump	Visited doctor 7-90 days after discovering lump
'I felt sheer panic, I freaked out' (1 day)	*'I felt fine'* (7 days)
'I was worried – my hands were shaking' (1 day)	*'I'm not a worrier – sometimes I'm too relaxed'* (90 days)
'Scared stiff' (3 days)	*'Just a little bit worried'* (14 days)
'Scared – I even cried' (1 day)	*'Just 'oh', a lump'. I was fairly blasé'* (7 days)
'I felt bad – panic and worry' (2 days)	*'I didn't think anything of it really'* (7 days)
'I was scared, nervous and sweaty' (3 days)	*'I wasn't really bothered'* (21 days)

(adapted from Petrie and Pennebaker, 2004)

a person interprets the panic attack as being linked to a particular situation they will be highly anxious when put in that situation again and may become phobic. For example, if a patient has a panic attack in an MRI scanner they are likely to get more anxious when having another MRI, which in turn increases the likelihood they will experience another panic attack.

In a nutshell, the meaning that people attach to their experience of panic can result in them becoming anxious about being anxious, which becomes a self-fulfilling cycle. However, although the cognitive component is *necessary* for emotion it is not *sufficient* on its own. Emotions are rarely consciously initiated – we cannot force ourselves to feel panic, disgust, or anger. The physical response that accompanies emotion is an important part of how we feel.

2.3.2 PHYSIOLOGICAL COMPONENTS OF EMOTION

The physiological components of emotion are initiated in the brain from a number of structures that form the **limbic system** (see Chapter 7). Elements of the limbic system control the autonomic nervous system and endocrine responses (see Chapter 3), and are involved in learning and modulating emotion. For example, the amygdala is particularly important in fear. If the amygdala is damaged, animals are unable to learn fear when exposed to a threatening object. In people, imaging studies have shown the amygdala is activated during fear (Lang and Davis, 2006).

Emotion also involves areas of the **frontal cortex**. It is thought that the limbic system provides a fast initial response and the cortex then provides a slower, secondary response that regulates this initial response (Le Doux, 1996). This would explain why we often react or 'feel' before we think. The role of the cortex in inhibiting emotional and behavioural responses was first suspected in the case of Phineas Gage in Box 2.3. Research has since

---

BOX 2.3   The case of Phineas Gage

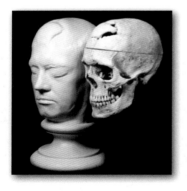

Phineas Gage was working on the railroads in 1848 when a gunpowder explosion drove a large metal rod straight through his head. The rod entered below his left cheek bone and passed through the frontal cortex before exiting and landing many metres behind him. A model of the injury he sustained is shown here. Remarkably he survived his injury and was conscious moments later.

After his injury, Gage is reported to have changed from a hardworking, kind and likeable man to an impulsive, inconsiderate person who used frequent profanities. Up to this point, the frontal lobes were not considered to affect personality or social interaction. Gage became the first case to indicate the frontal lobes were important. Although there is some controversy over whether the damage was exclusively to the left frontal lobe or involved both lobes, it was apparent that the frontal lobe was involved in the inhibition of inappropriate emotional responses.

Image reproduced courtesy of the Warren Anatomical Museum, Francis A. Countway Library of Medicine.

indicated that the orbitofrontal cortex, in particular, plays an important role in inhibiting emotional and behavioural responses. For example, damage to the orbitofrontal cortex is associated with increased anger, anxiety, pride, depression, inappropriate crying or laughing, and the impaired filtering of emotional information (Beer and Lombardo, 2007).

2.3.3 BEHAVIOURAL COMPONENTS OF EMOTION

The behavioural component of emotion can be divided into:

- action tendencies – the potential or drive to act;
- nonverbal responses – e.g. posture, gestures;
- facial expression.

It is thought that the behavioural components of emotion are part of its purpose. In other words, emotion makes us want to do something (Frijda, 1986). Emotions intrude on what we are doing and take priority. This can be clearly seen in Figure 2.3. on the faces of people observing the attack on the Twin Towers on 9/11. Thus emotions are early warning signals that there may be something we need to attend to. Research shows that negative emotions lead to a narrow focus of attention on whatever prompted the negative emotion. Conversely, positive emotions lead to a broadening of attention and more reliance on simple heuristics in how we respond to events.

Emotions therefore direct our attention. The physiological response equips our body for action – and action tendencies provide us with ways to cope with the situation, such as fight or flight if we are under threat. The fight-flight response is certainly observable in extreme

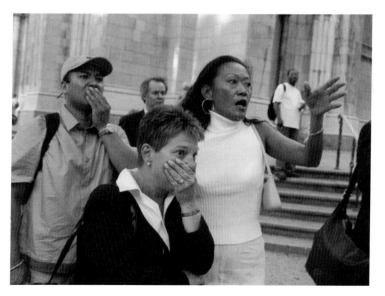

FIGURE 2.3   Observers of 9/11
Photograph reproduced courtesy of Associated Press

situations, but people do not always respond in this way. For example, inside the Twin Towers there were reports of people walking in a calm and orderly fashion to get out. Thus, people's responses to threat are more complicated and influenced by social circumstances and norms. Consequently, there has been a substantial amount of research that has examined how people regulate their emotions, and the coping strategies they use to deal with challenging circumstances. We shall return to this in the section on emotion and health on page 38.

The behavioural component of emotion also includes the nonverbal expression of emotion (for example, body posture or clenched fists) and facial expression. Studies of facial expression suggest that this affects the way we label our emotions. Research where people have been asked to tense certain facial muscles in ways that resemble a 'smile' has shown that people will report more positive emotion in response to stimuli, such as a film clip or photographs. According to the **facial-feedback hypothesis,** signals from muscles in the face are used by the brain to interpret which emotion is being felt (Izard, 1991).

ACTIVITY 2.3   FACIAL-FEEDBACK HYPOTHESIS

Raise your eyebrows and try to be angry.
- What happens?
- Why do you think this is?

2.3.4 THEORIES OF EMOTION

Early theories of emotion concentrated on the relationship between different components of emotion. In a chicken and egg type of debate, theorists argued about whether physical responses preceded appraisal or not. The current consensus is that appraisal processes initiate our physiological, behavioural, and conscious experience of emotion. These appraisal processes can be preconscious or conscious, which fits with the view that the limbic system is a fast processing system (preconscious appraisal), that can be moderated later by the frontal cortex (conscious appraisal).

Substantial evidence confirms that preconscious processing occurs and influences our mood and behaviour. For example, Chartrand et al. (2006) flashed positive words (e.g. friends, music), negative words (e.g. war, cancer), and neutral words (e.g. plant, building) very quickly on a screen so

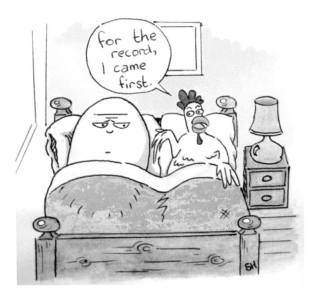

people could not consciously 'see' them. They found that even though people could not 'see' the words, they reported a more negative mood after being shown negative words. Other experiments have shown that if we 'see' something preconsciously we are more likely to prefer it or feel good if it is shown to us so we can consciously see it (Monahan et al., 2000).

Theories of emotion vary in focus. One way to conceptualise emotion is to divide it into positive and negative affect (Watson and Tellegen, 1985). Thus all emotions can be plotted according to whether they are positive (e.g. pleasurable) or negative (e.g. distressing), and on a second dimension according to intensity (high versus low) as shown in Figure 2.4. This has the advantage of simplifying emotions so it is easier to look at relationships between emotions, health, and illness. It also accounts for the *intensity* of emotion which may be important in the effect emotion can have on health. It is quite reasonable to assume that emotion at a low level of intensity (e.g. irritation) will have a different physiological effect and influence on health from a high intensity emotion (e.g. extreme anger).

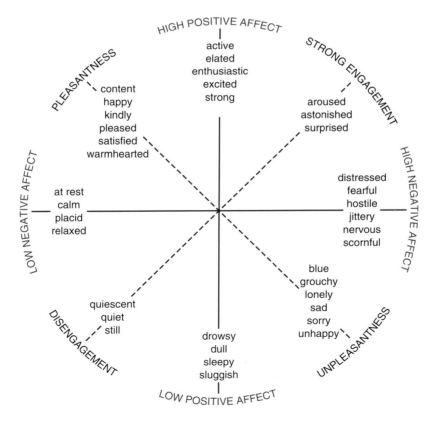

FIGURE 2.4   Model of positive and negative affect

2.4 EMOTION AND HEALTH

A good example of the link between emotions and health is the association of psychological disorders such as clinical depression with an increased risk of morbidity and mortality (Kisely et al., 1997). Here, the nature of the relationship between emotions and health is considered in three main ways:

1 The association between normal emotions and health.
2 The influence of emotional dispositions on health.
3 The effect of how people regulate and express their emotions on health.

2.4.1 NORMAL EMOTIONS AND HEALTH

Laboratory studies show that any acute, strong, or extreme emotion is associated with increased physiological arousal regardless of whether that emotion is positive or negative. This physical arousal has potentially negative effects on health through influencing systems such as the cardiovascular and immune system. However, studies of people's moods in day-to-day settings suggest that positive emotion in natural settings produces less negative physiological responses than negative emotion (Pressman and Cohen, 2005).

Large-scale epidemiological and survey studies of mood and health generally find that being happy is associated with better health. People with high positive affect report fewer symptoms or pain and have fewer illnesses, such as strokes, colds, and accidents. In people aged 55 and over, positive affect is associated with longer life (Pressman and Cohen, 2005). However, the association between happiness and health does not mean that one causes the other. Better health may mean people are more likely to be happy: happier people may be more likely to *say* they are healthier, have a stronger support network, be more likely to carry out good health practices, etc.

The role of negative emotions in health has been extensively researched with mixed results depending on which outcomes are examined. There is now substantial evidence that some types of negative emotion are associated with specific illnesses. The main examples of this are associations between hostility and cardiovascular disease (Miller et al., 1996), depression and cardiovascular disease (Steptoe, 2006), and anxiety and a slower recovery from surgery or illness (Johnston and Vogele, 1993). Depressive disorders are associated with a range of illnesses and with mortality. For example, depressed people are between 50 per cent and 100 per cent more likely to develop cardiovascular disease than healthy people (Lett et al., 2004). However, it is difficult to determine whether depression causes illness, illness causes depression, or whether depression is a symptom of illness. The role of hostility and depression in cardiovascular disease is discussed in more detail in Chapter 12.

In summary, there is evidence that positive emotions are associated with health and that specific negative emotions are associated with certain illnesses, but there are many ways in which one may influence the other. This is often the case with links between psychosocial and biological phenomena and explains why we use terms such as **association** or **relationship**, rather than **cause** or **predictor**. For example, the association between

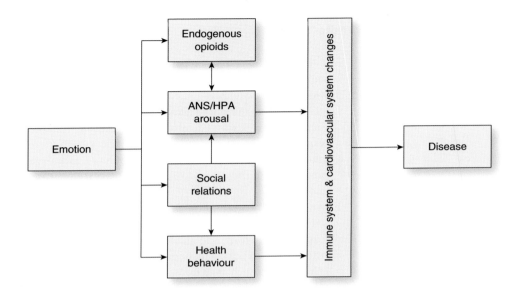

FIGURE 2.5   Pathways between emotion and health (adapted from Pressman and Cohen, 2005)

emotion and health could in part be explained by biased attention leading to a greater focus and reporting of symptoms or, alternatively, mood influencing the way people interpret their symptoms. Possible pathways between emotion and health are summarised in Figure 2.5. The important point to note is that emotion could influence our health through biological, behavioural, and/or social mechanisms.

2.4.2 EMOTIONAL DISPOSITIONS AND HEALTH

Emotional dispositions are personality-like tendencies towards experiencing certain emotions. There are five main personality traits: openness to new experience, conscientiousness, extraversion, agreeableness, and neuroticism (as shown in Box 2.4). Of these, conscientiousness and neuroticism are considered more fully here because they are most consistently linked with health (Stone and McCrae, 2007). **Conscientious** people are defined as having self-discipline and being efficient, organised, reliable, responsible, etc. Evidence suggests conscientious people live longer, although this is probably due to the fact that conscientious people are more likely to practise positive health behaviours, such as exercising, and less likely to practise negative health behaviours, such as smoking. However, conscientiousness is not associated with particular emotions.

Neuroticism is the personality trait with the most obvious emotional component. People who are high in neuroticism experience a wide range of negative emotions, such as low mood, anxiety, guilt, hostility, and fear. People high in neuroticism report more somatic symptoms and are more at risk of psychological disorders (Contrada and Goyal,

---

BOX 2.4 Five main personality traits (OCEAN)

Openess to new experiences	Intellect and interest in culture. Includes characteristics such as artistic, curious, imaginative, insightful, having wide interests, and being unconventional.
Conscientiousness	Dependable with the will to achieve. Includes characteristics such as self-disciplined, efficient, organised, reliable, responsible, dutiful, and thorough.
Extroversion	Outgoing. Includes characteristics such as talkative, gregarious, enthusiastic, seeking excitement, assertive, and active.
Agreeableness	Loving, friendly, and compliant. Includes characteristics such as sympathetic, appreciative, trusting, kind, forgiving, generous, and altruistic.
Neuroticism	Tendency to experience negative emotions. Includes characteristics such as anxious, tense, self-pitying, worrying, self-conscious, hostile, and vulnerable.

2005). However, it is difficult to know whether this is due to the personality trait of neuroticism or to components of neuroticism such as negative affect, depression, anxiety, and hostility. There is also no consistent link between neuroticism and measures of chronic morbidity such as heart disease, cancer, or mortality (Stone and McCrae, 2007).

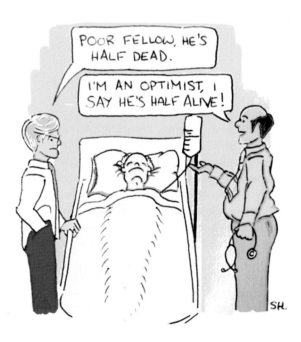

Emotional dispositions associated with psychological health are **optimism** and **pessimism**. Optimism is a general disposition toward expecting good things to happen in the future and pessimism is expecting bad things. These are not mutually exclusive and it is possible to be generally optimistic about most things but pessimistic about others. The most widely used measure of optimism and pessimism is shown in Box 2.5.

Optimism is associated with better psychological wellbeing and with some measures of physical wellbeing, such as better recovery from myocardial infarctions and heart surgery (Smith and MacKenzie, 2006). However, as with other dispositions or traits, it is difficult to distinguish the mechanisms involved or to be sure what role, if any, emotions play. As with conscientiousness, evidence shows that optimism is also associated with positive health behaviours, healthier coping strategies, and increased social support, which could in turn affect our responses to illness or stress (Contrada and Goyal, 2005). The mechanism through which optimism affects physical health is unclear. Some immunological studies show that in mild or moderately stressful events optimists have a better immune function compared to pessimists. However, in highly challenging or difficult events optimists show poorer immunological functioning (Segerstrom, 2005). This may be because optimists will engage with stressful situations and try to resolve them. Hence difficult circumstances might lead to greater physiological strain for optimists than for pessimists who disengage.

BOX 2.5   Measuring optimism

The Life Orientation Test (Revised)

Please be as honest and accurate as you can throughout. Try not to let your response to one statement influence your responses to other statements. There are no 'correct' or 'incorrect' answers. Answer according to your own feelings, rather than how you think 'most people' would answer.

4 = I agree a lot
3 = I agree a little
2 = I neither agree nor disagree
1 = I DISagree a little
0 = I DISagree a lot

1	In uncertain times, I usually expect the best.	
2	It's easy for me to relax.	[filler]
3	If something can go wrong for me, it will.	[reverse]
4	I'm always optimistic about my future.	
5	I enjoy my friends a lot.	[filler]
6	It's important for me to keep busy.	[filler]
7	I hardly ever expect things to go my way.	[reverse]
8	I don't get upset too easily.	[filler]
9	I rarely count on good things happening to me.	[reverse]
10	Overall, I expect more good things to happen to me than bad.	

Scoring

To calculate your score, ignore the fillers (items 2, 5, 6, 8). Reverse your score on negatively worded statements (items 3, 7, & 9). Then total your score. Scores range from 0 to 24: high scores indicate optimism, low scores indicate pessimism.

Source: Scheier, M.F., Carver, C.S. and Bridges, M.W. (1994) 'Distinguishing optimism from neuroticism (and trait anxiety, self-mastery, and self-esteem): A re-evaluation of the Life Orientation Test', *Journal of Personality and Social Psychology*, 67, 1063–1078. Copyright ©1994 by the American Psychological Association. Reproduced with permission.

2.4.3 EMOTIONAL EXPRESSION, EMOTIONAL REGULATION, AND HEALTH

Research into emotional expression raises a few puzzles. On the one hand, there is a view that not expressing strong emotions is bad for you. Research has found that the suppression of emotion is associated with poorer health, but the evidence is inconsistent (Garssen, 2004). In contrast, we have already seen that anger and hostility, which both involve some expression of these emotions, increase the likelihood of heart disease.

A particularly interesting area of research has looked at the effect of writing about negative or traumatic events on health. This research shows that writing about negative events leads to better health in normal samples, and a small (but significant) positive effect on health in people with illnesses (Slachter and Pennebaker, 2007). Research Box 2.1 shows how emotional expression is associated with better wound healing.

It is not clear why emotional expression in this way leads to better health. Various explanations have been put forward including that people find more meaning in the experience, expect to feel better when they have talked or written about it, are more likely to talk about it again with others, or that other people are more supportive when told about the event.

Emotion regulation may take two forms. There is intrinsic regulation, where we regulate our own emotions, and extrinsic regulation, where we regulate someone else's (as, for example, when a doctor soothes a patient). Emotion regulation can involve conscious, automatic, or unconscious processes. An example of ways to regulate emotions and how this is relevant to managing illness is given in Case Study 2.3, which illustrates how emotion regulation techniques can help people manage chronic illness more effectively.

CLINICAL NOTES 2.2

Emotions and medicine

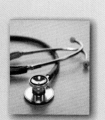

- Emotional disorders cost society billions every year and mental illness is responsible for 40 per cent of disability.
- How people respond to illness is initially determined by how they appraise it.
- Helping people appraise things more positively can reduce negative emotions and help people cope.
- Humour and smiling (even when feeling low) have the potential to lift people's mood and may also have an indirect influence on health.
- Negative emotions such as anxiety, anger, and depression are associated with chronic illnesses such as heart disease. Treating people with these dispositions early could prevent later illness.

- Encouraging optimism could help people if they are facing an essentially controllable or modifiable illness.
- Getting people to write about stressful or traumatic events has the potential to improve their health.

RESEARCH BOX 2.1   Emotional expression and wound healing

Background

In the research literature there is some inconsistency as to the health effects of the expression or suppression of emotions. This study examined how the expression of stress-related emotions affects one aspect of immune function.

Methods and findings

36 men were randomly allocated to the experimental group which wrote for 20 minutes a day for three days about traumatic experiences in their life, or a control group focusing on time management.

Two weeks later all men were wounded using a 4mm punch biopsy that removed skin from their arm. Healing of the wound was monitored over three weeks.

Men who wrote about traumatic events healed much quicker than men who wrote about time management.

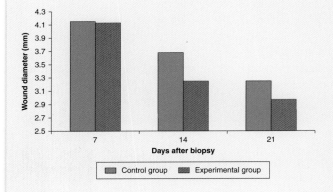

Significance

The use of punch biopsies to study wound healing is significant because it means all the men had comparable wounds. Therefore, any differences in healing were more likely to be due to the experimental condition. Previous studies using punch biopsies had shown that stress was associated with a longer time for a wound to heal. The significance of this study was that it showed a simple intervention to help people deal with traumatic events through writing about them had an effect on wound healing over the next 2-3 weeks. This was a clear example of the influence of psychological factors on physical processes.

Weinman et al. (2008). Enhanced wound healing after emotional disclosure intervention, *British Journal of Health Psychology, 13*: 95–102.

CASE STUDY 2.3   Regulating emotion and managing chronic illness

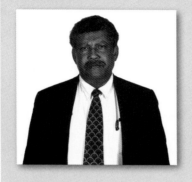

Clive is 62 years old and has Type 2 diabetes which means he needs regular injections of insulin. Clive is not managing his diabetes well and has been hospitalised twice in the last three months. He does not like needles and cannot face injecting himself. When nurses try to do the injections, he gets very worked up and distressed.

How can Clive regulate his emotional reaction to needles?
Select situations that make things less negative: Distraction is useful for dealing with needle anxiety, so it might help for Clive to have his injections in a situation where he can be distracted by something he really enjoys, such as a film, music, or something else he finds interesting.

Modify the situation: the situation could be changed in many ways including (i) finding an alternative mode of delivering insulin; (ii) changing the timing of injections so he has less time to get anxious beforehand; (iii) having a healthcare professional do the injections; (iv) bringing a friend who can support him and help him stay calm.

Focus attention away from the situation or emotion: Clive should be encouraged to concentrate on something else whilst the injection is being done, by distracting him, asking him to focus on another object, or talking about a happy event. Helping him cope is much more effective than empathy, which usually increases distress.

Change the way a situation or emotion is appraised or labelled: Clive's appraisals need to be changed from negative (e.g. the injection will hurt, he won't cope, the nurse will think he's stupid) to positive (e.g. the injection will be over very quickly, he's managed it before, after the injection he will feel better).

Regulate physical, behavioural, and emotional responses: there are many things Clive could adopt to help regulate his responses in injections. For example, he could do physical exercises before the injections to make him more physically relaxed. Before and during the injection he could use relaxation techniques such as focusing on his breathing. He could also use positive self-statements to cope.

(based on Gross and Thompson, 2007)

Summary

- Emotion includes affect, moods, and impulses.
- Emotion has cognitive, physiological, and behavioural components. Behavioural components include action tendencies, nonverbal behaviour, and facial expression.

- Appraisal processes initiate the physiological, behavioural, and conscious experience of emotion.
- Positive emotions are associated with good health and negative emotions, such as anger and depression, are associated with certain illnesses. However, the mechanisms or causes underlying this association are not clear.
- Emotional dispositions of optimism and neuroticism are positively and negatively associated (respectively) with psychological health as well as with some measures of physical health.
- Research into emotional expression is double-sided: expressing emotions such as hostility is bad for physical health, yet expressing other emotions, such as those attached to traumatic events, is good for health.

CONCLUSION

This chapter has looked at how motivation and emotion can have an important influence on our behaviour, health, and sometimes illness. There is substantial overlap between these different areas and their implications: motivation drives us to act while emotions also include impulses and action tendencies. Appraisal is important in determining how we feel and respond to different stimuli. In this chapter we have concentrated on the effect of motivation and emotion on health and the possible pathways this works through, including cognitive and behavioural changes. A good example of the interplay between appraisal, emotion, cognition and behaviour, and how this affects our health, is what happens when we are stressed. This is the subject of the next chapter.

FURTHER READING

Ayers, S. et al. (eds) (2007) *Cambridge Handbook of Psychology, Health and Medicine*. Cambridge: Cambridge University Press. This contains short chapters on emotional expression and health, and personality and health.

Ryff, C.D. & Singer, B. (2001) *Emotion, Social Relationships and Health*. Oxford: Oxford University Press. This is a good book if you want to know more about how social relationships and context affect emotions and health. It includes chapters on immunity, common colds, and breast cancer.

Steptoe, A. (2006) *Depression and Physical Illness*. Oxford: Oxford University Press. A comprehensive text on the effect of depression on physical illness.

? REVISION QUESTIONS

1 Describe motivation and give examples of different types of motives.

2 Outline and evaluate three different theories of motivation.

3 Describe the main components of emotion.

4 What are the six basic emotions that are expressed similarly across different cultures?

5 Discuss how the different components of emotion might interact to determine our emotional experience.

6 Outline the effect of positive and negative emotions on health.

7 How may the expression of emotion affect health?

8 Outline the two-factor model of positive and negative affect.

9 Distinguish the various pathways through which emotion may influence health.

10 What emotional dispositions have been associated with health?

3 STRESS AND HEALTH

LEARNING OBJECTIVES

This chapter is designed to enable you to:

- Define stress and outline aspects of stress, including (a) appraisal and (b) stress responses.
- Describe physical responses to stress and discuss variations, (a) between individuals and (b) between situations, in how we respond physically to stress.
- Discuss the relationship between stress and physical health, and outline the factors that protect us or make us more vulnerable to illness following stress.
- Understand some of the main psychological consequences of stress, including burnout.

Most people know that stress is bad for us. In fact, stress is *not* always bad for us – a small amount of stress is necessary for us to rise to challenges such as competitions or exams. However, long-term stress is indeed negative in its effects: there is a lot of evidence linking stress to adverse outcomes like depression, burnout, and cardiovascular disease. Stress is also associated with infections, slower recovery, and a worsening of symptoms in illnesses such as asthma, herpes, and rheumatoid arthritis (Steptoe and Ayers, 2005). In this chapter we look in more detail at stress, our physical responses to it, how it can affect our physical and mental health, and what can protect us against stress.

3.1 WHAT IS STRESS?

The concept of stress originated in mechanics where it is used to describe the internal forces in a system caused by external pressures, such as the pressure of water or wind on a bridge. Over time the word **stress** has become widely used to mean many things, including a negative situation, a feeling of pressure, tension, or negative emotion. According to the psychological definition, stress occurs when demands are appraised as exceeding a person's resources to cope.

Like emotion, stress has many components and first it is necessary to distinguish between stressors and stress responses. **Stressors** are external or internal events that trigger stress responses. If, for example, you feel stressed because you are sitting an exam, we may say that the exam is acting as an external stressor. If, on the other hand, you feel stressed because you are torn between helping a good friend who needs you and revising for that exam, the stress is caused by an internal stressor (your conflicting desires). Stressors can be further divided according to their type or duration, such as acute events (e.g. the death of a friend), chronic stressors (e.g. caring for a sick relative), daily hassles (e.g. problems getting to work), traumatic stressors (e.g. an assault), and role strain (e.g. balancing home and work roles).

Stress responses are the various ways we respond to a stressor. These can be divided into cognitive, affective, behavioural, and physiological responses. Interestingly, there is not always a strong association between these different responses. In other words, it is possible for a person to have a strong physical response to stress but not report feeling emotionally stressed. This is very apparent in people who have a repressive coping style who, when put under stress, will report little or no emotional distress but show strong physiological responses (Furnham et al., 2003).

3.1.1 THE PHYSICAL RESPONSE TO STRESS

Understanding physical responses to stress is critical if we are to explain the link between stress and disease. Our understanding of physical responses to stress initially comes from research in the 1950s detailing the fight-flight response. The **fight-flight response** involves the sympathetic branch of the **autonomic nervous system** as a fast, first wave response; and the endocrine pathways of the **hypothalamic-pituitary-adrenal (HPA)** axis as a slower, second wave response. The sympathetic and HPA responses are illustrated in Figure 3.1. The sympathetic nervous system directly activates body systems to prepare the body for immediate action. The adrenal medulla is stimulated to produce stress hormones such as **adrenaline** (epinephrine) and **noradrenaline** (norepinephrine). This causes stimulation of the heart and lungs and the diversion of energy away from unnecessary functions such as saliva production, digestion, and reproduction.

At the same time, the HPA axis is activated so the hypothalamus releases corticotrophin releasing factor (CRF), which then sets off a cascade of endocrine events culminating in the release of cortisol and other hormones from the adrenal cortex. **Cortisol** is a steroid and is a critical stress hormone. It results in an increase in blood sugar levels and metabolic rate, hence further supporting the body in the need for fight or flight. It also influences the regulation of blood pressure, the immune system, and the inflammatory response. Normally, the HPA axis works as a negative feedback loop so the presence of cortisol in the blood stream triggers the hypothalamus to stop producing CRF. Thus cortisol will usually return to normal levels 40 to 60 minutes after a stressful event. However, under prolonged periods of stress the HPA axis can become dysregulated and result in chronically elevated levels of cortisol. In the long term this will have negative effects, such as the accumulation of abdominal fat and the wasting of bone and muscle tissue. The effects of excess cortisol are illustrated by **Cushing's syndrome** – a syndrome where there is overproduction of cortisol (hypercortisolism). People with Cushing's syndrome have large amounts of fat on their abdomen and face, sweating, thinning of the skin, stretch marks, and facial hair. In some cases it also leads to sleep problems, reduced sexual function, reduced fertility, increased depression, and anxiety.

Selye (1956) proposed that physical responses to stress can be understood as a **general adaptation syndrome** with three stages:

1 *Alarm*: an immediate physical response to stress that prepares us for fight-flight.
2 *Resistance*: our body attempts to resolve the stress and return to normal, but if the stressor continues we will remain in a physiologically active state.
3 *Exhaustion*: if the stressor continues indefinitely the physical strain on our body will lead to exhaustion, illness, or death.

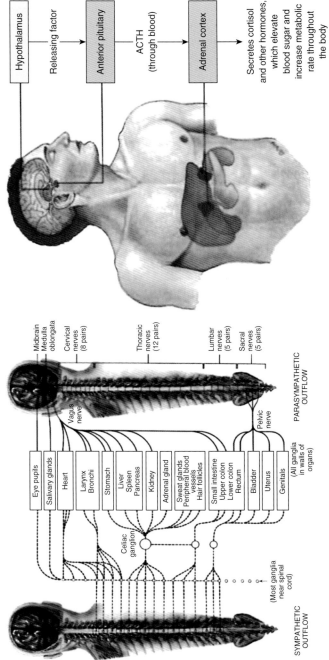

Physical stress response

FIGURE 3.1 Fight-flight responses to stress

Source: Kalat, *Biological Psychology,* 4E. © 1992 Wadsworth, a part of Cengage Learning Inc. Reproduced by permission. (www.cengage.com/permissions)

Research provides some support for the general adaptation syndrome but our understanding of physical responses to stress has developed substantially since these were first proposed. We now know that physiological responses to stress will vary according to the characteristics of a situation, especially if the situation is novel, unpredictable, or uncontrollable. Evidence shows that stronger physical stress responses will occur in situations that are novel. For example, a novice jumping out of a plane with a parachute will have much stronger cardio-vascular and autonomic responses than an experienced parachutist (Schedlowski and Tewes, 1992). Similarly, unpredictable events can lead to greater physical stress responses. For example, a study of commuters found that those who rated aspects of their journey as unpredict-able reported more stress and had higher cortisol levels (Evans et al., 2002).

The other important characteristic of situations is whether they are controllable. Research generally indicates that a lack of control is associated with greater stress and a more negative impact on health (Walker, 2001). This has led to the view that it is impor-tant to empower patients and encourage them to have as much control as possible. Though this is usually true, it is worth noting that if a situation is essentially uncontrollable, encouraging someone to strive for control might result in more strain on the person. In experiments where people are told they can prevent an obnoxious loud alarm going off if they perform well enough at a task, people often have stronger physiological responses than if they are told they cannot control the noise (Manuck et al., 1978). The evidence for this is not consistent but, if this is the case, it has important implications for uncontrolla-ble situations in healthcare, such as births that involve obstetric complications women cannot predict or control. In these circumstances it may be unhelpful to encourage women to strive for control and perhaps more emphasis should be placed on supporting them through such events.

Therefore, the characteristics of a situation will affect how we respond to stressors. Individuals will also vary in how they respond. Some individuals will be more physi-cally responsive than others. This is called **stress responsivity.** Studies of twins indicate that stress responsivity may be partly genetically determined (Hewitt and Turner, 1995) or established very early on in development. Babies of mothers who have high levels of stress and anxiety during pregnancy are more responsive to stress, show more anxiety and fearfulness, and are more likely to have cognitive and attentional problems (Talge et al., 2007). This makes sense from an evolutionary perspective, because offspring born into a stressful or dangerous environment will need exaggerated stress responses to survive.

The environment is also important in shaping infants' stress responses. Animal studies show that offspring of more nurturing mothers have reduced HPA axis responses through less CRF and enhanced negative feedback (Champagne and Meaney, 2001). Thus, indi-viduals will vary in their levels of stress responsivity and this is determined by nature *and* nurture. Individuals will also vary in their pattern of physical responses to stressors. One person may have high blood pressure responses to stress and another person may show a stronger inflammatory response. Research Box 3.1 gives an example of ethnic differences in responses to stress and support.

The physical fight-flight response and the general adaptation syndrome thus provide the basis of our understanding of physical stress responses. However, the matter is more complex than this. In particular, there is more variation between individuals than the above explanations imply. For example, there is emerging evidence that the fight-flight response may be more relevant to males, while females may be more likely to show **tend-befriend responses,** where they will turn to the group for safety and to protect their young (Taylor et al., 2000). It is possible that oxytocin is the underlying biological mechanism for this and indeed there is some evidence to support this. If male animals are injected with oxytocin and then put in a stressful situation they are more likely to nurture any young animals present (Taylor et al., 2000). This illustrates the notion that physical responses to stress will differ according to circumstances, the individual differences present, and the group involved.

CLINICAL NOTES 3.1

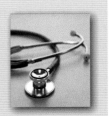

Stress and health

- In uncontrollable circumstances such as an emergency situation it may be more helpful to support people through it rather than encourage them to strive for control.
- Severe or chronic stress is associated with poor health, so helping people manage and reduce their stress has the potential to reduce illness in the long term.
- The physical symptoms of stress will vary between individuals–some may experience cardiovascular symptoms, such as palpitations, whereas others may experience gastro-intestinal symptoms.

RESEARCH BOX 3.1   Culture, social support, and stress

Background

People's responsiveness to stress is determined by both nature and nurture. This study aimed to examine the influence of culture and ethnicity on stress responses.

Methods and results

This study investigated how support influenced stress as reported by students from an Asian or European background before and after they performed a public speech. Before the speech students were asked to write about one of the following:

1. A group they were close to and things about that group that were important to them (indirect support).
2. People they were close to and what advice and support they would ask from them for the public speech (direct support).
3. Campus landmarks (control group).

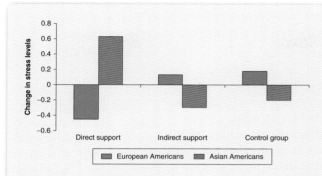

Measures of stress and cortisol were taken before and after the tasks.

Students from European or Asian backgrounds were completely different in the types of support that helped reduce their stress. As shown in the figure, direct support reduced stress for European students but increased stress for Asian students. In contrast, Asians were least stressed when asked to imagine indirect support.

Significance

This study demonstrates the individual differences in stress responses, by showing the interaction between ethnicity, stress, and different types of support in students.

Taylor, S.E. et al. (2007) Cultural differences in the impact of social support on psychological and biological stress responses, *Psychological Science, 18(9)*: 831–837.

3.1.2 STRESS AND THE IMMUNE SYSTEM

Stress will have various effects on the immune system, depending on the demands of the situation. Both the sympathetic nervous system and the HPA axis affect the immune system. The sympathetic nervous system increases immune system activity, particularly large granular lymphocyte activity such as natural killer cells. However, the HPA axis suppresses some immune activity through the production of cortisol, which has an anti-inflammatory effect and reduces both the number of white blood cells and the release of cytokines (see Chapter 11).

Different types of stressful events will make different demands on the body and the immune response to stress has developed to reflect this. Short stressors, such as giving a presentation, will lead to an acute immune response such as the one described above to provide an immediate defence against injuries and the broad risk of infection. This response is very rapid and the immune system will quickly return to baseline levels. Stressors that continue for a few days, such as studying for exams, will have a different effect on the immune system and will influence the *function* of the immune system more than the relative distribution of different types of immune cells. Increases in cytokine production mean the body will be more able to co-ordinate responses against infections. This might explain why students often get sick after exams – because during the stressful revision period they have increased immunity against infections which largely disappears when exams are over. Chronically stressful events, such as bereavement or work stress, will have a negative impact on almost all aspects of immune functioning, with poorer immune function overall. This makes a person more likely to get ill, particularly if they are already vulnerable (e.g. elderly people) or have pre-existing disease.

3.1.3 THE ROLE OF LIFE EVENTS

Life events are usually measured with a checklist of different types of stressful events, such as divorce, bereavement, marriage, or financial problems. The advantage of this approach is that it distinguishes the stressor from the stress response and provides a pseudo-objective measure of stress. The disadvantage is that it assumes the same event is equally stressful for all people, which is clearly not the case. A muscle injury will potentially be much more stressful for a professional athlete than for an office worker.

The life events approach to stress has therefore been widely criticised because (a) it fails to account for individual differences in events that are perceived as stressful and (b) the measurement of stress by checklists is likely to be affected by recall biases. For example, people who are ill are much more likely to search for a cause of their illness and attribute it to stress. Therefore they are more likely to recall stressful events than people who are healthy. Alternative measures of stress, such as the one shown in Box 3.1, focus on

---

BOX 3.1   Perceived stress scale

How often have you ...	never	almost never	sometimes	fairly often	very often
been upset because of something that happened unexpectedly?	0	1	2	3	4
felt that you were unable to control the important things in your life?	0	1	2	3	4
felt nervous and 'stressed'?	0	1	2	3	4
felt confident about your ability to handle your personal problems?	4	3	2	1	0
felt that things were going your way?	4	3	2	1	0
found that you could not cope with all the things that you had to do?	0	1	2	3	4
been able to control irritations in your life?	4	3	2	1	0
felt that you were on top of things?	4	3	2	1	0
been angered because of things that were outside of your control?	0	1	2	3	4
felt difficulties were piling up so high that you could not overcome them?	0	1	2	3	4

Scoring: Add your scores together. Scores range from 0–40. The average score for people aged 18–29 is around 14; aged 30–44 is 13; >45 years is approximately 12.

Source: Cohen, S., Kamarack, T. & Mermelstein, R. (1983) A global measure of perceived stress. *Journal of Health and Social Behaviour*, 24: 385–396. Copyright © 1983 American Sociological Association. Reproduced with permission.

appraisal and stress responses. These improve on life event measures but conversely suffer from a lack of clarity between stressors, stress responses, and coping responses.

ACTIVITY 3.1

- Can you remember how many stressful events you have been through in the last year?
- How accurate do you think you can be – are there things you might have forgotten?
- What do you think affects whether you remember stressful events or not?

Despite the difficulties with the life events approach, there is a plenty of evidence to show that more life events are associated with various illnesses and even death. For example, studies of bereavement show that older people are more likely to die in the year after their spouse dies than other people of the same age and health (Subramanian et al., 2008).

3.1.4 PUTTING IT TOGETHER: STRESS AS A PERSON-ENVIRONMENT INTERACTION

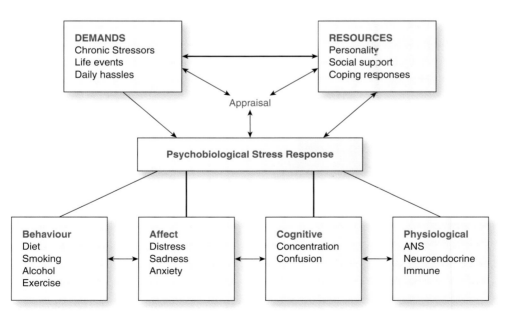

FIGURE 3.2 Interactional approach to stress

Stress occurs when the demands of a situation are appraised as greater than a person's ability to cope. Appraisal processes are central and explain the variation in people's responses to stress. Examples are given of behavioural, affective, cognitive and physiological responses to stress.

It is now widely accepted that how we respond to stress depends on the interaction between a person and their environment. Interactional explanations of stress provide a more complete account of the different processes involved in stress. A model of an interactional explanation is shown in Figure 3.2. This approach argues that stress occurs when a person appraises the demands of a situation as being greater than their ability to cope with these (Lazarus and Folkman, 1984). Appraisal processes are central and explain why there is so much variation in how people respond to stressful circumstances.

There is a wealth of evidence on the importance of appraisal in stress responses. Experiments carried out by Lazarus would stress people by showing them gruesome films and changing the instructions or information given to participants to alter their appraisal. One experiment showed people a series of real accidents in a saw mill, which included limbs being severed. People watching the film either thought it was real (control group); real but shown for educational purposes (intellectualisation); or acted (denial of reality). This and similar experiments typically show that people who can either intellectualise or deny the reality of the film will have smaller stress responses (Lazarus et al., 1965; Steptoe and Vogele, 1986).

The interactional approach proposed by Lazarus and colleagues outlines three processes of appraisal:

1 *Primary appraisal*: the demands of a situation are evaluated as benign, challenging, or stressful/threatening.
2 *Secondary appraisal*: a person evaluates their resources and capacity to cope.

BOX 3.2   Appraisal and stress

Trigger	Skin rash	Skin rash
Primary	*'It's meningitis'* (threatening)	*'It's probably nothing'* (benign)
Secondary	*'I can't cope with this on my own'*	*'I'll just leave it'*
Feelings	Stressed	Calm
Coping	Visit doctor – find out it's eczema	Keep an eye on it
Reappraisal	*'The cream the doctor gave me should make it better'* (can cope)	*'It doesn't seem to be getting worse so I'll wait a bit longer'*
Feelings	Calm	Calm

3   *Reappraisal*: a person reconsiders the situation once they have tried to cope with it. This may lead to reappraisal of a situation as less or more stressful than originally thought, depending on the effect of their coping responses.

The importance of primary appraisal is illustrated throughout this book (see, for example, the discussion in Chapter 2 of responses to discovering a breast lump). Box 3.2 gives examples of primary and secondary appraisal, and reappraisal. A strength of the interactional approach is the recognition of the appraisal-coping-reappraisal cycle. This constant interplay between appraisal, coping, and reappraisal means stress is conceptualised as a dynamic process.

Summary

- The stress process involves (a) stressors and (b) stress responses.
- Stress responses include physiological, behavioural, emotional, and cognitive changes.
- Stress occurs when the perceived demands of a situation are appraised as exceeding a person's perceived resources and ability to cope.
- Appraisal is therefore central to whether a person feels stressed or not.
- Physical stress responses involve the sympathetic nervous system, HPA axis, and immunological changes.
- Physical stress responses will vary according to the characteristics of the situation, e.g. novelty, predictability, and control.
- Individuals will vary in the strength and nature of their physical responses to stress (stress responsivity).

3.2 STRESS AND HEALTH

3.2.1 LINKS BETWEEN STRESS AND HEALTH

The impact of stress on physical health varies between illnesses. There is good evidence that stress results in increased episodes of infectious illnesses like colds (see Research Box 3.2), cardiovascular disease and slower wound healing, and worsens auto-immune conditions such as asthma, rheumatoid arthritis, inflammatory bowel disease and HIV/AIDS. Examples of research in these areas can be found throughout Section III of this book. Similarly, the association between stress and poor mental health is well-recognised. Chronic or severe stress can lead to a number of mental health problems, including anxiety, depression, stress burnout, and post-traumatic stress disorder (PTSD).

However, as with our emotions it is difficult to establish the definitive pathways between stress and health. There are three main issues. The first is the huge variation in how people respond to stress. Why is it that if we put two people in the same circumstances,

RESEARCH BOX 3.2   Stress and the common cold

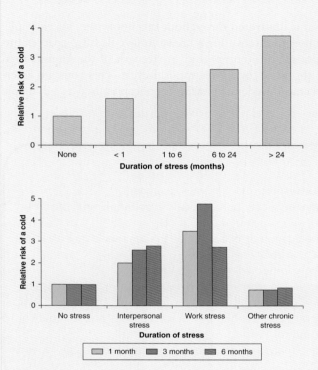

Background

Research shows that stress increases susceptibility to the common cold. This study examined the effects of stress on susceptibility expressed in terms of immune response and symptoms.

Methods and findings

276 healthy adults were kept in quarantine for six days and given cold viruses through nasal drops. Beforehand, measures were taken of stressful life events in the previous year. Pre- and post-measures were taken of blood, urine, respiratory symptoms, and nasal mucous. Other potential influences on health were also measured: sex, age, education, health behaviour, personality, body weight, and social support.

The risk of catching a cold and developing symptoms increased with the length of time a person had been stressed. This effect remained when controlling for other factors such as antibody status at baseline.

People who reported chronic work stress were most affected and were 2–5 times more likely to develop symptoms of a cold than people without chronic stress. Interpersonal stressors had the next strongest impact with people 2–3 times more likely to catch a cold.

Significance

This study confirmed that stress increases susceptibility to the common cold. The real significance of this research, however, was in showing that stress affects whether people catch cold viruses (through an examination of immune antibodies) and also whether they then display the symptoms of a cold (through an examination of coughs, mucus, etc). This was one of the first well-designed studies to show that the effect of stress is strong enough to be clinically relevant.

Cohen, S. et al. (1998) Types of stressors that increase susceptibility to the common cold in health adults, *Health Psychology, 17(3):* 214–223.

one person becomes stressed and the other does not? Or that one person develops heart disease and another remains healthy? Some of these differences can be accounted for by differences in appraisal, but the effect of stress is also moderated by many other factors, such as situational characteristics, coping responses, and social support.

The second issue is that it is usually not possible to say whether an illness is due (a) entirely to stress or (b) entirely to other factors (i.e., not at all to stress). Illnesses will usually have multiple causes, ranging from the genetic and biological to the environmental. The role of stress will also vary widely in different illnesses. A traumatic stressor may cause PTSD but only exacerbate the symptoms of asthma. The contribution of stress to illness will therefore vary widely between individuals, circumstances, and illnesses.

A third issue is that the effect of stress on health can be due to behavioural, emotional, or physical responses to stress. For example, people who are stressed are also more likely to smoke, drink alcohol, and have a poor diet (Wardle et al., 2000). The physical response to stress is therefore not the only pathway between stress and disease.

Thus stress will contribute to the development of disease in a variety of ways, including a person's physical vulnerability, psychosocial vulnerability, environment, coping responses, etc. This can be summarised by the **vulnerability-stress model** (sometimes called the diathesis-stress model) as shown in Figure 3.3.

3.2.2 FACTORS THAT PROTECT AGAINST STRESS

The effect of stress on individuals is influenced by range of factors, as indicated above. We have already seen that characteristics of a stressor, such as novelty, predictability or control, will make a difference to the impact of an event. Other moderators of the effect of stress on health include (a) personality, (b) the methods a person uses for coping, (c) how much social support they have, and (d) whether they take physical exercise. These are examined in more detail below.

Personality

The dimensions of personality that have most effect on how a person responds to stress are those involving negative emotions, such as neuroticism or a predisposition towards negative

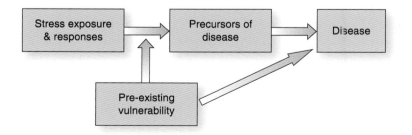

FIGURE 3.3   Pathways between stress and disease (vulnerability-stress model)

affect. Neuroticism is a personality trait that involves high symptoms of anxiety, depression, hostility, and emotional instability. People high in neuroticism will generally report more pain and symptoms. The reasons for this are examined in more detail in the next chapter on symptom perception. However, there is also a consistent association between neuroticism and a range of health problems, including arthritis, diabetes, asthma, coronary artery disease, headaches, kidney or liver disease, and ulcers (Friedman and Booth-Kewley, 1987; Goodwin et al., 2006). A large prospective study of 21,676 adult twins in the USA who were followed up over twenty-five years found that, after controlling for genetic vulnerability in twins, those who were high in neuroticism were significantly more likely to report musculoskeletal pain, headaches, migraine, chronic fatigue, colitis, irritable bowel syndrome, gathroesophageal reflux disease, and cardiovascular disease twenty-five years later (Turk Charles et al., 2008).

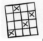

ACTIVITY 3.2

- Do you know anyone who gets stressed very easily?
- Which kind of factors do you think influence why they are like that?
- How much of it is due to circumstances, personality, or coping strategies?

Coping

As we saw earlier when looking at the interactional model of stress, coping is a vital part of the stress process. How we cope with stressors will partly determine our physical and emotional responses. People who appraise an event as challenging will have smaller cortisol responses than people who appraise it as stressful. Research looking at coping defines it as *any* attempt to cope with a stressor, irrespective of whether this is successful or not. This covers a huge range of coping actions and there has been an extensive debate over how to best conceptualise different coping strategies. Categories that are widely used distinguish between emotion-focused and problem-focused coping; or between approach and avoidant coping. **Emotion-focused strategies** are those that concentrate on reducing distress (e.g. not thinking about it; eliciting emotional support); whereas **problem-focused strategies** concentrate on dealing with the problem (e.g. information seeking; problem solving).

For medical practice the distinction between approach coping and avoidant coping may be more useful. **Approach coping** strategies try to deal with the situation pro-actively and thus share some overlap with problem-focused strategies. **Avoidant coping** strategies try to avoid the problem (e.g. denial; not wanting to talk about it). The important point for medical practice is that a person who is predominantly an avoidant-coper may find it very difficult to discuss their illness, the side-effects of treatment, or any potential complications. Conversely, an approach-coper will want to know everything about it and may come to consultations armed with extensive information gleaned from the internet!

In general, coping strategies that enable a person to feel more in control, increase positive mood, and decrease negative mood are associated with better health. One meta-analysis of longitudinal research found that positive affective states (e.g. emotional wellbeing, positive mood, joy, and happiness) and positive personality dispositions (e.g. hopefulness, optimism, humour) were associated with reduced mortality in healthy people and better outcomes in people with chronic illnesses, including renal disease and HIV (Chida and Steptoe, 2008). However, it is not as simple as saying one coping style is better than another. Avoidant coping strategies are very good for reducing anxiety and distress in the short term. Before an operation this can be helpful because it keeps anxiety levels down and once the operation is over the stress of this is gone. However, for someone with a chronic illness, avoidance can lead to a lack of adherence to treatment regimens and compound illness problems.

ACTIVITY 3.3

- What kind of coping strategies do you tend to use?
- Can you think of anyone who is clearly an avoidant-coper or an approach-coper?
- How well does this approach work for them in different situations?

Social support

Interpersonal relationships are vital to our quality of life and health. Negative relationships involving abuse or conflict are some of the most potent stressors. Traumatic events that involve intentional harm from another person, such as rape, assault, or torture, are much more likely to cause PTSD than natural disasters (Charuvastra and Cloitre, 2008). Social relationships also shape the way we respond to stress. As we have seen, early mothering influences the developing HPA axis of young animals. In humans, social bonds are very influential in shaping a child's stress responses. Attachment theory (see Chapter 8) proposes that babies are born with an instinct to turn to their parents or significant others when they are stressed or in danger. In extreme situations, such as children being abandoned or abused, children are more likely to develop insecure and chaotic responses to stress. Even with secure attachments, however, parents will continue to shape children's responses to stress. Studies of parents and children exposed to the same stressor show that their responses are very similar. There is also increasing evidence that anxious parents raise anxious children through having controlling parenting styles (Van der Bruggen et al., 2008). Conversely, a study of college students found that those who felt supported by their parents coped better with stressful events by using more active coping and positive reappraisal (Valentiner et al., 1994).

For adults, social support can dramatically reduce the impact of stress. People who have a lot of social support are less likely to get stressed in the first place and, when they do become stressed, are more likely to cope with it successfully (Taylor, 2007). Laboratory experiments that induce stress by asking people to undertake social speaking or hard arithmetic tasks show that having someone present can reduce sympathetic and HPA axis responses, although this does vary according to gender and the nature of the relationship (Phillips et al., 2009). This has also been observed with pets being present (Allen et al., 2002). Thus, social support during a stressful event buffers people against the effects of stress. Social support also has a direct effect on health. A huge number of studies have reported a relationship between social support and disease progression, recovery from illness, and mortality (Wills and Ainette, 2007). It is therefore a critical factor in both stress and health.

Physical activity

It is well known that physical activity is good for health. People who have active lifestyles are at lower risk of obesity, cardiovascular disease, breast cancer, colon cancer, depression and diabetes, and live longer (Owen et al., 2007). People who are physically active are also less likely to smoke, more likely to have a healthy diet, and more likely to have social support. Using exercise as a method of coping with stress therefore has independently positive effects on health. There is evidence that exercise reduces anxiety, depression, and is associated with increased self-esteem and self-confidence (Ussher, 2007). Exercise intervention programmes have been used and evaluated for a wide range of conditions, including cardiovascular disease, depression, learning disabilities, dementia, arthritis, back pain, Parkinson's, cancer, and schizophrenia.

CLINICAL NOTES 3.2

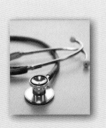

Coping styles and clinical practice

- Consider people's coping styles when giving information in clinical practice.
- People with avoidant coping styles may not want information and may become anxious or distressed if given information.
- Conversely, people with approach coping styles will want information and may become distressed if not given information.
- Exercise has a positive effect on physical and mental health so it is worth encouraging exercise for patients and yourself!
- Social support is critical to wellbeing so it is important to identify those patients who are socially isolated and encourage/help them to increase their support networks.

Summary

- Severe or chronic stress is associated with a range of illnesses and mortality.
- Variability in how we respond to stress makes it difficult to establish causal pathways between stress and disease.
- A vulnerability-stress approach explains how stress may interact with an existing vulnerability to affect health.
- Factors that moderate the relationship between stress and health include neuroticism, coping, physical activity, and support.
- Interpersonal relationships and social support are critical in shaping how we respond to stress, in buffering the impact of stress, and for our general wellbeing.

3.3 STRESS IN MEDICINE

Medicine is an inherently stressful profession: it involves dealing with health crises and making life and death decisions. As we have already seen, stress is associated with negative psychological states, including anxiety, depression, burnout, and PTSD. **Stress burnout** is experienced by approximately 18 per cent of adults and has three main symptoms:

1 *Emotional exhaustion*: involves feelings of physical exhaustion, being depleted, worn out.
2 *Depersonalisation*: involves having an unfeeling, impersonal approach to co-workers or patients, cynicism, and a lack of engagement with the job or people.
3 *Reduced personal accomplishment*: involves a poor sense of effectiveness, involvement, commitment and engagement and a poor belief in one's ability to change or improve work patterns or environment.

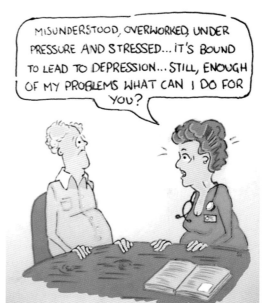

Burnout leads to high job dissatisfaction, absenteeism, and staff turnover. Symptoms of exhaustion are associated with many other physical symptoms such as headaches, gastrointestinal disorders, hypertension, colds or flu, and sleep disturbances (Leiter and Maslach, 2000). The workplace is critical to whether people develop burnout (see Box 3.3) and this is particularly relevant for healthcare professionals. A survey of 882 hospital consultants in the UK found that 27 per cent reported burnout and

---

BOX 3.3 Workplace and burnout

Evidence suggests burnout is more likely in jobs that involve:

- A high workload.
- A lack of control.
- Insufficient rewards.
- An absence of fairness.
- Value conflicts.
- A poor sense of community.

(*Source*: Maslach, 2007)

---

psychological problems, which were associated with feeling overloaded, poorly managed, poorly resourced, dealing with patients' suffering, and having problems outside work. Burnout is also more common in consultants who feel poorly trained in their communication and management skills (Ramirez et al., 1996). Areas such as intensive or palliative care tend to have higher rates of burnout e.g. a meta-analytic review of people working in oncology found that 25 to 36 per cent of them had symptoms of burnout (Trufelli et al., 2008).

Medical students also face many stressors. These include constant evaluation by exams, staff, and patients; dealing with death, suffering, and difficult ethical issues; performing intimate examinations of others at a young age; and a demanding number of work hours. Longitudinal studies that have followed medical students over a number of years have found a few characteristics that are associated with stress and burnout later in life. Medical students who are disorganised, have poor time management, feel overwhelmed, and who are unsure of the demands of different tasks are more likely to report stress and burnout in their thirties (McManus et al., 2004). Students who are self-critical, neurotic, perfectionists, report feeling like an 'imposter', and if female are also more likely to suffer from stress and burnout later in their career (Firth-Cozens, 2001). Learning positive ways to manage stress is therefore extremely important for healthcare professionals. These include accessing appropriate support and learning positive stress management techniques. Case Study 3.1 shows how the interactional model of stress could be used to help a medical student cope with exam stress.

3.4 MANAGING STRESS

Understanding the processes of stress provides the basis for helping people manage stress more effectively. There are six main approaches to stress management: relaxation; physical fitness; cognitive restructuring; meditation; assertiveness training; and stress inoculation (see Chapter 19). Interventions such as **stress inoculation** are based on exposing people to potentially stressful situations so they become 'inoculated' against them. For example, paramedic training will

CASE STUDY 3.1   Managing stress in medicine

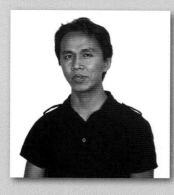

Kamal is a medical student approaching the end of his first year. Before medical school Kamal was a straight-A student. At medical school his results have varied. He has passed everything but has lost confidence. He is particularly worried about the Clinical Examinations where he has to demonstrate clinical skills with a patient in front of an examiner. Kamal is very anxious and not coping well. He is convinced he is going to freeze up, look stupid in front of the examiner, and fail the exam.

Kamal finds the constant examination and evaluation of medical school really hard. He feels tired, tense, and is finding it difficult to concentrate on his studies. He is beginning to doubt whether medicine is the right career for him.

Stress management

Stress management involves education about stress and coping, exploring each person's unique way of dealing with stress, and facilitating more adaptive coping. When based on the interactional model, stress management looks at demands, resources, appraisal, and coping as follows:

Demands

The demands of medical school on Kamal may be explored in order to make them explicit. For example:

- *What are the triggers to this situation?* e.g. Clinical examinations.
- *What demands does it place on Kamal?* The exams make Kamal feel evaluated, not good enough, and he has lost confidence.
- *How real are these demands?* Are they based on fact or Kamal's fears?

Appraisal

This stage would look at his appraisals and how they are affecting his feelings and coping, such as:

- *When he is feeling unable to cope, what thoughts are going through his head?* This would emphasise the role of appraisal in how Kamal feels. Current appraisals include: '*I am going to fail*'; '*I will freeze up and look stupid*'; '*Maybe medicine isn't right for me*'.

(Cont'd)

- *How could he think differently to help him feel and cope better?* This would highlight appraisals and coping strategies that might be more adaptive: *'Exams are hard but I have got through them before'*; *'It's not only me that finds exams hard'*; *'If I freeze up it's not the end of the world'*, etc.

Resources to cope

This stage would involve exploring with Kamal which resources he can use to cope. This includes helping him learn new coping strategies and draw on existing ones. For example:

- *What support is available?* Including other students, teachers, friends, family, and healthcare professionals. *How can he use this now?*
- *How has he coped with situations in the past?* This would hopefully raise his awareness of which coping strategies are available to him.
- *What worked and what didn't work?* This would help Kamal realise what might be adaptive and maladaptive coping in different situations.
- *How can he use these strategies to cope now?* This could help Kamal realise he has the resources to cope now. This should reduce his feelings of helplessness, increase his confidence, and encourage him to use strategies that will help him feel better.
- *What new ways of coping might help him now?* This encourages Kamal to learn and use new ways of coping.

Managing stress

Drawing on the previous stages, you can explore practical steps and strategies that may help Kamal manage his exam preparation now and in the future. To some extent this is very individual. For example, Kamal might realise that talking to other students really helps because it normalises a certain amount of anxiety and worry. He might find that working with a group of students to revise and practise together boosts his confidence. Or he might realise that in a previous stressful situation he was able to think about it differently and 'talk' himself out of his fears.

often include rehearsals or 'mock ups' of major road traffic accidents in order that when paramedics are in a real accident situation they are equipped with the right knowledge and actions to deal with it. However, reviews suggest that cognitive behavioural techniques, such as cognitive restructuring, will have the largest and most enduring effect on reducing stress (van der Klink et al., 2001). Delvaux et al. (2004) found that stress management intervention with oncology nurses led to less stress, better communication skills with patients, and more patient satisfaction with the nursing care up to six months later. There is some evidence these interventions may improve physiological states, such as immune function (see Chapter 11).

Cognitive-behavioural stress management programmes focus on appraisals and coping responses to help people manage their stress better. These can be very useful to assist people coping with illness. These kinds of stress management techniques have therefore been widely implemented and evaluated for people with cardiovascular disease, cancer, and chronic headaches – but with mixed results. The evidence suggests stress management has positive effects on psychological outcomes, such as reducing depression and increasing self-esteem, but the impact on physical morbidity or mortality is mixed. Early studies showed stress management programmes led to decreased mortality from heart disease (Friedman et al., 1986) and cancer (Spiegel et al., 1989). However, recent studies have failed to replicate this effect (e.g. Berkman et al., 2003). Cognitive-behavioural techniques are looked at in more detail in Chapter 19.

One particular type of stress management, critical incident debriefing, has proved controversial. Debriefing was initially developed to help people deal with very stressful or traumatic events and prevent the development of PTSD. Debriefing programmes do vary but they will usually involve one session within four weeks of the event, during which a person is encouraged to talk about their thoughts and feelings during the event and their symptoms since the event. The therapist will then educate the person about responses to traumatic events, in an attempt to normalise these experiences. A number of studies have shown that debriefing has little effect on symptoms of PTSD or depression, and one study of using debriefing with burns patients found it made them worse (Bisson et al., 1997). Clinical guidelines therefore explicitly recommend *against* using debriefing interventions.

CLINICAL NOTES 3.3

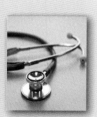

Looking after yourself

- Studying medicine and working in healthcare can be very stressful. It is therefore really important that you are aware of your own stress levels and take steps to look after yourself.
- Recognise the signs and symptoms of stress in yourself and take steps to manage your stress.
- Avoid trying to 'go it alone'. Use formal and informal support available to you such as student counsellors (at university) and colleagues (in practice). Some areas have Balint groups where doctors can talk through stressful or difficult issues in medical practice (www.balint.co.uk).
- If you have symptoms of burnout or other psychological problems, then get help as soon as possible, before the problem becomes chronic or severe.
- Skills in organisation, time management, and finding positive ways of dealing with stress are worth developing early on in your career.
- Perfectionism and self-criticism will increase the stress you put on yourself.

CONCLUSION

It is clear that we need to take a more sophisticated approach than thinking there is a simple dose-response relationship between stress and illness. As we saw in the chapter on emotion, some negative emotions like depression and anger are associated with illnesses such as heart disease. However, as this chapter on stress has shown, we need to account for individual differences in many factors, including a pre-existing vulnerability, exposure, health behaviour, and coping, in determining whether a person will become ill and the type of illness they may suffer.

In the last two chapters we have concentrated on the effects of motivation, emotion, and stress on health. In trying to explain the mechanisms underlying the association between emotion, stress, and health we have primarily concentrated on physical and behavioural pathways. However, emotion and stress will also influence symptom perception, help-seeking, and illness behaviour. In the next chapter we shall examine the role of symptom perception and illness beliefs in more detail.

Summary

- Severe or chronic stress is associated with psychological problems such as anxiety, depression, stress burnout, and PTSD.
- Burnout occurs when people feel exhausted, depersonalised, and have a poor sense of personal accomplishment.
- Health professionals are at increased risk of burnout and stress-related psychological problems, particularly in demanding specialities such as intensive and palliative care.
- Understanding stress processes is important in developing interventions to help people manage stress more effectively.
- Stress management interventions increase psychological wellbeing, but evidence of their effect on physical health is mixed.

📖 FURTHER READING

Ayers, S. et al. (eds) (2007) *Cambridge Handbook of Psychology, Health and Medicine*. Cambridge: Cambridge University Press. This book includes brief chapters on many topics in this chapter including 'Stress and health', 'Support and health', 'Coping assessment', 'Psychoneuroimmunology' 'Social support and health' and 'Burnout in health professionals'.

Sutton, S., Baum, A. & Johnston, M. (eds) (2004) *SAGE Handbook of Health Psychology*. London: SAGE. This book includes a comprehensive chapter on stress, health, and illness.

? REVISION QUESTIONS

1 How is stress defined in psychology?

2 Outline the different elements of the interactional model of stress.

3 Describe the physiological responses to stress.

4 What factors affect a variation in how we respond physiologically to stress?

5 Outline the vulnerability-stress explanation of how stress influences health.

6 Discuss four factors that moderate the effect of stress on health.

7 Define 'coping' and describe two different ways in which coping strategies have been classified.

8 Outline the evidence that social support affects health.

9 What is stress burnout and how does it affect healthcare professionals?

10 Describe two types of stress-management interventions and briefly discuss the evidence that they are effective.

4 SYMPTOMS AND ILLNESS

Research boxes

4.1   Intervention to help manage diabetes
4.2   Listening to prozac and hearing placebo
4.3   Self-management intervention for MI

LEARNING OBJECTIVES

This chapter is designed to enable you to:

- Discuss the role of different psychological factors in physical symptoms.
- Describe the multidimensional nature of pain and the role of psychological factors in the perception of pain.
- Outline the placebo and nocebo effects and how they affect illness and recovery.
- Describe different representations of illness and understand how these impact on the psychological and physical outcomes of illness.
- Understand how these principals can be used in clinical interventions to improve outcomes.

Understanding symptoms is fundamental to providing good healthcare. Symptoms are a sign that something might be wrong, they motivate people to seek help from healthcare services, help doctors diagnose the problem, and give an indication of whether a treatment is working and people are getting better. All of this would be fairly straightforward if there were a simple relationship between having symptoms and having a disease, or the severity of a symptom and disease. In reality, however, the relationship is not simple or straightforward.

First, symptoms are remarkably common – indeed studies suggest that most people experience two to three symptoms a week (Broadbent and Petrie, 2007). Population surveys show that in a two-week period 38 per cent of people reported headaches, 29 per cent of people reported aches and pains, and 16 per cent reported sleep disturbances (Petrie and Pennebaker, 2004). Similarly, 20 to 40 per cent of people report feeling tired all the time (Lewis and Wesseley, 1992).

A second complication is that most people with symptoms do not consult doctors, preferring to ignore the symptoms, treat themselves, or rely on a natural recovery. Research suggests that people see their doctor for fewer than 5 per cent of new symptoms that they experience (Campbell and Rowland, 1996). In addition, approximately one third of those who do attend a doctor will not receive a medical diagnosis for their symptoms (Kroenke, 2003b).

Thus symptoms are remarkably common and also ambiguous: they are strongly influenced by psychological factors, such as the degree of attention paid to symptoms, how they are interpreted, and how beliefs about illness and healthcare can affect subsequent actions. The previous chapters have described how the perception of symptoms is influenced by emotion and stress, and how motivation determines whether people will act and in what way. In this chapter we examine more specifically how people perceive symptoms and illness, including pain, which is a primary symptom in many disorders. Placebo and nocebo effects demonstrate the importance of beliefs in the perception of symptoms and illness. People recover because they believe they will recover, or feel ill because they believe they will get ill.

Symptoms are not only a sign of the *onset* of illness but also indicate the *progression* of illness. Chronic illnesses, such as rheumatoid arthritis or multiple sclerosis, involve remitting or slowly worsening symptoms and disability. Perhaps unsurprisingly, beliefs about symptoms play an important role in how people adjust to chronic illness and predict further symptoms, distress, and disability. For example, a person who believes their illness is uncontrollable, incurable, and disrupts every area of their life will be highly distressed and focused on their symptoms, worrying about whether the disease is getting worse. In contrast, a person who believes their illness is controllable and requires adjustment but does not disrupt every area of their life will be less distressed and less focused on their symptoms. As we have seen in previous chapters, distress such as anxiety or depression is in turn associated with poorer health and slower recovery. Thus negative beliefs, distress, and negative interpretation of symptoms can become a vicious downward cycle. This is often seen in chronic pain patients. This chapter therefore examines the perception of symptoms, pain, placebo and nocebo effects, and finally looks at how beliefs about symptoms and illness can influence the experience and progression of chronic illness.

4.1 SYMPTOM PERCEPTION

A **symptom** can be thought of as any variation in a physiological or emotional state that is interpreted as unusual and labelled as potentially harmful. Therefore, as with emotion and stress, appraisal and interpretation are central. For example, a racing heartbeat just before giving a presentation could be interpreted either as nerves (unusual, transient, not harmful) or as a possible heart problem (unusual, potentially chronic, harmful). Symptoms of a myocardial infarction (MI) are often interpreted as gastro-instestinal symptoms, particularly by women who often do not believe they are at risk of heart problems. This affects how women respond to these symptoms – which may cost them their life if medical treatment is delayed. Evidence shows women suffering a heart attack can take up to twice as long to get to hospital as men (Walsh et al., 2004).

How people appraise and interpret symptoms is therefore critical. Unfortunately people are generally not very good at interpreting their physical state accurately. This has huge implications for treatment. For example, people with asthma are expected to monitor their symptoms and use inhaler medication when they need it. However, up to 60 per cent of asthmatic patients are unable to detect changes in their lung function reliably

(Kendrick et al., 1993). Similarly, people with hypertension are not able to detect consistently when their blood pressure goes up, although 90 per cent of them believe they can (Meyer et al., 1985). There are a few exceptions to this. Some individuals are more accurate at detecting symptoms than others, and most people can accurately perceive extreme symptoms or physical changes that need immediate action, such as a bad injury or strong pain.

4.1.1 HOW DO PSYCHOLOGICAL FACTORS AFFECT SYMPTOMS?

Psychological factors can affect the perception and interpretation of symptoms in a number of ways including (a) the role of *attention* in whether people notice their symptoms, (b) the effect of the *environment* on symptom perception and interpretation, (c) *individual differences in the interpretation* of symptoms, and (d) the *influence of emotions* on symptom perception and interpretation.

Attention and the environment

The degree of attention we pay to our internal physical state has a strong influence on the perception of symptoms. Most theories of attention assume we have a limited capacity to pay attention to different stimuli at the same time. Therefore, changes in our internal states have to compete with what is going on around us for attention. There are many examples of injured soldiers fighting on and not feeling the injury, or of sports men and women continuing to play with serious injuries (see Case Study 4.1). This can be explained on different levels. Physiologically, the release of endogenous opioids like endorphin will reduce the level of pain we feel. Psychologically and socially the demands of an immediate situation mean people are less likely to attend to their physical symptoms.

ACTIVITY 4.1 DOES ATTENTION INFLUENCE SYMPTOM PERCEPTION?

- Close your eyes and focus completely on the sensations in the tip of your right middle finger for one minute.
- Did you notice any change in sensation from how it usually feels?

Research evidence confirms the importance of attention in the perception of symptoms. People are more likely to report symptoms if they are in boring environments. More symptoms are reported by people who are unemployed, living alone, or who are

CASE STUDY 4.1   Claire Markwardt: running through the pain

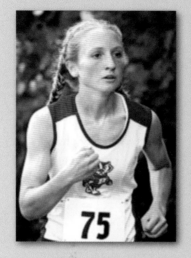

Claire Markwardt was competing in the Ohio State high school cross country championships when she broke her leg in two places. Two miles around the course she was running at her personal best. About 400m from the finish line she heard her left leg crack. Claire thought she'd pulled or torn a muscle so continued to run for the finish:

'There was a runner from one of our rival schools right in front of me - I kept staring at the back of her jersey and pushing myself to catch her.'

200m further on her leg cracked again and gave out. She fell to the ground but a team mate encouraged her to get up and continue. She tried, using her right leg. But as soon as she shifted weight to the left, her leg cracked again loudly and gave out again:

'At that point, I knew that my leg was hurt. I had a suspicion it was broken, but I also thought it might be a muscle. It was such a short time I wasn't overly analyzing it, but I knew I couldn't get up again so I started crawling.'

She said she didn't think of her coach, her parents, or team mates, but just of the many stories she had heard about runners who collapsed before the end of a race and somehow found the courage to cross that last line. She managed to crawl to the finish line and was only 18 seconds under her personal best time.

Reproduced courtesy of Claire Markwardt; image reproduced courtesy of Carl Chrzan

put in boring situations in laboratory research (Broadbent and Petrie, 2007). People will also report more symptoms if they are instructed to attend to their internal physical stimuli rather than external stimuli. For example, one study asked people to run on a treadmill and listen to either the sound of their own breathing or other distracting sounds. Those who listened to their own breathing reported more tiredness and symptoms than people listening to other sounds (Pennebaker and Lightner, 1980). The implications of this for healthcare are that taking a person's attention away from internal stimuli by using strategies such as distraction can lower the perception of symptoms. Distraction is therefore useful for managing symptoms like pain. (Attention is covered in more detail in Chapter 10.)

Individual differences in the interpretation of symptoms

Individuals will differ in the amount of attention they pay to internal states and also in which types of symptoms they are more likely to attend to. Most people will have sets of beliefs, or **schemas**, about which illnesses they are vulnerable to, which symptoms indicate potential illness, and which illnesses comprise a threat to their overall health. Schemas are mostly developed during childhood and are not always rational. Events in adulthood may lead to schemas changing or being modified. Schemas people have about their health and illness will therefore be influenced by their past experience of illness and others' attitudes to illness – particularly parents.

Schemas will usually operate unconsciously to influence what symptoms people attend to and how they interpret them. For example, in one study students were tested for a fabricated illness and were informed of the risk factors for this. One group was told they had the illness and another group was told they did not have it. Students who believed they had the illness reported far more of the risk factors than students in the non-illness group (Croyle and Sande, 1988). A similar phenomenon was apparent in the finding that up to a third of medical students worry they have an illness they have just studied. This is probably because they scan their symptoms for any that fit with the illness they are learning about (Broadbent and Petrie, 2007).

Thus the perceived cause of symptoms is important. In the example above, medical students were more likely to think a serious disease they had just learned about had caused their symptoms. This process of interpreting the cause of something is called **attribution**. At a very simple level, people can attribute the cause of their symptoms to somatic causes, psychological causes, or environmental causes. If a middle-aged woman feels hot and faint she could attribute this to the menopause (somatic), being upset or embarrassed (psychological), or the room being too hot (environment). Within each category there are potentially many explanations. Which explanation a person adopts will affect the action they then take. For example, an aching muscle could be attributed to exercise (somatic but benign) or to the start of flu (somatic, threatening) and this will influence whether someone seeks help for a symptom.

Research into attribution indicates that people can have different **attributional styles**. Individuals might be more or less likely to attribute events internally (to themselves) or externally (to the environment or others). In relation to symptoms it is possible that some individuals who have an internal/somatic attribution style may also have increased healthcare use in response to symptoms.

Influence of emotion

Emotion is strongly associated with the perception and reporting of symptoms, which was partly covered in Chapter 2. Strong emotion is accompanied by physiological changes that can be misinterpreted as symptoms. There is a large amount of evidence that negative emotions or negative emotional dispositions are related to increased reports of symptoms,

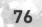

pain, disability, and psychological distress. In part this is due to negative emotions making people more likely to notice symptoms and interpret them as threatening. Research into anxiety has established that this results in a narrowing of attentional focus and a bias towards the perception of threat. Anxiety will therefore make people hypervigilant, in which case they will scan themselves and the environment for any potential threat (Bar-Haim et al., 2007).

This is also the case for symptom perception and interpretation. Research that induces negative moods in people, usually by showing upsetting films or asking people to recall difficult episodes from their past, finds people report more symptoms and think they are more vulnerable to illness when they are in a negative mood. People are also more likely to attribute the cause of symptoms to illness. For example, one study looked at people a week after a vaccination and found that those with high negative affect reported more symptoms from the vaccination than people who were low in negative affect (Petrie et al., 2004).

CLINICAL NOTES 4.1

Symptoms

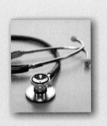

- There is no straightforward linear relationship between the extent of reported symptoms and disease.
- Because most people are bad at detecting physical changes, *do not* rely on self-reported measures of physical processes such as lung function or blood pressure.
- Getting patients to focus on external stimuli (e.g. distraction) is a useful technique for reducing symptoms such as pain. It is particularly useful for brief painful procedures such as injections or venepuncture.

4.1.2 EFFECTS OF SYMPTOM PERCEPTION ON HEALTH

The main effects of symptom perception on health are through the misperception and interpretation of symptoms. The misperception of symptoms potentially compromises the effectiveness of healthcare services through:

- A delay in seeking help if symptoms are interpreted as nonthreatening.
- The overuse or underuse of healthcare services if symptoms are interpreted wrongly.
- Compromised treatment if people self-treat or do not adhere to a treatment because they misattribute the cause of symptoms.

For example, someone might stop taking medication, such as antibiotics, because they feel a bit better but are not 'cured'. This is an obvious waste of resources and undermines

RESEARCH BOX 4.1   Intervention to help manage diabetes

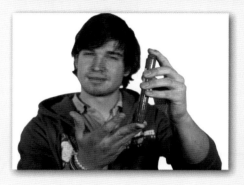

Background

Appraisal and interpretation of symptoms influence whether people seek and receive appropriate treatment. This is important in chronic illnesses such as diabetes. People with insulin-dependent diabetes have to make important self-care and treatment decisions based on their blood glucose levels or they can become hyper- or hypoglycaemic.

Many patients will rely on subjective judgements of blood glucose levels to do this, such as how they are feeling and how much food they have eaten. These types of judgement are usually very inaccurate.

Methods and findings

39 people with diabetes were randomly allocated to one of three interventions:

1 *Blood Glucose Awareness Training (BGAT)* – Seven weekly classes where patients worked through a manual giving information about blood glucose, symptoms, and estimating blood glucose levels. Patients also completed daily diaries recording symptoms, estimated blood glucose and actual blood glucose levels.
2 *Intensive BGAT* – as above but patients were also brought into hospital where their blood sugar levels were altered to put them into hypoglycaemia and hyperglycaemic ranges. During this procedure, patients were asked to focus on internal cues and record their experiences and estimate their blood glucose levels. This was followed by immediate feedback on their actual levels.
4 *Placebo control group* – seven weekly meetings with presentations on topics relevant to diabetes. Patients also kept diaries of daily stress and self-care behaviours.

Standard BGAT increased accuracy of estimates of blood glucose levels by 15 per cent (from 41 per cent before training to 56 per cent after training). Intensive BGAT was slightly more effective, increasing accuracy by 22 per cent. It also resulted in better metabolic control.

Significance

This was one of a few studies that showed how fairly simple interventions based on education and changing people's perceptions of symptoms can improve the self-management of chronic conditions like diabetes.

Cox, D.J. et al. (1991) Intensive versus standard glucose awareness training (BGAT) with insulin-dependent diabetes: mechanisms and ancillary effects, *Psychosomatic Medicine, 53*: 453–462.

effective treatment. (Factors influencing adherence are discussed in more detail in Chapter 17.)

Understanding the processes that affect symptom perception can therefore help us to design more effective interventions, particularly for chronic illnesses where people have to adhere to intensive treatment regimes. Research Box 4.1 gives an example of an intervention for people with diabetes, which includes education about symptom recognition, biases, and management. This led to a better metabolic control of diabetes than a standard educational intervention (Cox et al., 1991). Next we shall look at the symptom of pain and how psychological knowledge and research can help design effective treatments for chronic pain.

Summary

- Understanding symptoms is fundamental to good healthcare.
- Symptoms are any variation in our physiological state that are interpreted as unusual and labelled as potentially harmful.
- Symptoms can be a sign of the onset and progression of a disease. However there is not a straightforward relationship between symptoms and disease.
- How people appraise and interpret their symptoms is critical to whether they act and receive appropriate treatment.
- Psychological factors affect the perception and interpretation of symptoms though variables such as degree of attention, beliefs, or schemas about illnesses and individual vulnerability.
- Negative mood is associated with increased symptom perception.

4.2 PAIN

Pain is a common symptom and often an important signal that the body has been damaged or something is wrong. In rare cases of congenital insensitivity to pain, children have a reduced ability to feel pain and will be unable to recognise physical damage or danger. These children are at risk of a range of problems, including biting off parts of their tongue, being prone to eye infections following damage by foreign objects, and suffering broken bones or fractures.

Acute pain is therefore necessary to protect us from damage or infection. **Chronic pain** is somewhat different. In the general population chronic pain is common and thought to affect around 20 per cent of adults. An Australian survey of over 17,000 people found that 17 per cent of men and 20 per cent of women reported experiencing pain every day for at least three months (Blyth et al., 2001). In the USA, back pain is the sixth most common reason for attending a physician and accounts for 17.4 million visits every year (Cherry et al., 2001). Prolonged aches or pains are usually a signal that a part of our body is damaged or healing. However, if pain continues for three months or longer it is possible that the original physical damage has healed but that pain pathways have become over-sensitised or dysregulated so that pain is still felt in the absence of physical injury. Research has shown that after three months of stimulation to a pain pathway molecular changes occur in the RNA in the neurons of the spinal cord. Thus pain neurons adapt and change in the face of constant stimulation. Similarly, imaging research has shown extensive corti-cal reorganisation in response to chronic pain and that some maladaptive coping strategies, such as thinking the worst, can affect this (Gracely et al., 2004). This has implications for the treatment of chronic pain. Rather than taking a 'wait and see' approach, early interven-tion is important to prevent changes to the neural pathways.

How we view pain has implications for understanding and treatment. Biological explana-tions of pain assume pain results from physical damage. Treatment will therefore comprise analgesia to numb the pain and, if possible, surgery to repair the damage. However, as we have seen above, there can be many instances where pain occurs or continues in the absence of physical injury. Pain is increased by negative emotion, cognitive processes, and behaviour, such as inactivity. Studies of the influence of psychological factors on pain will typically use pain tolerance tasks under different conditions. For example, Rhudy and Meagher (2000) used electric shocks to create conditions where people would feel different emotions. In the anxiety group people were told 'You may or may not receive brief, surprising, and painful electrical shocks' so were anxious but not shocked. In the fear group people were given the same instructions and three electric shocks. In the neutral group people were told they would not receive any surprising negative stimuli. Pain tolerance was examined before and after the different conditions by asking participants to hold their hand under an intense heat and measuring how long they could withstand it. In keeping with previous research they found that anxiety led to reduced pain tolerance. However, fear led to increased pain toler-ance, which is probably due to the release of endogenous opioids under physically stressful conditions. This indicates that emotional states are important in the perception and toler-ance of pain. The range of factors that can affect pain perception is illustrated in Box 4.1 on page 82. Overall, we may say that pain is highly subjective and influenced by many factors, including biological, psychological, and social factors.

A number of distinctions are important in understanding pain. First, it is important to distinguish between nociception, sensation, and suffering. **Nociception** is the stimulation of peripheral pain receptors, which send pain messages to the central nervous system. The **sen-sation** of pain is how this is interpreted and, as we have already discussed, this will be influ-enced by many factors including attention, schemas, emotion, etc. **Suffering** refers to the perceived pain, distress, and disability that can arise from pain and other related factors.

Secondly it is important to distinguish between pain threshold and pain tolerance. The **pain threshold** is the point at which a stimulus becomes painful and is similar for most people, regardless of their gender, race, or culture. **Pain tolerance** is the degree to which a painful stimulus can be tolerated and this varies widely between individuals, cultures, and contexts. Humour, for example, can increase pain tolerance. Research shows that simply watching a funny film increases pain tolerance but this is moderated by how cheerful an individual is generally (Zweyer et al., 2004). Thus the point at which a person complains of pain will vary according to their background and characteristics, what they have learned from others about pain expression, and their immediate context. The implication for healthcare professionals is that each person's pain should be treated *as needed*, without referring to stereotypes about how much pain they 'should' be in.

Recent literature emphasises the importance of a multidimensional understanding of pain like that shown in Figure 4.1. A multidimensional understanding acknowledges that pain occurs within a social context and that there are different aspects to it: nociception, sensation, and emotional, cognitive, and behavioural responses. In many ways, this is similar to the models of emotion in Chapter 2 in that it shows the interdependence between sensation, thoughts, and emotion. It very much reflects a biopsychosocial approach.

Theory has made a significant contribution to our understanding of how psychological and physical factors can interact in the perception of pain. The **gate theory of pain** (Melzack, 1999; Melzack and Wall, 1965) is based on the notion of a synaptic gate between peripheral nerves and neurons in the spinal cord as illustrated in Figure 4.2. Pain signals from peripheral nerves compete with other neural signals to get through the gate. The gate can be open or closed by physical factors (e.g. stimulation from other peripheral nerves, endogenous opioids) or by psychological factors (e.g. attention, downward stimulation from the brain, moods). This theory therefore provides a good basis on which to understand the interplay between physical and psychological factors in pain. It also accounts for the phenomenon of pain being reduced through touch, such as when a child is hurt and their parent 'rubs it better'.

The advantage of gate theory is that it provides a physiological explanation for how psychological factors affect pain perception. It also makes it clear that pain is not simply physical or psychological, but a combination of both. However, evidence for this theory is mixed. There is a large amount of supporting evidence showing how psychological factors can influence pain

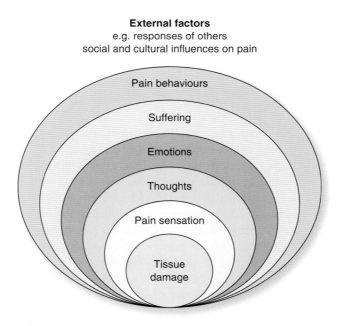

FIGURE 4.1 Multidimensional model of pain

ACUTE PAIN PROCESSES

CHRONIC PAIN

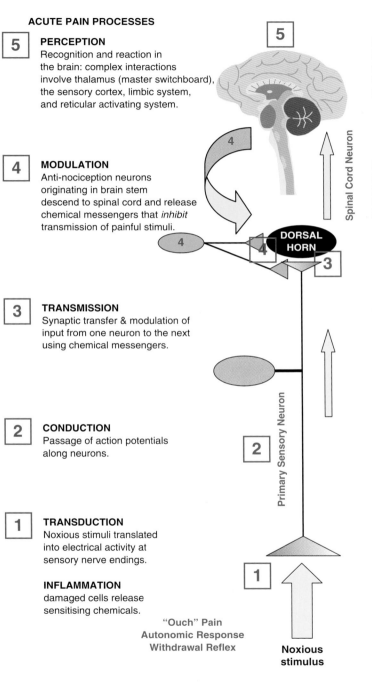

5 **PERCEPTION**
Recognition and reaction in the brain: complex interactions involve thalamus (master switchboard), the sensory cortex, limbic system, and reticular activating system.

MENTAL OVERLOAD
Possible neurochemical link between pain and memory. High incidence of depression, anxiety. Suffering increases perceived pain.

4 **MODULATION**
Anti-nociception neurons originating in brain stem descend to spinal cord and release chemical messengers that *inhibit* transmission of painful stimuli.

LOSS OF CONTROL
Normally innocuous stimuli become painful. Once activated, even small movements/deformity of tissues becomes painful.

DORSAL HORN

Spinal Cord Neuron

3 **TRANSMISSION**
Synaptic transfer & modulation of input from one neuron to the next using chemical messengers.

SENSITIZATION:
Repeated pain signals produce changes in the nervous system. Pain becomes more painful.

2 **CONDUCTION**
Passage of action potentials along neurons.

DAMAGED NERVE:
Damaged sensory nerves may send constant pain signals like an alarm bell that won't shut off.

Primary Sensory Neuron

1 **TRANSDUCTION**
Noxious stimuli translated into electrical activity at sensory nerve endings.

NEUROGENIC INFLAMMATION:
Increased prostanoid production at site of pain produces allodynia and hyperalgesia and generates spontaneous pain.

INFLAMMATION
damaged cells release sensitising chemicals.

"Ouch" Pain
Autonomic Response
Withdrawal Reflex

Noxious stimulus

FIGURE 4.2   The psychophysiology of pain
Reproduced courtesy of Christine Whitten MD (Whitten et al., 2005)

but the physiological evidence for gate theory is less consistent. Nonetheless, gate theory is an important and useful part of pain management programmes because it helps people with chronic pain understand that their mental attitude and behaviour can influence their pain. This

---

BOX 4.1   Factors that open or close the pain 'gate'

	Factors that tend to open the gate	Factors that tend to close the gate
Physical	Further injury	Appropriate use of medication
	Inactivity/poor physical fitness	Heat/cold
	Long term drug and alcohol use	Massage
Behavioural	Poor pacing of activity i.e. doing too much	Exercise
		Relaxation training
	Poor sleep	Meditation
Emotional	Anxiety, depression	Laughter/humour
	Stress, distress	Love
	Hopelessness/helplessness	Pleasure/happiness
Cognitive	Focusing on the pain	Focusing on other things e.g. hobbies
	Worrying about the pain	
	Catastrophising (thinking the worst)	Distraction
	Focusing on the negative consequences of pain	Positive coping strategies
	Wishing it would go away	

---

can help them feel less helpless and more in control. It provides them with knowledge about the things that can open or close the gate, such as those shown in Box 4.1, so they can actively work to reduce their pain by increasing those things in their life that will close the gate.

4.2.1 MANAGING CHRONIC PAIN

Because pain is multidimensional, effective interventions for chronic pain need to tackle the physiological, psychological, and social factors involved in pain. Chronic pain management programmes will therefore involve physicians, physiotherapists, psychologists, and specialist nurses who work together to use pharmacological, behavioural, and psychological techniques to help people with chronic pain. The aim of these programmes is to assist people in effectively *managing* their pain so they can lead a functional and positive life. These programmes are very effective, particularly if they involve a psychological component. Psychological components include educating patients about the different dimensions of pain and how vicious cycles can arise such as that shown in Figure 4.3. Patients are encouraged to take control of their life and through a process of empowerment to become more active. This can then lead to a positive cycle of less anxiety, less focus on the pain, and therefore less pain.

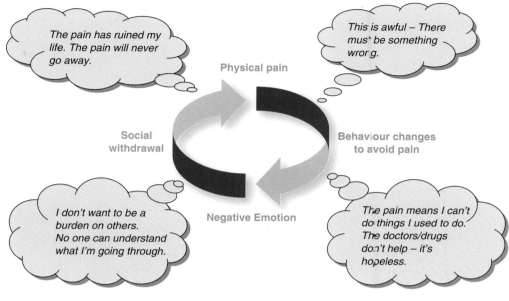

FIGURE 4.3 Vicious cycle of pain

CASE STUDY 4.2 Treating chronic back pain

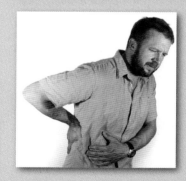

Bob is a 40 year old man who works as a laboratory technician and has chronic lower back pain. The pain started following a work-related accident three years ago. In the last six months the pain has become constant and seems to get much worse when Bob is driving or sitting. Bob's back occasionally 'goes into spasm'. When this happens he feels semi-paralysed and has to lie down on the floor until the attack passes. This has only happened twice but Bob is very anxious about the possibility of another attack.

Bob is on long-term sick leave and may have to transfer onto disability benefits. He does not go out very much because he is worried he will have another attack and collapse.

Bob is depressed and says the pain has taken over his life. He uses a number of pain relief medications every day but says it doesn't help. He is physically inactive.

(Cont'd)

TREATMENT

In a typical pain management programme Bob would be seen by a physician to rule out any physical cause for his pain and agree an effective approach to analgesia. A physiotherapist would examine Bob and teach him exercises to strengthen his back. The physiotherapist might also help Bob increase his activity levels each week.

Psychological treatment may involve education, deconstructing the pain problem, and reconstructing more adaptive ways of coping.

Educating Bob about psychological aspects of pain may help him understand how his actions and thoughts affect his pain. He would be encouraged to manage his pain, rather than allowing it to manage him.

Deconstructing the pain involves monitoring and increasing the awareness of pain processes. Bob might complete a pain diary to identify any pattern to his symptoms, the effect it is having on his life, and how his pain is linked to triggers like stress, thoughts, emotions and general activity levels. Maladaptive thought processes or behaviours would be identified and Bob would be encouraged to change these.

Reconstructing beliefs and coping to be more adaptive may involve teaching Bob strategies such as relaxation techniques (there are many CDs available that do this), positive self-talk, and setting and achieving goals. By this stage Bob should be exercising and going out more often, which should be eroding his fear and avoidance of activity, and helping him feel more in control of his pain. Providing him with positive coping strategies may consolidate Bob's feelings of control and empowerment and eventually result in him returning to work and leading a happier and more productive life.

Pain management programmes are very effective and can result in less pain, depression or other negative emotion, and abnormal pain behaviour. They can also lead to more successful coping, increased activity, and improved social functioning (Morley, 2007). Programmes vary widely in their specific approach. Case Study 4.2 illustrates a broad approach.

Summary

- Pain is a common symptom: up to 20 per cent of the adult population is estimated to suffer from chronic pain.
- Pain is multidimensional: it involves nociception, pain sensations, thoughts, emotions, pain behaviours, and suffering.
- Attention, anxiety, and distress are associated with increased pain.
- The gate theory of pain provides a physiological explanation for the influence of psychological factors on pain.
- Pain management programmes help patients cope better with chronic pain. They are often effective at reducing pain, depression, negative emotion, negative coping, and maladaptive pain behaviour; and increasing activity, positive coping, and social functioning.

4.3 PLACEBO AND NOCEBO EFFECTS

Placebo and nocebo effects provide clear examples of the effect of beliefs on symptoms. The term 'placebo' is Latin for *I shall please*. A **placebo effect** is when people are given a fake treatment that has no active ingredient yet report an improvement. Placebo effects are not limited to fake drugs but can also occur in response to fake surgery (Moseley et al., 2002). An example of research showing a placebo effect is given in Research Box 4.2.

Some people will respond more strongly to placebos than others, and some illnesses are more amenable to placebos. Evidence suggests that placebo effects are most powerful for conditions with psychological components such as pain, depression, asthma, and insomnia. Placebos however are not effective for disorders with a clear biological basis, such as anemia and infections (Wampold et al., 2005). Characteristics of the placebo will affect how well they work. For example, injections have a larger effect than pills; fake morphine has a larger effect than fake aspirin; placebo effects are larger if the doctor expresses a belief it will work; and so on.

RESEARCH BOX 4.2   Listening to prozac and hearing placebo

Background

Meta analysis is a technique used to synthesise the results of several studies to give a statistical summary of the findings. However to produce the most accurate information, meta analysis should be based on published and unpublished research.

Method and findings

Information from published and unpublished randomised controlled trials of the most widely used antidepressant medications (SSRIs) was collected. Thirty-five trials were found involving 5,133 people with major depressive disorder. All trials compared the effect of SSRIs with a placebo drug.

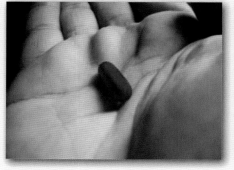

For most patients, the effect of SSRIs was so small it was not clinically significant. A placebo could duplicate 80 per cent of the effect of antidepressants.

In patients with extremely severe depression, antidepressants had a small effect on recovery, but this seemed to be mainly due to these patients being less responsive to placebos rather than being more responsive to antidepressants.

(Cont'd)

Significance

Previous meta-analyses of published research had found more positive results, with small effects of some SSRIs on depression. This meta-analysis was the first to include unpublished evidence and clearly shows that SSRIs are no better than a placebo for treating mild or moderate depression. SSRIs are therefore only clinically useful for the treatment of very severe depression.

Photograph reproduced courtesy of Clix (stock.xchng)

Kirsch, I. et al. (2008) Initial severity and antidepressant benefits: a meta-analysis of data submitted to the Food and Drug Administration *PLoS Medicine, 5(2)*: 260-268.

The **nocebo effect** is less well known. The term 'nocebo' is Latin for *I shall harm*. The nocebo effect occurs when people develop symptoms that will fit their beliefs when they have not been exposed to a pathogen. For example, Lorber et al. (2007) asked students to inhale an inert substance, which they said was a toxin that could result in particular symptoms. In addition, half the students watched another person, who was secretly a research confederate, inhale the substance first and show these symptoms. All students who inhaled the placebo reported the symptoms they were told they might have. Women were particularly influenced if they saw the confederate display symptoms.

What underlies these placebo and nocebo effects remains the subject of much debate. Explanations here include classical conditioning, modelling, and the effect of expectations. **Classical conditioning** occurs when a stimulus (in this case an active drug or treatment) is paired with a response (an improvement in health) and over time becomes associated with a neutral stimulus that also occurs in this context (pills, injections, doctors' actions). The neutral stimulus then becomes a conditioned stimulus, which results in some of the changes observed to the initial active stimulus. **Modelling** occurs when one observes the effect in someone else and learns it. These types of learning are outlined in more detail in Chapter 10.

Another explanation is that placebos work by altering a person's **expectations** – they expect to get better, so they do. There is evidence that both classical conditioning and expectations can contribute to the placebo effect, that these are not incompatible. Classical conditioning may also lead to altered expectations about the effect of the conditioned stimulus (Kirsch, 2007).

4.3.1 USING THE PLACEBO EFFECT IN CLINICAL PRACTICE

The placebo effect has many clinical implications. The first is that the effect of many active drugs can be increased by the way they are presented – both in form, such as a pill or injection; and in manner, such as with enthusiasm and conviction. A doctor who encourages patients to believe treatments will work can harness the placebo effect in addition to the drug. The second implication is that placebos can result in a positive change without any negative side effects, so are useful treatments for those conditions that are amenable to placebos, such as depression. In fact, up to 60 per cent of physicians and nurses report already using placebos to treat patients (Nitzan and Lichtenberg, 2004). However, if we use these strategies we must be mindful of the ethical issues. People should be encouraged to have positive expectations, but within realistic limits. The dilemma when using placebos is how to do so without employing deception. Kirsch (2007)

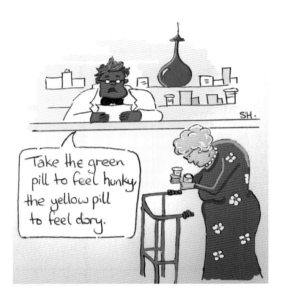

CLINICAL NOTES 4.2

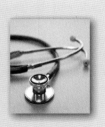

Pain and placebo

- Pain is subjective so each person's pain should be treated *as needed*, without reference to stereotypes about how much pain they 'should' have.
- Chronic pain results in extensive neural changes that are difficult to reverse so we should intervene as early as possible to avoid these.
- Placebo effects can duplicate 80 per cent of the effect of antidepressants in people with mild or moderate depression.
- Use the placebo effect to increase the effect of treatment: express confidence that treatments will work to increase patients' positive expectations.
- Conversely, if you tell patients to expect side-effects or negative symptoms they will be more likely to experience them (the nocebo effect).

recommends looking for treatments that do not have active components but where there is some evidence they might be effective, such as some complementary therapies or physical exercise.

Summary

- A placebo effect occurs when someone's health improves in the absence of any active substance or treatment.
- A nocebo effect occurs when someone reports symptoms because they expect or believe they will have them.
- These effects can account for a substantial proportion of recovery, particularly in illnesses with strong psychological components, such as asthma and depression.
- The extent of the placebo effect varies between individuals.
- Placebos are thought to work through a combination of expectations, classical conditioning, and modelling.
- The placebo effect can be used in clinical practice to aid recovery.

4.4 ILLNESS BELIEFS AND REPRESENTATIONS

Earlier in this chapter we looked at the effect of unconscious schema on the perception of symptoms. In addition to this, people hold conscious beliefs about illness which will shape their behaviour in response to symptoms. Beliefs about illness will determine the action a person chooses to take, which information they give to a doctor, the kind of treatment they want, whether they adhere to that treatment, and their emotional, behavioural, and cognitive responses to the illness. Illness beliefs are not necessarily accurate or coherent. **Illness representations** are people's organised sets of beliefs about the experience, impact, effect and outcome of an illness. They are unique to each individual and will be shaped by many factors, including their personal history, experience of different illnesses, and social and cultural learning.

Five main dimensions of illness representations have been established: identity, timeline, cause, control, and consequences (Leventhal et al., 1984). Here we will outline each of these in more detail. The concept of **illness identity** refers to the way a person labels the illness and symptoms, such as what multiple sclerosis is and what it involves. People will have mental models of which symptoms go with different illnesses. The more various symptoms match a person's model of a particular illness the more likely it is they will diagnose themselves as having that illness. For example, a headache could be due to many things like a hangover, tension, migraine, a brain tumour, or meningitis. A self-diagnosis of meningitis is more likely if a person experiences a headache, stiff neck and a rash. Making a self-diagnosis is important in seeking help. Research shows that people are more likely to attend a doctor if they have self-diagnosed a specific illness (Cameron et al., 1993).

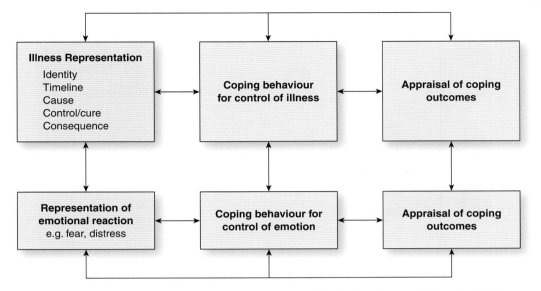

FIGURE 4.4   Self-regulation model of illness cognition and behaviour (Leventhal et al., 1984)

CASE STUDY 4.3   The self-regulation model and chest pain

The self-regulation model illustrates how symptoms, such as chest pain, will be perceived and interpreted by a person on the basis of their illness representations, which in turn will influence their coping behaviour. The symptom will also evoke an emotional reaction that will lead to coping strategies to control that emotion. Both the emotional and cognitive strands will influence each other. Coping and reappraisal can then lead to an adjustment of beliefs, emotions, and coping responses and so on, as illustrated below.

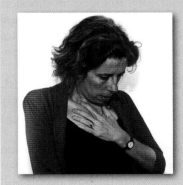

Tanya is 48 and has a pain in her chest one evening after she has eaten a large dinner and had a heated argument with her husband. Tanya's uncle died of a heart attack a few years ago, aged 65. Tanya thinks that men are particularly vulnerable to heart attacks but women are not (identity). Tanya knows that indigestion or heartburn can also cause pain in the chest (cause). She also knows that arguments and stress can lead to an upset stomach (cause). She therefore interprets this pain as indigestion, which will pass if she relaxes (consequences). She makes herself a calming cup of tea and goes to lie down (coping response).

(Cont'd)

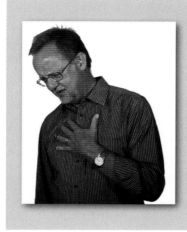

Tom is 48 and has a pain in his chest one evening after he has eaten a large dinner and had a heated argument with his wife. Tom's uncle died of a heart attack a few years ago, aged 65. Tom knows that men in their 40s are particularly vulnerable to heart attacks (identity) and that they can be caused by stress (cause). He therefore immediately interprets this pain as a possible heart attack with potentially fatal consequences (consequences). He becomes very anxious and upset and feels his heart pounding. He calls an ambulance to take him to hospital immediately (coping response).

The **timeline** is the length of time that a person believes the illness will last and the pattern it will take e.g. chronic, acute, remitting, or cyclical. This will affect their adjustment to the illness and adherence to treatment. For example, people who believe their illnesses are chronic will report more disability and distress compared to other people with the same illness who believe it is acute or cyclical (Millar et al., 2005).

The **cause** is what a person thinks caused their symptoms or illness. This overlaps with the attributions and interpretation of symptoms discussed earlier (see page 75): however they may not be medically accurate. For example, stress is commonly believed to cause a range of illnesses including cancer, diabetes, multiple sclerosis, and arthritis (Cameron and Moss-Morris, 2004).

Beliefs about **control** concern whether the person believes their illness can be prevented, controlled or cured. People who think their illness is controllable are more likely to take an active part in their treatment and rehabilitation. Conversely, thinking an illness is uncontrollable is associated with using passive coping strategies (e.g. avoidance) and increased hospital admissions (Scharloo et al., 1999). In a chronic or terminal illness, we should therefore encourage people to focus on those aspects of their illness they can control, such as their symptoms, disability, and the timeline.

Beliefs about **consequences** are concerned with the effect of the illness e.g. physical, psychological, social, and economic effects. Perceived consequences are usually closely linked to the severity of someone's symptoms. Therefore asymptomatic illnesses, such as hypertension, are often viewed as having no consequences.

The diagram in Figure 4.4 shows how illness representations can affect the way a person copes with their symptoms, illness, and treatment (Leventhal et al., 1984). This is known as the **self-regulation model of illness behaviour** because it accounts for how people will self-manage their illness as a result of their personal beliefs. The strengths of this model are that it recognises the importance of appraisal, emotion, and coping in managing illness.

Case Study 4.3 illustrates how illness beliefs can affect perceptions of chest pain. A difficulty with the illness representations model is that severe illnesses like cancer are more likely to result in negative illness representations e.g. being chronic, uncontrollable, and having severe consequences. A key question is therefore whether illness representations can affect a person's adjustment over and above the severity of the illness itself Many studies have shown that this is the case. Beliefs about the consequences of chronic diseases such as rheumatoid arthritis and multiple sclerosis are associated with poorer psychological outcomes, reports of more symptoms, and an increased use of health services (e.g. Jopson and Moss-Morris, 2003).

ACTIVITY 4.2   ILLNESS REPRESENTATIONS

- Think of a patient you have seen who was particularly upset by their illness.
- What sort of beliefs did they have about their illness identity, timeline, cause, control, and consequences?

RESEARCH BOX 4.3   Self-management Intervention after a myocardial infarction

Background

Self-management interventions focus on patients' illness representations and coping skills in order to promote effective self-management for a range of illnesses. This study compared a self-management intervention to standard care for MI patients.

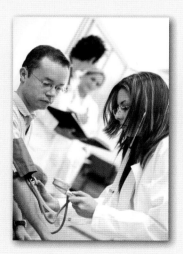

Methods and findings

Sixty five people who had had an MI were randomly allocated to receive a self-management intervention or standard care while in hospital. Patients were assessed before and after the intervention and followed up three months later. The self-management intervention involved three half-an-hour sessions:

- *Session 1*: educating about MI and exploring patients' beliefs about the cause of their MI; challenging the common perception that an MI is largely caused by stress; educating patients about the importance of lifestyle (e.g. exercise and diet).

(Cont'd)

- *Session 2*: exploring patients' perceptions of the timeline and consequences; encouraging patients to develop beliefs of control. Developing an individualised written illness management plan to minimise future risks and encourage returning to normal levels of activity.
- *Session 3*: reviewing the action plan from session 2 and educating about distinguishing normal symptoms of recovery from symptoms that might indicate another MI.

People who had the self-management intervention did much better. They felt more prepared for leaving hospital, had a better understanding of MI, were less distressed at discharge, were more likely to attend cardiac rehabilitation, viewed their MI more positively, and had more positive beliefs about control, consequences, and the timeline of MI. Three months later, patients in the self-management group had returned to work quicker and reported fewer symptoms of angina.

Significance

This study shows how a brief intervention in hospital based on the principles of illness representations helped patients understand and manage their MI better, return to work quicker, and have fewer symptoms in the long term.

Photograph © Andres Rodriguez/Fotolia

Petrie, K.J. et al. (2002) Changing illness perceptions after myocardial infarction: an early intervention randomized controlled trial, *Psychosomatic Medicine, 64*: 580–586.

4.4.1 APPLICATION TO CLINICAL PRACTICE

Illness representations have many implications for clinical practice. Managing an illness which is abstract is harder than managing an illness when a person has concrete experience of it. In other words, people are less likely to adhere to treatment for an illness where there are no concrete symptoms. This can be the case in asymptomatic illnesses like hypertension, or illnesses that do not have regular symptoms such as diabetes or HIV. This links to the issue of motivation: if people do not have symptoms, they may be more likely to favour an immediate reward (such as sugary food for diabetics) over the long-term consequences.

People can also have beliefs and representations about treatment procedures which will affect how likely they are to adhere to particular treatments. For example, the use of corticosteroids will not be effective if a person associates it with the steroids used by body builders and is put off by this. Some people may also worry about the addictive properties of certain drugs and will therefore not take them. For example, one study found 78 per cent of people believed antidepressants were addictive (Priest et al., 1996). For this and other reasons, between 30 and 60 per cent of people on antidepressants will not take them as prescribed (Demyttenaere, 2001).

The self-regulation model of illness beliefs can therefore be useful when treating patients. By exploring and changing a person's illness beliefs we can maximise the chances of them managing their illness appropriately, both through changing their lifestyle and adhering to treatment. These types of intervention are broadly referred to as **self-management interventions** because they target patients' beliefs and coping in order to help them manage their illness and treatment effectively. Research has shown that self-management interventions are usually effective at promoting the positive self-management of diabetes, asthma, HIV, and cancer (Petrie et al., 2003). Research Box 4.3 gives one example of a study that used a self-management intervention with patients following MI. This was found to be very effective at reducing patients distress, symptoms, and increasing their return to work.

Summary

- Beliefs about illnesses will affect how people appraise symptoms; interpret symptoms; whether they seek help; and their adherence to treatment.
- Illness representations can include illness identity, timeline, cause, control, and consequences.
- Illness representations are associated with both the psychological and physical outcomes of illness.
- The self-regulation model explains how illness representations can interact with coping to determine health outcomes.
- Illness representations can be used to develop effective self-management interventions for chronic illnesses that will help people cope with and manage their illness and treatment more effectively.

CLINICAL NOTES 4.3

Illness representations

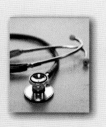

- How a person thinks about their illness will affect their distress, symptom perception, and disability.
- Self-management interventions can educate patients and help them think about their illness in more adaptive ways.
- To help people manage their illness better we need to help them:

  o Correct any misperceptions about the cause of their illness (and therefore future risk).
  o Focus on an aspect of their illness that they can control – such as treatment adherence or symptom management.
  o Reduce their perceptions of severe consequences through education and joint treatment plans. In cases of terminal illness this may involve tackling worries about pain relief and dying.

CONCLUSION

In this chapter we have seen how the perception of symptoms is strongly influenced by psychological factors including attention, emotions, beliefs, and environmental factors. The importance of psychological factors in the outcome of illnesses has been illustrated by placebo and nocebo effects, which can be substantial. Research and theory in this area are therefore highly relevant to clinical practice and have been used to develop effective treatments such as pain management programmes and self-management programmes in order to help people manage their symptoms and illness more effectively.

FURTHER READING

Ayers, S. et al. (eds) (2007) *Cambridge Handbook of Psychology, Health and Medicine* (2nd edition). Cambridge: Cambridge University Press. This book includes many relevant chapters, including some short chapters on pain, pain management, placebos, and illness representations.

Cameron, L.D. and Leventhal, H. (2003) *The Self-Regulation of Health and Illness Behaviour*. London: Routledge. This book has more in-depth information on illness beliefs and self-regulation, with chapters on the theory of self-regulation, illness representations, social and cultural influences, and interventions.

Sutton, S., Baum, A. and Johnston, M. (eds) (2004) *The SAGE Handbook of Health Psychology*. London: SAGE. This book has a useful chapter on 'Living with chronic illness' which gives more details about illness representations and self regulation in chronic illness.

? REVISION QUESTIONS

1   What is a symptom? How accurate are people at detecting changes in physiological states (e.g. blood pressure)?

2   Discuss the role of two psychological factors in the perception of physical symptoms.

3   What is the difference between a person's pain threshold and pain tolerance? Briefly outline the role of psychological factors in both.

4   Outline the gate theory of pain and discuss how it has extended our understanding of the interplay between psychological and physical factors.

5   What is the multidimensional model of pain? What implications does it have for treatment?

6   What is a placebo effect? What factors affect how strong it is?

7   What is a nocebo effect? What is the evidence it affects symptom perception?

8   Outline three different explanations for why placebo and nocebo effects might occur.

9   Describe the five main dimensions of illness representations.

10 Describe a self-management intervention based on the self-regulation model.

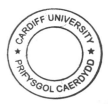

5 HEALTH AND BEHAVIOUR

LEARNING OBJECTIVES

This chapter is designed to enable you to:

- Discuss the importance of health behaviour and of health behaviour change.
- Outline the different models of health behaviour.
- Understand how to apply these models in clinical practice to help people change.

Understanding and changing health behaviour effectively would do more than anything else to reduce morbidity and mortality in our society. In the UK the top three causes of death are cardiovascular disease, which accounts for 30 per cent of all deaths, respiratory infections (11 per cent) and lung cancer (6 per cent). This pattern is similar in most developed countries (WHO, 2008). All of these illnesses can be caused or exacerbated by smoking, which has been labelled the number one cause of preventable illness and death (Office of the Surgeon General, 2004). Most people know cigarette smoking is bad for their health, yet approximately one out of every four or five people smoke. Even when they are in hospital some patients will continue to smoke, despite often having to stand outside to do so.

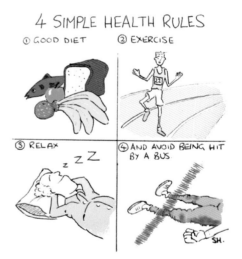

5.1 PREDICTING AND CHANGING HEALTH BEHAVIOUR

5.1.1 WHAT ARE HEALTH BEHAVIOURS?

It is not only risky behaviours like smoking that have an impact on our health. In a famous longitudinal study of almost 7,000 people living in Alameda County in the USA, it was

---

BOX 5.1   Behaviours associated with long life

Not smoking
Being physically active
Moderate weight
Moderate alcohol consumption
7–8 hours sleep a night
Eating breakfast regularly
Not snacking

(Belloc, 1973; Kaplan et al., 1987)

---

found that the seven behaviours listed in Box 5.1 were associated with a longer life. These included eating breakfast and getting eight hours sleep a night.

Thus our health is affected by a range of behaviours, which can be categorised as (a) health protective behaviours and (b) health risk behaviours. **Health protective behaviours** consist of things like exercise, a good diet, sleep, and dental care. It also includes **screening behaviours** such as attending regular screening checks for chlamydia, cervical cancer, hypertension, and dental checks. **Health risk behaviours** include things such as smoking, substance misuse, unsafe sex, and risky driving. Behaviours particularly pertinent to morbidity and mortality include smoking, diet, physical activity, alcohol consumption, screening behaviour (particularly for cancer), sexual behaviour, and driving behaviour.

CLINICAL NOTES 5.1

Smoking and health

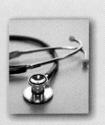

- Smoking is the number one cause of preventable illness and death.
- Every single person you help to give up smoking reduces a lot of morbidity and mortality – not only for them but also potentially for their children too.
- Doctors' advice is one of the most effective triggers for people to give up smoking.
- Even *brief* advice from a doctor makes it more likely a person will give up smoking and remain non-smoking a year later.

We need to understand why people choose to behave in ways that will harm their health in order to help them change. This is not simple: behaviour is determined by many factors, including individual differences, social surroundings and influences, and cultural aspects. In order to have effective health promotion programmes we need to know the main causes of specific behaviours in different groups of people. For example, young people might be more motivated to eat a low-fat diet and regularly brush their teeth to improve their appearance rather than to improve their health, so emphasising the health benefits of these behaviours would not result in significant change in this group. The range of factors that influence health behaviour is shown in Box 5.2. Research and theories of health behaviour try to identify the strongest or proximal causes of behaviour so intervention can target those factors which are most likely to result in change.

BOX 5.2   Factors that influence health behaviour

Biological factors	Heredity (i.e. genetic factors)
	Sex
	Age
Psychological factors	Operant conditioning
	Modelling
	Emotional state
	Cognitive factors
Social factors	Demographic factors
	Social factors
	Financial/employment status
Cultural factors	Legislation
	Economics
	Healthcare provision
	Systems of provision

5.1.2 THEORIES OF HEALTH BEHAVIOUR

Many theories of health behaviour have been proposed. In recent years, **social-cognition models** have been most successful at explaining health behaviour. These models include the interplay between social and cognitive factors, such as social pressures, social norms, beliefs and attitudes. These models are based on an *expectancy-value* principle. This assumes that a behaviour is most likely to be maintained or changed if (a) a person expects it to result in certain outcomes and (b) the person values these outcomes as important or positive. These models account for up to a third of the variance in people's behaviour. Other theories integrate aspects of social-cognition models with other factors, such as an individual's readiness or motivation to change.

This chapter discusses four models of health behaviour: two social-cognitive models and two integrative models. We examine the evidence for these models and explore how we can use them in clinical practice to help people change their behaviour. This is illustrated by a case study that shows how each model could be adopted to help a young woman stop smoking.

Predicting and changing health behaviour

The social-cognition models that have been most widely used in the study of health behaviour are the Health Belief Model and the Theory of Planned Behaviour. Examples of integrative approaches are the Transtheoretical Model and PRIME Theory. These models do not necessarily compete. Although one model may be more successful at predicting a particular type of behaviour, aspects of all these models can be used in clinical practice.

5.2 THE HEALTH BELIEF MODEL

The Health Belief Model (HBM) was developed by a team of social psychologists in the US Public Health Service to understand why the uptake of tuberculosis (TB) screening programmes in the 1950s was so low (Rosenstock, 1974; Strecher et al., 1997). The HBM is shown in Figure 5.1 and suggests that the likelihood of someone changing their behaviour is primarily determined by the **perceived threat** of their current situation, coupled with an **evaluation of the outcome** if they change. Perceived threat is thought to be influenced mainly by the **perceived susceptibility** to negative consequences and the **perceived severity** of these consequences for the person. For example, if a person thinks they are not susceptible to TB then obviously TB will not be a threat to them so they are unlikely to attend screening. Another person might think they are susceptible to TB but that TB is not severe enough to do anything about. Perceived susceptibility and severity then combine to produce a level of perceived threat that motivates people to take action or change their behaviour.

However, even when the perceived threat is high, people might still not change their behaviour. There is another factor here that influences behaviour, namely how a person evaluates the outcome. This evaluation is affected by **perceived benefits** and **perceived barriers.** Perceived benefits are what a person thinks they will gain from the behaviour or behaviour change. This can be the removal of negative as well as positive factors. For example, attending TB screening can mean the threat of the illness is removed or the illness is treated in its early stages before it causes a disability. Perceived barriers are things that make it difficult for a person to carry out the behaviour. For TB screening this might include not being able to take time off work, the screening clinic being a long distance away, difficulty in finding childcare, a lack of transport, etc.

The HBM is the only model that explicitly recognises the importance of **cues to action** that will prompt people to change. These cues can be internal (such as perceived symptoms), or external (such as health promotion, the advice of a doctor or nurse, or the illness or death of a known person). The illness or death of a public figure can provide strong cues to act that may be wide reaching through extensive media coverage. For example, when Linda McCartney died of breast cancer, the media coverage resulted in many women being screened and treated who might not have accessed this service otherwise. More recently, the death of celebrity Jade Goody from cervical cancer resulted in a 20 per cent increase in the number of women having cervical screening in the UK.

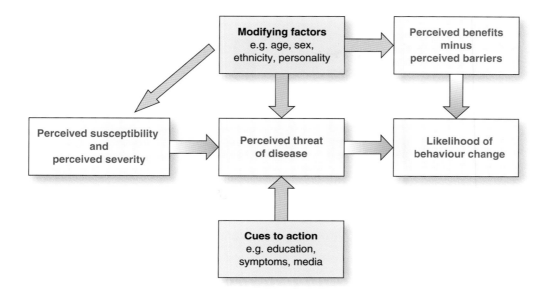

FIGURE 5.1   The Health Belief Model

Cues to action can take many forms. Smoking research has indicated that one of the most effective triggers in persuading someone to quit smoking is for a doctor to tell a patient they should give up. Even brief simple advice from a physician can make it more likely a smoker will quit and remain a non-smoker 12 months later (Stead et al., 2008). However, cues to action are not always necessary for change. If an individual has a suffi-cient perceived threat and positive evaluation of the outcome of change then they will often change without needing a cue. In other cases cues can be the final trigger that will tip the balance between a perceived threat and barriers and will prompt someone to act.

Later versions of the HBM have included **health motivation** as a factor. This relates to how much a person is concerned about their health and prepared to consider behaviour change. Surprisingly, health motivation and cues to action have been relatively ignored by research. Consequently there is little evidence available on whether these are important. From the limited evidence we do have it seems that health motivation might have a small but significant effect on behaviour (Abraham and Sheeran, 2007).

The HBM is one of the longest-standing models of health behaviour. It has been researched in relation to many health behaviours, including breast self-examination, flu vaccinations, diabetes management, medication for hypertension, and cancer screening (Janz and Becker, 1984). Reviews of the evidence for the HBM have been generally positive and find that perceived barriers are often the most important factor in preventing change (Harrison et al., 1992; Janz and Becker, 1984). The importance of the HBM for different categories of health behaviour is shown in Figure 5.2. It can be seen that screening behav-iours are most influenced by perceived barriers and susceptibility. When changing risky

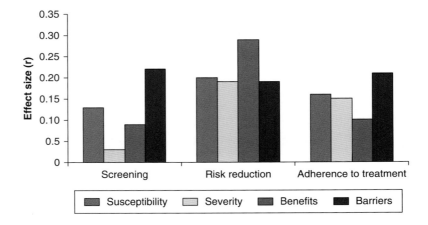

FIGURE 5.2   The Health Belief Model and different types of behaviour (adapted from Harrison et al., 1992)

behaviours it is the perceived benefits that are most important. Adherence to medical treatment is most affected by perceived barriers to the treatment.

Interventions using the Health Belief Model

To use the HBM in clinical practice we should explore patients' perceived susceptibility, severity, benefits and barriers, as well as any cues. People's perceptions of threat and benefits can be improved through education. Problem-solving and action plans could be used to reduce perceived barriers. Using the HBM to design interventions has proved very effective. For example, Yabroff and Mandelblatt (1999) looked at 63 interventions designed to increase breast cancer screening through mammograms. Interventions based on the HBM were 23 per cent more effective than the usual care.

ACTIVITY 5.1   YOUR OWN HEALTH BEHAVIOUR

Think back to the last time you:

- Went to the doctor.
- Checked yourself for breast or testicular lumps.

How much (if at all) was your behaviour affected by the perceived severity, susceptibility, benefits, and barriers in these different situations?

Case Study 5.1 shows how we might use the HBM to help a young woman give up smoking. This illustrates how the model may be implemented as a guide if we wish to help people change a risky health behaviour.

CASE STUDY 5.1 Smoking cessation using the Health Belief Model

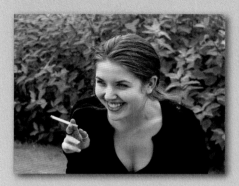

Jenny is a 22 year old woman who has smoked 20 cigarettes a day since she was 15 years old. She coughs every morning and gets breathless easily. She has a strong family history of asthma although she has never been checked for asthma herself.

Cues to action

Explore whether anything has triggered her to consider giving up smoking:

- *Has anything made you think about giving up smoking?*

If so, capitalise on this by reinforcing it. Give her positive feedback if she has thought about giving up smoking.

Health motivation

Explore how motivated or concerned she is about her health:

- *How concerned are you about your health?* (abstract health concern)
- *How important is it to you to stay healthy/not to get ill?* (concrete health concern)

Susceptibility and severity

Explore the perceived susceptibility and severity:

- *How do you think smoking is affecting your health?* (current susceptibility)
- *How might it affect your health in ten years' time?* (future susceptibility)
- *What would it be like if that happened to you/you got [illness]?* (severity)

Educate about the negative effects of smoking to increase the perceived susceptibility and severity:

- *If you smoke you are more likely to have heart disease, a stroke, circulation problems, lung cancer, and many other cancers.*
- *Every cigarette you smoke contains over 4000 chemicals.*
- *The toxins in cigarettes put huge strain on your body.*
- *Other effects of smoking are that your skin ages quicker, teeth become discoloured, gum disease, poor sense of smell, reduced fertility, and blindness.*
- *Smoking is therefore the single most preventable cause of illness and death.*

(Cont'd)

Perceived benefits and barriers

Explore the perceived benefits and barriers:

- *What are the pros and cons of smoking for you?* (current benefits & costs)
- *Is there anything stopping you from giving up?* (current barriers)

Problem solving to reduce barriers:

- *How can you/we change this? What steps can you/we take to help you give up?* (reducing current barriers and focusing on taking action)

Educate about the positive benefits if they give up smoking now, to increase the perceived benefits:

- *If you give up smoking you will improve your health and live longer.*
- *Your risk of heart disease drops dramatically in the first year after quitting.*
- *You will feel healthier and, as smoking damages the skin, you might look better too.*
- *You will save a huge amount of money! Someone who smokes 20-a day will spend around £1600 ($2600) a year on cigarettes.*

5.3 THE THEORY OF PLANNED BEHAVIOUR

The Theory of Planned Behaviour (TPB: Ajzen, 1988) originated from social psychology and was first proposed to explain all kinds of behaviour not just health behaviour. This theory is shown in Figure 5.3. It starts from the assumption that the strongest predictor of behaviour will be a person's **intentions** – in other words, how a person intends to behave will be the strongest determinant of how they will actually behave.

Intentions are thought to be determined by two factors. The first is a person's **attitudes** towards the behaviour (see Chapter 9). This is influenced by their *beliefs about the outcomes of the behaviour* (e.g. the pros and cons) and their *evaluation of these outcomes* (e.g. whether these are positive or negative). Consider our case study. If Jenny believes smoking will keep her slim and reduce stress (pros), and that these outcomes are the most important to her (her evaluation of outcome), then she will be motivated to quit.

The second factor that determines intentions is the **subjective norm**. This is the perceived social norm about the behaviour in a person's environment. This is influenced by the *perceived beliefs of others* about the behaviour and the person's *motivation to comply* with these beliefs. For example, young people are often most motivated to comply with the norms of their friends. Family-based interventions for young people are therefore less likely to be successful than interventions targeted at peer groups.

ACTIVITY 5.2   SOCIAL NORMS VERSUS ATTITUDES

Has there ever been a time when you have been persuaded to do something against your better judgement because everyone else was doing it? For example:

- Drinking and driving.
- Drinking too much.
- Smoking or other drug use.

What do you think is more powerful: your own attitudes or social pressure/group norms? Why is this?

A strength of the TPB is that it takes account of the importance of social pressures and norms as well as how much control a person believes they have over their behaviour. Research has shown that control is indeed important in behaviour change (Wallston, 2007). The TPB accounts for control quite broadly in the form of **perceived behavioural control**. The link between perceived behavioural control and intentions is via the amount of overall control people believe they have over their behaviour and changing this behaviour. If a person believes they do not have any control over their smoking then they will not intend to quit. The direct link between control and behaviour is thought to be due to an *actual* lack of control over the factors needed to support or change a behaviour, rather than a *perceived* lack of control. An actual lack of control might

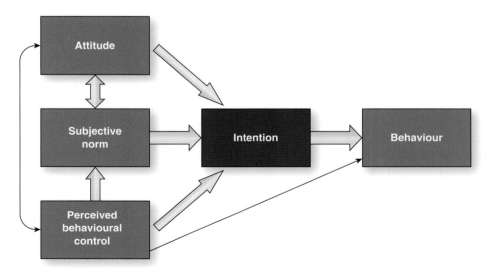

FIGURE 5.3   The Theory of Planned Behaviour

involve not having suitable transport to attend a smoking cessation clinic, not being able to afford nicotine replacement therapy, or living in an environment where many other people also smoke.

There are numerous ways in which we can look at control. For example, we can distinguish between an internal **locus of control**, where people believe they can control their behaviour or the outcome of events, or an external locus of control, where people believe that other people or fate are controlling the outcome of events (see Chapter 9). This will differ between different situations but is very relevant to medicine. For example, a patient with an external locus of control is more likely to expect medical professionals to control or sort out their illness. A patient with an internal locus of control will be more proactive and likely to make lifestyle changes or adhere to treatment because they believe they have control over the outcome of their illness. This is a useful characteristic to look out for in clinical work because it can help to develop a more effective treatment plan for each individual. For example, a person with diabetes who has an external locus of control might be more effectively treated with regular outpatient appointments to monitor their progress and adjust their medication.

The TPB therefore proposes that attitudes, subjective norms, and perceived behavioural control are the major determinants of intentions. The relative importance of these three factors will vary according to different behaviours and individuals. There is evidence that the TPB predicts between 55 per cent and 71 per cent of intentions for a wide range of health behaviours, including smoking, testicular self-examination, exercise, abortion, condom use, diet, and oral hygiene. The TPB is therefore very good at explaining people's intentions to act in certain ways. However, while many of us intend to live healthier lifestyles – especially at New Year – this does not always mean we will do so! The TPB is slightly less successful at predicting actual behaviour. Researchers are therefore endeavouring to improve the theory by adding such factors as **anticipated regret** about changing a behaviour, **moral norms**, and **action implementations** i.e. how a person plans to take action to change. These additions have appeared to be useful, particularly the action implementations. However, they have not added greatly to the predictive power of the model.

CLINICAL NOTES 5.2

Changing a health behaviour

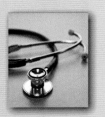

- Information (education) from a healthcare professional is a strong trigger for a behaviour change.
- Models of health behaviours are useful guides for clinical practice when helping someone change their behaviour (see case studies).
- It is important to identify the barriers to change: even when people are motivated to change, the perceived barriers can prevent it happening.

- Explore how a person's social environment and norms may facilitate or prevent a behaviour change.
- If a person thinks they have no control over a behaviour they will not attempt to change. Re-education and support can help increase a person's perceived control.
- Helping someone develop a plan for how they will change their behaviour makes it more likely they will succeed.

Interventions using the Theory of Planned Behaviour

Interventions based on the TPB appear to be effective, although there have only been a few methodologically rigorous research studies available to date. The results of these studies have been mixed, although most support the positive effect of these interventions for changing behaviour (Hardeman et al., 2002). One recent, well-designed study used the TPB to develop a leaflet to encourage school children to exercise more. This study found that children who received the intervention reported changes in their attitude towards exercise, subjective norm, behavioural control, and intentions. They were also more likely to have increased their exercise than children in the control group (Hill et al., 2007). The study design and leaflet are shown in Research Box 5.1.

RESEARCH BOX 5.1   Leaflet intervention based on Theory of Planned Behaviour

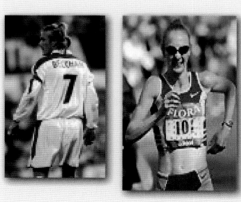

Background

The Theory of Planned Behaviour (TPB) suggests that healthy behaviour can be promoted by changing attitudes, normative beliefs, and feelings of control over behaviour. This study looked at whether a leaflet based on the Theory of Planned Behaviour would increase exercise in teenagers.

Methods and findings

503 school children were randomly allocated to receive either a:

(Cont'd)

- Leaflet.
- Leaflet + motivational quiz.
- Leaflet + implementation intention prompt.
- No leaflet (control group).

The leaflet was designed to improve:

- *Awareness* of different types of exercise
- *Attitudes* towards exercise – e.g. 'exercise will enhance your self-esteem and confidence', 'exercise can stop you putting on weight'
- *Normative beliefs* by highlighting others' exercising and approval of exercise – e.g. 'people are impressed by others who look fit and healthy'; 'It's cool to be fit'
- *Behavioural control* – e.g. 'It's easy to do one more session of exercise than you do at the moment', 'exercise such as jogging is free'
- *Intentions* – e.g. 'build exercise into your daily routine'.

The leaflet listed different sports activities and encouraged children to increase their exercise programme by one session each week.

Children were followed up three weeks after being given the leaflet. All children who had received a leaflet had increased their intentions to exercise and were doing more exercise – regardless of the type of leaflet.

Significance

This study tested a carefully designed leaflet that directly mapped onto aspects of the Theory of Planned Behaviour. The results suggest that such leaflets could be a simple, cost-effective intervention to increase exercise in children.

Leaflet reproduced courtesy of Charles Abraham

Hill, C. et al. (2007) Can theory-based messages in combination with cognitive prompts promote exercise in classroom settings?, *Social Science and Medicine, 65*: 1049–1058.

Case Study 5.2 illustrates how the TPB might be used as a guide for intervention in clinical practice. Next we look at a completely different model, which focuses on the *processes* of change rather than on the factors that determine behaviour.

CASE STUDY 5.2   Smoking cessation using the Theory of Planned Behaviour

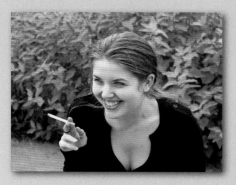

Jenny is a 22 year old woman who has smoked 20 cigarettes a day since she was 15 years old.

Attitudes

Explore her attitudes towards smoking:

- *What do you think about smoking?* (general attitude)
- *Is smoking a good or bad thing for you? In what way?* (evaluation of attitude/behaviour)

Educate about negative effects of smoking to try to change the attitude from positive to negative.

Social norms

Explore the norms of important people around her:

- *What do your friends/family/partner think about smoking?* (general norm)
- *What do your friends/family/partner think about you smoking?* (specific norm)
- *Whose opinion is most important to you?* (who she is motivated to comply with)
- *Would you like to give up smoking for [person]?* (motivation to comply with norms)

Discuss the pros and cons for her if she were to comply with the person or group norms she values most.

Intentions

Explore whether she intends to quit smoking:

- *Have you ever thought about giving up smoking?* (previous intention)
- *Do you intend to give up smoking in the next few months?* (current intention)

Perceived behavioural control

Explore how much control she thinks she has over quitting smoking.

- *Do you think you can give up smoking?* (perceived control over quitting)

If low control, explore the reasons e.g.

- *What makes you think you can't give up?*

(Cont'd)

Normalise the difficulty in quitting:

- *Many people find it hard to give up*

Increase the perceived control:

- *most people are successful if they keep trying*

Explore the actual control:

- *Is there anything in particular that stops you from trying to quit?*

Action implementations

If she is ready to try quitting, discuss the steps she can take to give up smoking:

- *What steps are you going to take to give up smoking?* (concrete plans)

Discuss how these can be changed or added to in order to increase chances of success:

- e.g. nicotine replacement, smoking cessation groups
- setting personal goals about quitting, and setting rewards for not smoking

5.4 THE TRANSTHEORETICAL MODEL

The Transtheoretical Model (Prochaska and DiClemente, 1983) was an early attempt to integrate models of health behaviour and psychotherapy to produce an effective model for smoking intervention. This model is often referred to as the 'Stages of Change' model. The stages that characterise this model are illustrated in Figure 5.4. It includes four components: (1) the stages of change, (2) decisional balance, (3) confidence and temptation, and (4) processes of change.

The **stages of change** are a series of stages that people are thought to go through when changing their behaviour. In *precontemplation* a person is not even considering changing their behaviour. In *contemplation* they begin to consider changing. This leads into *preparation* where the individual prepares to change. The final two stages are *action* and *maintenance* where the person makes the change in the short term (action) and this behaviour change is consolidated and maintained in the long term (maintenance).

An important aspect of this model is the inclusion of relapse, based on the recognition that people can relapse back to previous behaviour at any point and that they may have to go through the cycle a few times before the new behaviour becomes permanent. The advantage of this is that it normalises relapse and encourages people not to see this as a failure but to keep trying to change their behaviour. In clinical practice a healthcare professional could emphasise this and explore what a person has learned from a relapse and how this can be used to increase chances of success next time.

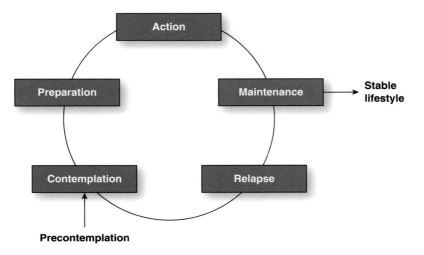

FIGURE 5.4 The Transtheoretical or 'Stages of Change' Model

Decisional balance involves the relative pros and cons of changing the behaviour. People are asked to write down the pros and cons of changing their behaviour in a decisional balance task. This helps them to clarify whether there are more pros than cons (or vice versa) and might prompt a person to consider changing their behaviour (i.e. move from precontemplation into contemplation).

Confidence refers to the confidence a person has in their ability to change. This overlaps with perceived behavioural control from previous models. **Temptation** is which factors will tempt a person to continue with an unhealthy behaviour in particular circumstances. For example, in our case study Jenny may want to give up smoking but finds it difficult to resist smoking when out with friends. The fourth aspect of the model is that it specifies ten processes of change which can be used to help people change their behaviour. These are consciousness raising (raising awareness), reinforcement management (helping a person to plan rewards if they change their behaviour), stimulus control, counter-conditioning, re-evaluation of self or environment, dramatic relief, social liberation, self-liberation and helping relationships.

ACTIVITY 5.3 CHANGING YOUR OWN BEHAVIOUR

- Do you have a bad habit or behaviour you would like to change?
- If so, what stage do you think you are at?
- How could you use the Transtheoretical Model to help yourself change that behaviour?

The strengths of the Transtheoretical Model are that it recognises people are at different stages of readiness for change and that interventions should be tailored to their particular stage. For example, if in our case study Jenny had never thought of giving up smoking (precontemplation) there is little point in trying to develop an action plan with her. It might make more sense to educate her about the dangers of smoking and encourage her to think about quitting (contemplation). Another strength is the inclusion of relapse. This is particularly important in addictive behaviour where relapse is common. However, the model has been criticised on the grounds that people do not necessarily move through the various stages consecutively. People might move backwards and forwards through the stages or miss out other stages completely.

CLINICAL NOTES 5.3

Working with resistance and relapse

- Whether a person is ready to change or not will affect the type of approach you should take.
- If a person has not considered changing, educate them about the negative impact of their current behaviour and encourage a change.
- Looking at the pros and cons of the current behaviour can also get people thinking about changing.
- Help them plan how they are going to change and build in rewards to reinforce the new behaviour.
- Relapse is a common part of behaviour change and not a failure. Explore why this happened and work out how to avoid it happening again the next time.

Interventions using the Transtheoretical Model

Evidence for the Transtheoretical Model is surprisingly weak. The majority of supporting evidence for the model comes from the research group who developed the model in its application to smoking cessation (e.g. Prochaska et al., 2001). Reviews of the evidence have concluded that there is, at best, weak evidence and, at worst, no evidence that interventions targeting people in particular stages are more effective than interventions that do not target such stages (Sutton, 2007). This is not to say an intervention based on the model has been completely unsuccessful, but rather that targeting stages does not significantly *improve* on interventions developed from other models such as the Theory of Planned Behaviour. The Transtheoretical Model at least provides a way to think about how the other different models of behaviour may operate at different stages. In other words, this is not an alternative to other models but a framework in which to place them. Case Study 5.3 illustrates how we might use the Transtheoretical Model in clinical practice.

CASE STUDY 5.3   Smoking cessation using the Transtheoretical Model

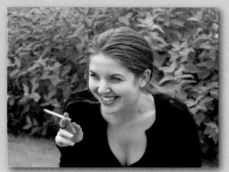

Jenny is a 22 year old woman who has smoked 20 cigarettes a day since she was 15 years old.

Stage of change

Identify which stage she may be at:

- *Have you ever thought about giving up?* (contemplation)
- *Have you ever planned to give up or tried to give up?* (preparation and action)

Decisional balance

Explore her perceived pros and cons of smoking. This is best done by writing them down and then looking at the list together:

- *What are the positive things for you about smoking?* (pros)
- *What are the negative things for you about smoking?* (cons)
- *Looking at this list, what does it make you think about your smoking?*

Confidence

Explore how confident she is that she can control her smoking:

- *Do you think you can control your smoking?*
- *How confident are you that you could reduce or quit smoking?*

Temptation

Explore which situations are particularly tempting for her to smoke and how this might affect a relapse:

- *Are there certain times or situations when you find it difficult not to smoke?*
- *How can you prevent this affecting you if you give up smoking?*

Processes of change

Use any of the processes to plan with her how she can quit smoking. For example:

- *Is there someone who can help you quit, or give up with you?* (helping relationships)
- *Can you do something instead of smoking that distracts you and makes you feel better, e.g. something relaxing, or exercise?* (counter-conditioning)
- *It's important to reward yourself regularly in the beginning to encourage you to continue not smoking. What would be a good reward for you?* (reinforcement management)

5.5 PRIME THEORY

A difficulty with many theories of health behaviour is that they tend to assume people will think rationally about their behaviour. Very few theories consider the role of emotions, or why people behave without thinking or in ways that they do not intend. **PRIME Theory** (West, 2006) is an attempt to incorporate motivation, emotions, impulses, and cognitive factors into one model.

The structural elements of PRIME Theory are shown in Figure 5.5. These consist of five factors thought to determine health behaviour:

> *Plans*: conscious representations of future actions including a commitment to act.
> *Responses* that are starting, stopping, or modifying any action.
> *Impulses* or inhibitory forces that are experienced as urges.
> *Motives* that are experienced as desires.
> *Evaluations* or evaluative beliefs.

As illustrated in Figure 5.5, momentary responses are influenced by external stimuli such as triggers, and internal states such as arousal and emotion, and then directly

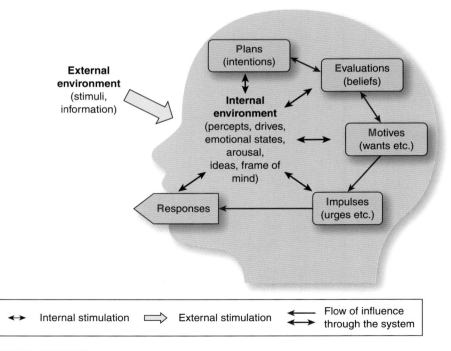

FIGURE 5.5   PRIME Theory
Image reproduced courtesy of Robert West

moderated by impulses and inhibitions. Impulses and inhibitions are in turn influenced by motives and evaluations. Motives and evaluations can be consciously experienced but not necessarily so. It is only at this level that beliefs and higher thought processes will come in. Finally, plans are cognitive intentions for future action that moderate motives and evaluations.

PRIME Theory is based on four assumptions about motivation and health behaviour. The first assumption is that we need to understand the moment-to-moment control of health behaviour before we can understand the long-term influences on behaviour. The second assumption is that the system has **plasticity** (is able to be modified or changed by experience). The third assumption is that **self-identity** is highly important to behaviour, our motives, and our plans (see Chapter 9). The fourth is that a system can appear complex but still be determined by relatively simple processes. For more detailed information see www.prime.co.uk.

One strength of PRIME Theory is that it integrates motivation (e.g. arousal, drives, motives) and emotion (emotional states, impulses) with cognitions (e.g plans, evaluations) in a theory of health behaviour. Also, the model includes self-identity, something which is rarely considered in other models. A difficulty with PRIME Theory is that there is little evidence available on whether it is effective at explaining health behaviours. However, PRIME Theory can still be used in clinical practice to help people change their behaviour, as is illustrated in Case Study 5.4.

ACTIVITY 5.4   HELPING OTHERS CHANGE

- If you wanted to help a friend stop binge drinking how would you use these models?
- What four things do you think would be most appropriate and useful for this person?
- How would you incorporate this into a behaviour change programme?

CASE STUDY 5.4   Smoking cessation using PRIME Theory

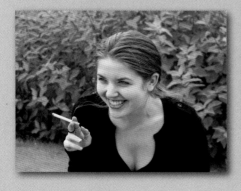

Jenny is a 22 year old woman who has smoked 20 cigarettes a day since she was 15 years old.

Plans

Explore whether she plans or intends to give up smoking:

- *Have you ever thought about giving up smoking?* (previous intention)
- *Do you intend to give up smoking? If so, when?* (intention and timeframe)

(Cont'd)

Evaluations/beliefs

Explore her beliefs about smoking and evaluation of it:

- *What do you think about smoking?* (beliefs)
- *Is smoking a good or bad thing? In what way?* (evaluation of smoking)

Educate about the negative effects of smoking to try to change her attitude from positive to negative.

Motives

Explore her motives and motivation to quit:

- *Do you want to quit? If so, how badly do you want to do this?*
- *What motivates you to give up?*
- *How important is that to you?*

Impulses

Explore the positive and negative impulses:

- *Are there times when you have strong impulses to quit?* (positive impulses)
- *What triggers this, or when do you feel this?* (triggers to positive impulses)
- *How can you make the most of this to help you quit?* (harnessing these impulses)
- *Are there times when you have strong impulses to smoke?* (negative impulses)
- *What triggers this, or when do you feel this?* (triggers to negative impulses)
- *How can you avoid this or change it?* (harnessing these impulses)

Responses

Explore her responses in these situations:

- *How do you usually respond to these (positive) impulses/circumstances?*
- *How do you usually respond to these (negative) impulses/circumstances?*

Self-identity

Examine her self-identity and how this is affected by smoking:

- *How does smoking affect how you feel about yourself?* (self-identity)
- *Do you think being a smoker affects how other people see you?* (perceptions of others)
- *How would you feel about yourself if you quit smoking?* (develop new positive self-identity)
- *How do you think other people would see you if you were a non-smoker?* (develop the reinforcing views of others)

CONCLUSION

Overall, there is good evidence that the Theory of Planned Behaviour and Health Belief Model can account for some of the factors that will determine health behaviour and that interventions based on these models are effective at changing behaviour. There is limited evidence to support the effectiveness of interventions based on the Transtheoretical Model. PRIME Theory has not yet been tested empirically, so it is not clear how effective it actually is at predicting behaviour and behaviour change.

From this chapter it should be clear that all of these models have various strengths and weaknesses. It should also be apparent that, although the models possess different concepts and underpinnings, many of the questions in the different case studies are similar and overlap. Thus, in clinical practice aspects of all these models can be mixed and used effectively to encourage people to change unhealthy behaviours. It is probable that different aspects of these models will work better for different clinicians and patients. However, a common implication is that we will need to explore each person's beliefs and reasons for behaving in the way they do in order to be most effective in helping them to change and develop an appropriate plan of change.

Summary

- Social-cognitive models of health behaviour take an expectancy-value approach and include the Health Belief Model and the Theory of Planned Behaviour.
- The Health Belief Model states a health behaviour change is determined by the threat of illness (perceived susceptibility and perceived severity) balanced by the perceived benefits and barriers to change. Triggers or cues to action can also be important in some cases.
- According to the Theory of Planned Behaviour a health behaviour is determined by intentions, which in turn are determined by attitudes towards the behaviour, social norms, and perceived behavioural control.
- The Transtheoretical Model of behaviour change is an integrative theory that focuses on the stages and processes of change, rather than the determinants of health behaviour.
- PRIME Theory is a recent attempt to integrate motivational and health behaviour theories to explain moment-to-moment behaviour. This theory focuses on plans, responses, impulses and inhibitions, motives, and evaluations as determining behaviour.
- There is evidence that the Theory of Planned Behaviour and Health Belief Model can explain some health behaviours, and that interventions based on these models are effective at changing behaviour.
- There is limited evidence to support the effectiveness of interventions based on the Transtheoretical Model. PRIME Theory has not yet been tested empirically so it is not yet clear how effective it is.
- Each model results in slightly different approaches to intervention, but aspects of all these models can be combined in clinical practice to encourage behaviour change.

📖 FURTHER READING

Ayers, S. et al. (eds) (2007) *The Cambridge Handbook of Psychology, Health and Medicine* 2nd edition. Cambridge: Cambridge University Press. This book has short chapters on many psychological factors relevant to health behaviour. It also has chapters on specific behaviours such as smoking cessation.

Conner, M. & Norman, P. (eds) (2005) *Predicting Health Behaviour: Research and Practice with Social Cognition Models* (2nd edition). Maidenhead: Open University Press. This book provides a comprehensive and authoritative overview of psychological models of health behaviour, including many not covered here.

Scriven, A. & Orme, J. (eds) (2001) *Health Promotion: Professional Perspectives* (2nd edition). London: Palgrave. This book provides a comprehensive overview of health promotion theory and also examines health promotion in the health service, schools, the voluntary sector, and the workplace.

？ REVISION QUESTIONS

1   What are health behaviours and how have they been categorised?

2   What biological, psychological, social, and societal factors influence health behaviours?

3   What is the expectancy-value principle? How is this relevant to health behaviour change?

4   Outline the Health Belief Model. How effective is it for behaviour change?

5   Outline the Theory of Planned Behaviour. How effective is it for behaviour change?

6   What is locus of control? How might it be relevant to clinical practice?

7   Outline the Transtheoretical Model. How effective is it for behaviour change?

8   Outline PRIME Theory. How might it be used to promote health behaviour change?

9   Compare and contrast two models of health behaviour change.

10   Describe how you might use one model of health behaviour to help someone give up smoking.

6 CHRONIC ILLNESS, DEATH, AND DYING

LEARNING OBJECTIVES

This chapter is designed to enable you to:

- Learn more about the experience of chronic or terminal illnesses.
- Outline some of the psychosocial interventions to help people adjust and cope with chronic illness.
- Understand the difficulties of palliative care, in particular the tension between helping a patient have a good death and euthanasia.
- Describe the processes of normal bereavement and pathological grief.

As we become more successful at treating disease and delaying death the proportion of people living with long-term illnesses increases. In developed countries approximately one in three people at any given time have a chronic disease. In the UK where state support is available, approximately one in seven people claim disability or incapacity benefit (Office for National Statistics, 2002b). In fact, most of us will have a chronic illness at some point in our lives. Treatment of chronic illness presents healthcare professionals with a particular challenge: it requires a change from focusing purely on a cure to focusing on helping people manage their symptoms. The implications of this are examined later when considering quality of life for people with chronic and terminal illnesses. Chronic illnesses raise some of the most difficult ethical issues in medicine. For example, how do we decide who gets a transplant and who does not, when should we stop resuscitation or turn off a life support machine, and what is the doctor's role in cases of assisted suicide?

Chronic diseases vary hugely. They include disorders such as epilepsy, arthritis, cancer, diabetes, chronic fatigue syndrome, asthma, hypertension, liver disease, and dementia. Chronic diseases account for approximately 80 per cent of deaths in developed countries. Figure 6.1 summarises death rates in the UK from key illnesses and disorders of different body systems. Cardiovascular disease and cancer are the largest killers, followed by respiratory diseases, disorders of the gastro-intestinal and genito-urinary system, and accidents. Interestingly, deaths that receive a lot of media attention, such as those from HIV or homicide, are much less likely. In the UK, homicide accounts for the deaths of seven men and two women in every one million people.

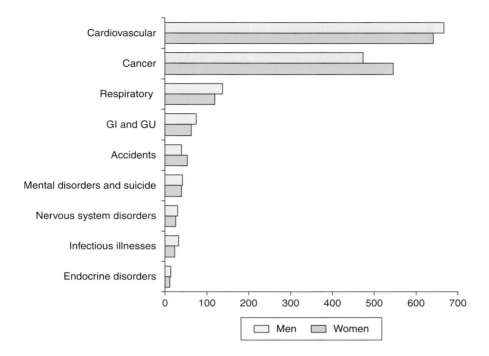

FIGURE 6.1   Causes of death in the UK. Death rates per 100,000 people in 2006 (adapted from WHO, 2009)

Given the wide range of chronic illnesses, it is difficult to generalise about the role of psychosocial factors. In previous chapters (Chapters 2, 3, and 5) we have seen how psychosocial factors such as lifestyle, stress, negative emotion, and support can affect the onset and prognosis of illness. We have also seen the importance of beliefs, attention, and behaviour in how we interpret symptoms and what we do about them (Chapters 2 and 4). The role of psychosocial factors in specific illnesses is covered in the chapters on different body systems in Section III. In this chapter we shall focus on the experience of chronic illness: the impact of chronic illness, how people adapt and cope, and whether psychosocial interventions can help. In the second half of the chapter we will look at the impact of terminal illness, coping with dying, the effect of death on others, bereavement, and dealing with death in medical practice.

6.1 CHRONIC ILLNESS

The onset and diagnosis of a chronic illness brings with it profound changes in a person's life which can lead to a reduced quality of life and wellbeing. The onset and diagnosis of chronic illness raise significant challenges, including:

- Adjusting to symptoms and disability.
- Maintaining a reasonable emotional balance.
- Preserving a satisfactory self-image and sense of competence.
- Learning about symptoms, treatment procedures, and self-management.
- Sustaining relationships with family and friends.
- Forming and maintaining relationships with healthcare providers.
- Preparing for an uncertain future.

The enormity of these tasks, coupled with the emotional distress brought on by chronic illness, mean patients are at high risk of depression. For example, studies of people with multiple sclerosis found between 16 and 54 per cent of them were severely depressed (Harrington and Ayers, 2008, unpublished). Compare this with postnatal depression, which is more commonly recognised but occurs in only 10 to 15 per cent of women.

The **crisis theory** of chronic illness (Moos and Schaefer, 1984) assumes that we need a social and psychological equilibrium which is similar to homeostasis. The diagnosis of an illness can put someone in an extreme state of disequilibrium, which is accompanied by negative emotions such as fear, anxiety, and depression. Because people cannot remain in a state of disequilibrium, some resolution must be found. People in disequilibrium are also more susceptible to outside influence, such as the actions of healthcare professionals. In chronic illness, people's equilibrium may be very fragile and can be destroyed at any moment by even small setbacks or other stressful events. This explains why patients may overreact to seemingly minor setbacks or difficulties.

Crisis theory is a useful analogy for the challenges of chronic illness. Theories of stress and coping (Chapter 3) are also useful in understanding people's responses. For example, the demands of illness are more likely to overwhelm a person if they have existing psychological problems, make negative or catastrophic appraisals, and have poor coping skills and resources. Case studies illustrating how stress theory can be used to help people cope with difficult events are given in Chapters 3 and 11.

6.1.1 IMPACT OF CHRONIC ILLNESS

Common emotional responses to illness are denial, anxiety, and depression. **Denial** is a psychological defence that allows people to avoid thinking about the illness and its consequences. Patients may refuse to accept that they have an illness, play down the severity of it, or insist they will recover and the illness will be cured. Denial is not helpful in the long term because it interferes with adherence to treatment and self-management. However, denial can be helpful in the short term – particularly if patients are physically weak and not able to cope with the full psychological consequences of the illness. In these circumstances, denial can help to keep fear and anxiety lowered until they have recovered and feel more able to cope with the emotional consequences of the illness. For example, denial is associated with faster initial recovery from a heart attack and fewer treatment side effects (Sirois, 1992).

Anxiety and depression are common in people with chronic illness. A review of heart disease, stroke, diabetes mellitus, asthma, cancer, arthritis, and osteoporosis found that depression was more common in people with these illnesses than in the general population. Anxiety is more common in people with heart disease, stroke, and cancer than in the general population (Clarke and Currie, 2009). Depression and anxiety can be a response to illness, present before illness, or both. As we saw in Chapter 2, there is strong evidence that negative emotion is associated with poor health. Both anxiety and depression have associated physiological states that might affect the course of chronic illness. Anxiety is associated with sympathetic nervous system and HPA axis arousal, while depression is associated with neuroendocrine changes that can affect inflammatory and immune pathways (see Chapters 3 and 11). For example, depression is associated with an increased risk of cardiovascular disease (Steptoe, 2006) and mortality from a wide range of other illnesses (Anstey and Luszcz, 2002). Anxiety is associated with more frequent or severe symptoms in disorders such as asthma or irritable bowel syndrome (see Chapters 12 and 13).

Though anxiety and depression are often comorbid (occuring together), they stem from different types of appraisal. Anxiety is a response to threat. In chronic illness this is likely to be a threat to a person's wellbeing, work, self-image, etc. Patients' anxiety significantly increases in medical settings because of potentially threatening events such as getting test results, having invasive procedures, dependence on healthcare professionals, and uncertainty about the disease course (Jacobsen et al., 1993). Depression, on the other hand, is usually a response to loss, failure, or helplessness. In chronic illness this will include a loss of health or physical capacity, a loss of social status, a failure to conform to healthy standards, and helplessness in the face of illness.

Learned helplessness occurs when people believe they have no control over events, become hopeless, helpless, and subsequently depressed (Seligman, 1975). This is particularly relevant to chronic illness. If people believe they have no control over their illness or outcome it can lead to detachment, withdrawal, and depression (see illness representations, Chapter 4). Self-management programmes and cognitive behaviour therapy (CBT) deal with this by encouraging people to identify and challenge maladaptive beliefs, educating them about the importance of psychosocial factors and empowering them to manage their illness.

In chronic illnesses the emphasis of treatment is on improving **quality of life** rather than curing the illness. However, there are tensions between improving quality of life on the one hand, and side effects of medical treatments that may decrease quality of life on the other. There is also the controversy of deciding the point at which gains in quality of life are worth expensive treatments, such as those for advanced cancer. Finding treatments that maximise physical wellbeing and quality of life can therefore be difficult. For example, NICE guidelines for dementia care aimed to combine best practice in social and physical care for dementia, but formulating these guidelines was so complex that the panel to publish information on how to do it (Gould and Kendall, 2007).

The measurement of quality of life in chronic illnesses is therefore critical to inform healthcare guidelines. However, it is also fraught with problems. Self-report measures typically ask people about pain, disability, restricted functioning or roles, mental health, energy, and overall ratings of health. Unsurprisingly, research using these measures has found that people with chronic illnesses report a poorer quality of life. Measures of quality of life are often not specific to the illness being studied and do not take into account changes in people's goals and priorities during illness. For example, standardised measures of pain may be interpreted differently by people with chronic illness. Similarly, some domains of life may be more or less important to someone with a chronic illness.

Specialised measures of quality of life have therefore been developed, such as patient-generated indexes, where people list the five domains of life that are important to them and then rate how much each domain has been affected by their illness. Research using this measure shows people generate a wide range of domains, including some not encompassed in traditional quality of life measures. Such domains include memory, writing, and sexual function. Domains will also change over time as patients adjust to continuing disease and incapacity. This type of measure is moderately related to global measures of quality of life, life satisfaction, and mental health, but only weakly associated with health and functional status (Wettergren et al., 2009). General quality of life is usually best predicted by psychological functioning (Arnold et al., 2004).

6.1.2 FINDING MEANING AND BENEFIT

So far, we have focused on negative aspects of chronic illness. However, many people with chronic illnesses report positive changes to their lives. This is referred to as **stress-related growth, post-traumatic growth** or **benefit-finding**. Three main types of positive change occur:

1 *Enhanced relationships* – patients need support from others and positive interpersonal experiences may strengthen their appreciation of relationships.
2 *A changed view of themselves* – people may develop a greater sense of personal resilience and strength, an acceptance of their vulnerabilities and limitations, or a heightened awareness of the fragility of life.
3 *Changed life philosophy* – the concern that illness might result in incapacity and a shorter life can lead to changes in priorities and values, a different approach to life, and a greater appreciation of living.

These positive changes can lead to a whole new approach to life (see Research Box 12.3). Reviews have shown that 60 to 90 per cent of people with HIV or cancer report positive growth. Growth is associated with less distress in the short term and better physical and mental health overall (Sawyer et al., 2010).

6.1.3 ILLNESS AS A STORY – NARRATIVES IN MEDICINE

The events of chronic illness, positive, and negative changes will become part of a person's story about themselves (Case Study 6.1). Books, internet sites and blogs provide millions of examples of people writing about their experiences of illness. Stories or narratives have a number of functions (Hydén, 1997). **Illness narratives:**

- Transform events and construct meaning from the illness.
- Help people reconstruct their history to incorporate the illness and reconstruct their identity to retain a sense of self worth in the face of illness.
- Help people explain and understand their illness.
- Relate the illness to their values and life priorities.
- Make illness a collective experience.

CASE STUDY 6.1   Narratives of illness

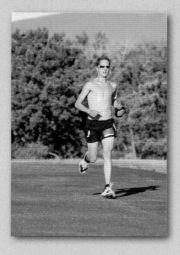

Fighter in the face of adversity

Brooks Williams was diagnosed with cystic fibrosis at 5 1/2 months old. He says, "when I was 21 I had a serious bout of pneumonia: my lung function was down to 40% and I was coughing up lots of blood. After I was released I was told that due to scarring in my lungs I might never make a full recovery. It made me realise how quickly my health could take an irreparable turn and this fear is what made me start running seriously. I started running to live and I attribute my improved health to running. My doctor told me not many people with cystic fibrosis try running marathons so I'm a guinea pig.

I have been running for six years now and have completed ten marathons and seven ultramarathons. I just completed a 100 mile ultramarathon in Texas in 17.5 hours and finished 12th overall. I think only half of finishing is down to your physical conditioning – the rest is down to mental fortitude."

(reproduced with the kind permission of Brooks Williams; photograph reproduced courtesy of Thomas Dewane)

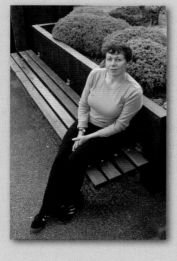

Reactions, struggles and changing priorities

Ten years ago I was diagnosed with multiple sclerosis – I was going blind and was scared to death. I had young kids and more than anything I was scared I would never see them again. All I knew about MS was the worst so I was convinced I'd become totally handicapped and have a terrible life. However, the treatment worked well and my sight came back, although I have other side effects to deal with. My hands and feet are numb and I am allergic to some drugs so can't take them – so it is an ongoing process of trying different drugs and finding out what works.

I try to look on the bright side – I have a great husband, good friends, and God. On good days I can see how wonderful life is. On bad days I try not to take anything for granted and concentrate on what I can do, rather than what I can't. I am excited by the new drugs they are working on and pray for a cure. I take each day at a time and am thankful for what I have.

(Cont'd)

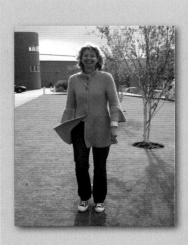

Acceptance of death – strength in existential issues

My dad died of cancer when I was young so I was really scared of cancer. When the doctor told me I had cancer I was shocked and frightened. I was so scared of dying – I had young children so was really worried about what would happen to them. It took a while to get my head around it but eventually I realised that we all have to die sometime. I can't run away from it – none of us can. I feel connected to all the people who died before me and those who will die after me. I am just a small part of a big circle of life.

I am doing everything I can to get rid of the cancer because I don't want to die, but I am not worried anymore. I enjoy my time with family and friends. I know my children will be OK because other people will be there for them. My experience of cancer has been a revelation and I have a very different perspective now. I'm not afraid of dying. I think nature has its own way of making it alright because who wants to live in pain? I see that my life has been good – it has been a privilege.

The importance of illness narratives is reflected in **narrative-based medicine** (Greenhalgh and Hurwitz, 1998) in which the emphasis is on listening to patient narratives and using these to improve clinical care. In diagnosis, narratives are useful because they provide an insight into someone's experience of ill-health and encourage empathy and understanding between doctor and patient. Narratives encourage a holistic approach to treatment. Talking through illness narratives can prove therapeutic or palliative for patients. In addition, it may suggest other treatment options. In patient education, narratives are memorable, grounded in experience, and encourage reflection. The use of narratives can therefore be helpful both for patients and doctors at many stages of illness (see Chapter 18).

ACTIVITY 6.1   USING NARRATIVES IN MEDICINE

Think about a patient you saw recently. How much do you remember about:

- the clinical details?
- the person and their story?

Summary

- Chronic illnesses affect approximately 33 per cent of people in developed countries and account for approximately 80 per cent of deaths.
- The onset and diagnosis of a chronic illness brings with it profound changes in a person's life which can lead to a reduced quality of life and wellbeing.
- Common emotional responses are denial, anxiety, and depression. Depression and anxiety may be a response to the illness, present before the illness, or both.
- The relationship between quality of life and physical health is not straightforward, which is partly due to variations between illnesses and the measurement of quality of life.
- People with chronic illness can report positive life changes such as enhanced relationships and a changed view of themselves and their philosophy of life.
- Illness narratives are important in how people make sense of their illness. Narrative-based medicine uses narratives to improve diagnosis, treatment, and the education of patients.

6.2 PSYCHOLOGICAL INTERVENTION

The previous section highlighted the importance of psychological factors in chronic illness. Psychological interventions for chronic illness are usually associated with improvements in psychological wellbeing, quality of life, the self-management of illness, and general functioning, as well as reductions in pain, symptoms, and healthcare use. However, there is little evidence that they affect morbidity or mortality. Information is given elsewhere on specialist interventions (CBT, stress management and support – see Chapter 19; self-management – see Chapter 4]. The interventions we look at here are expressive writing and relaxation, which are both easy to learn and use with patients.

Expressive writing interventions offer a simple and effective intervention for chronic and terminal illness. People are asked to write for 15 minutes every day for three or four days about things they find (or have found) stressful or very upsetting. It is important that people write about their thoughts and feelings and do not just describe factual events. Evidence has shown that this intervention has small but significant effects on psychological wellbeing, physical health, general functioning, and health service use. It is also especially beneficial during stressful periods (Frattaroli, 2006). For example, a study of people with end-stage renal cancer showed that those who wrote about their cancer slept better, longer, and had fewer problems with day-to-day living than those who wrote about neutral topics (de Moor et al., 2002). Writing interventions are easy to use in clinical practice with the instructions given above and some encouragement.

Relaxation training can take many forms, including physical relaxation techniques such as progressive muscle relaxation, mental relaxation techniques such as meditation, or a combination of both as shown in Box 6.1. Relaxation is useful for coping with pain (Kwekkeboom and Gretarsdottir, 2006), reducing anxiety and depression, and coping with nausea and the side effects from treatment (Luebbert et al., 2001; van Dixhoorn and White, 2005). However, relaxation training is not effective for all illnesses. For example, there is little reliable evidence that relaxation can have an effect on asthma (Huntley et al., 2002).

BOX 6.1   3-minute relaxation exercise

1   Make sure you are sitting comfortably and as relaxed as possible.
2   Ask yourself, **what am I experiencing right now?** What body sensations do you have? What thoughts are going through your mind? What sounds can you hear? Just observe all these experiences without trying to change them. (*1 minute*)
3   **Focus on your breathing.** Breathe slowly and deeply: count to 4 as you inhale, then count to 4 as you exhale. Focus on the physical sensations of breathing like the movement of your stomach as your breath goes in and out. Let all thoughts go. (*1 minute*)
4   **Expand your awareness** to the sensations throughout your body. If you have strong feelings it's OK, just allow yourself to feel them – breathe with the feelings. If you have worries try saying to yourself '*let it go*' when you breathe out. (*1 minute*)

(adapted from www.cci.health.wa.gov.au)

The internet can also be a significant resource for people with chronic illness. It provides easy access to information, blogs, and online support. This raises the possibility that many interventions could be accessed via the internet. Computerised cognitive therapy treatments for anxiety and depression are already widely used, with evidence showing these are effective (Proudfoot et al., 2003, 2004). Online support groups for illnesses are also widely available (e.g. www.dailystrength.org, www.mdjunction.com).

Summary

- Psychological interventions for chronic illnesses include expressive writing, relaxation, stress management, self management, and support interventions.
- Psychological interventions are associated with better psychological wellbeing, quality of life, the self-management of illness, less pain, reduced symptoms, improved general functioning, and reduced pain and healthcare use.
- There is no consistent evidence that a psychological intervention has an effect on morbidity or mortality.
- The internet has become a significant resource for people with chronic illness through access to information, blogs, and online support.

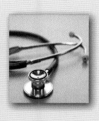

CLINICAL NOTES 6.1

Treating chronic illness

- As a clinician, you should be especially alert to depression or anxiety in patients with chronic illness and treat it appropriately.
- When adjusting to illness, people may have a fragile psychological equilibrium and react strongly to minor setbacks or difficulties.
- Reactions to illness vary hugely, so do not assume you know how a person thinks and feels about their illness.
- When diagnosed, people may use denial to avoid being emotionally overwhelmed. Do not challenge denial too much at this stage – it is only a problem if it continues long-term and interferes with treatment.
- Helping people consider any positive life changes since in illness can reduce distress.
- Listening to people's narratives will help us know them and treat them better.

6.3 DEATH AND DYING

The way we die has changed substantially. At the beginning of the twentieth century the majority of people died at home and their bodies were laid out for friends and family to see, touch, and mourn. By the 1960s two-thirds of deaths in the UK happened in hospitals and this still remains the case. Although most people would prefer to die at home the majority will die in an institution (Murray et al., 2009). Death is therefore much less on display in our society, which means it is perceived as less 'normal' or acceptable.

The fact that the majority of deaths in our society occur in hospitals raises a number of tensions and ethical issues. Medical staff are trained to save life rather than support death. Medical technology is rapidly advancing to help people live with severe disease. People have increasing expectations about their ability to survive, which can make it harder to come to terms with dying. As medics, it is often difficult to decide the point at which we stop prolonging life and allow someone to die. Which criteria should we base these decisions on, and how much autonomy does the patient have in decisions about dying? In this part of the chapter we shall look at death and bereavement from the perspective of the individual and family. We will then consider death in medical practice, including palliative care, assisted suicide, and deciding to end life.

6.3.1 DYING AND THE END OF LIFE

For most of us who are healthy, when and how we will die remain unknowns. Deaths in modern society can be divided according to three main patterns: a **gradual death** typified by a slow decline in ability and health; a **catastrophic death** through sudden and unexpected events; and **premature deaths** in children and young adults through accidents or illness (Clark and Seymour, 1999). With most terminal illnesses, people will be aware that they are going to die for some time before their actual death.

ACTIVITY 6.2   HOW LONG HAVE YOU GOT?

Life expectancy counters or 'death clocks' use a combination of questions about lifestyle to estimate your lifespan. These are just for entertainment as they are the technological equivalent of a crystal ball! See www.livingto100.com, www.deathclock.com

As illustrated in the case studies earlier, responses to illness are very individual. Box 6.2 summarises some of the main challenges of terminal illness for the individual. It is also common for honest and open communication between terminally ill patients, family, friends, and health professionals to break down because of taboos about death, worries that others do not want to talk about it, or finding it difficult to talk about. This combination of the impact of terminal illness and difficulties in communicating can result in reduced social interaction. Dying has subsequently been referred to as a 'falling from culture' as terminally ill patients become increasingly isolated (Seale, 1998).

Doctors also find it difficult to 'diagnose' death and discuss prognosis in terminal illness (see the research box) and patients may have a false optimism about their prognosis which

---

BOX 6.2   Challenges of terminal illness

Illness-related	Self-concept	Social
• Illness symptoms and disability • Continuous treatment and side effects • Possible invasive surgery • Decisions whether to continue treatment • Threat of death	• View of self as patient • View of self as terminally ill • Changes in physical function due to illness or treatment e.g. tremours, pain • Changes in appearance • Changes in mental function e.g. cognitive ability	• Depression or anxiety leading to withdrawal • Preparing for loss and withdrawing from others • Mental or physical decline leading to shame, embarrassment, or concern about the impact on others • Worries about being a burden on others • Feeling bitter, angry, or resentful of healthy people

RESEARCH BOX 6.1 Doctor-patient collusion about dying

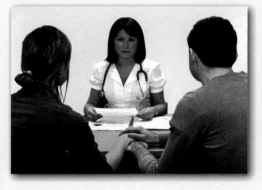

Background

This study stemmed from the clinical observation that many patients with terminal lung cancer had unrealistic optimism about their prognosis. The researchers wanted to discover why this was.

Methods and findings

A qualitative study of 35 patients with small-cell lung cancer who were followed from diagnosis to death over four years.

False optimism was put down to a 'collusion' between doctors and patients, where doctors focused on the benefits of treatment and this fed into patients' need to believe they could recover.

In keeping with this, false optimism was highest during chemotherapy treatment but disappeared when the tumour recurred. People became more realistic about prognosis as the disease progressed and by having contact with patients at a more advance stage. Below is the view of one of the consultants.

> "This is one of the most difficult things in my work. Just before the therapy I told him that his life expectancy was short and that this was the last thing I could do. He and his wife were crying all the time. Because they were very upset, I could not continue my explanation. That's why I wanted to talk to them again today. You saw what happened. They asked me again whether other therapies are available. Must I ruin their life by being honest? By telling things again that I have already told them? Or just leave it? That's a huge problem. I tell them once or twice what the situation is. If people want to know more, they must ask for it. I leave it to them."
>
> "Do you find it difficult to break bad news?" the researcher asks.
>
> "I think people must know what their situation is, but I find it difficult. What are the effects of what I say? That's my problem."

Significance

This study highlights the difficulty doctors face when discussing prognosis with patients and why it might be easier to collude with the patient. More research is needed to explore whether false optimism is helpful or unhelpful to the patient and their family.

The, A.M. et al. (2000). Collusion in doctor-patient communication about imminent death: an ethnographic study *British Medical Journal, 321*: 1376–1381.

helps them in the short term but makes it harder to accept death if it comes quickly. Barriers that make it hard for doctors to diagnose dying include:

- A hope that the patient will get better.
- The lack of a definitive diagnosis.
- Pursuing unrealistic or futile treatments.
- Disagreements about the patient's condition.
- A failure to recognise the severity of an illness.
- A lack of knowledge about specific care.
- Poor communication skills.
- Concerns about withholding treatment.
- A fear of foreshortening a patient's life.
- Concerns about resuscitation.
- Cultural and spiritual barriers.
- Medico-legal issues.

ACTIVITY 6.3   DIAGNOSING DYING

- What do you think patients should be told about their illness?
- Should people always be given a complete and honest prognosis?
- Are there reasons why we should withhold information?

6.3.2 RESPONSES TO TERMINAL ILLNESS

Death is the ultimate existential crisis when we are forced to confront our very existence. Existentialism assumes that most personal crises are prompted by realising our mortality. Therefore people will tend to question their purpose in life, the meaning of their life, the values they have held, the foundations of their life, their relationships with others, and their religious beliefs. This realisation of mortality may make people feel alone and isolated.

One of the most influential views of dying was put forward by the psychiatrist Kübler-Ross (1969), who proposed that people go through five stages:

1 *Denial*, where the person uses this to adjust to the fact they are dying without being emotionally overwhelmed.
2 *Anger*, which stems from a frustration at dying and is often directed at those closest to the person. Questions like 'why me?' are common. Understanding that the person is angry at dying (not at people, around them) can help carers to cope with angry outbursts.
3 *Bargaining*, where people try to make a deal with God or the medical professionals so they live, promising good behaviour in return for their life.
4 *Depression*, which occurs when the person realises there is nothing that can be done. This is seen as 'anticipatory grief' where people prepare for, and mourn, their own death.
5 *Acceptance*, where the person accepts their death with calmness and peace.

We now know that people with terminal illness do not go through discreet or consecutive stages of tasks or emotions. People may experience any of these feelings concurrently or move between them. Many patients never reach the stage of acceptance and anxiety and a fear of death are common. Patients fear death, pain and suffering, loneliness, and the unknown. Fear of death is higher in patients with poor physical health and a low life satisfaction or purpose in life, and those who have anxiety or depression (Fortner and Neimeyer, 1999).

6.3.3 BEREAVEMENT

Dying does not occur in isolation but affects family, friends, and the community. In this section we shall consider the process of bereavement, the impact of bereavement on health, and normal and pathological grief processes.

Process of bereavement

Bereavement involves loss, grief, and mourning. **Loss** occurs when a person or object we are emotionally attached to becomes permanently unavailable. Loss is an integral part of terminal illness – patients lose the ability to function physically, occupationally, and at home. **Grief** is a normal reaction to loss. It involves emotional reactions (e.g. anger, guilt, anxiety, sadness, despair), physical reactions (e.g. changes in appetite, sleep, somatic complaints) and social reactions (e.g. changes in social functioning, inability to work). **Mourning** is the process by which people adapt to loss.

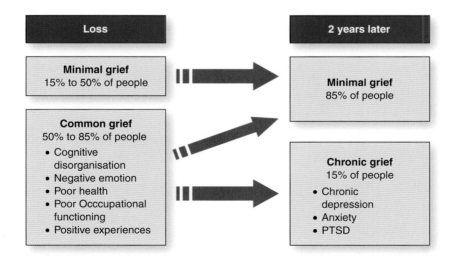

FIGURE 6.2 Responses to bereavement (adapted from Bonanno & Kaltman, 2001)

How we grieve and mourn is strongly influenced by cultural customs and rules. What happens after death is prescribed by society. For example, work regulations affect the process and length of mourning. In the UK, health service workers are allowed three days paid leave following a bereavement. Compare this with some specific cultural and religious values, such as Hindu funeral rituals, which can last for up to 13 days.

The symptoms that people may experience during bereavement are given in Box 6.3. Although there are individual differences in how people grieve, 85 per cent of people will usually adjust by the second year of bereavement (Figure 6.2). The duration and severity of a person's grief depend on:

- How attached they were to the deceased person.
- The circumstances of the death and situation of loss.
- How much time they had to work through anticipatory mourning.

Bereavement is associated with an increased risk of illness and mortality, particularly in older adults who lose their spouse. This is probably due to a range of factors such as stress (see Chapter 3), depression (see Chapter 2), and lifestyle (Chapter 5).

What we classify as 'normal' during bereavement will depend on the theoretical view we take. Traditional views focus on the *work* of grieving. Bereavement is seen as a time

---

BOX 6.3   Responses to loss

Physical	Behavioural	Emotional	Cognitive
• Fatigue	• Irritability	• Depression	• Lack of concentration
• Sleep pattern changes	• Restlessness	• Anxiety	• Shorter attention span
• Aches and pains	• Searching	• Hypervigilance	
• Appetite changes	• Crying	• Anger/hostility	• Memory loss
• Digestive problems	• Social withdrawal	• Guilt	• Confusion
• Shortness of breath	• Inability to fulfil normal roles	• Pining/yearning	• Preoccupation
• Palpitations		• Emotional loneliness	• Helplessness/hopelessness
• Restlessness		• Social loneliness	• Sense of disrupted future
• Increased vulnerability to illness		• Feeling detached or distant	• Search for meaning
			• Disturbances of identity

(adapted from Bonanno & Kaltman, 2001; Payne et al., 1999)

during which people work through unresolved conflict or issues to do with the deceased, accept the reality of their loss, adjust to life without them, and emotionally detach from them to continue living (Worden, 1991). Stage theories emphasise the different stages a person will go through such as numbness, yearning, despair, and recovery (Payne et al., 1999). Stress theories emphasise stress and coping with bereavement as a dynamic process involving changes in orientation toward loss or restoration (Stroebe et al., 2007). When people are orientated towards loss they will be preoccupied with their loss, think about and yearn for the deceased, and carry out behaviours such as seeking out common places or searching for the deceased. When orientated towards restoration people will adjust their lifestyle, cope with day-to-day life, build a new identity, distract themselves from painful thoughts, and take over the tasks and roles that the deceased used to do.

In pathological or chronic grief, people are severely affected and will develop mental health problems such as depressive or anxiety disorders. Pathological grief is more likely if the death was sudden or unexpected, if the deceased was a child, and/or there was a high level of dependency in the relationship. Risk is also increased if the bereaved person has had a history of psychological problems, poor support, and additional stress such as financial difficulties. Psychological interventions for bereavement appear to have little effect on depression, grief, or physical symptoms except for in high risk people (Jordan and Neimeyer, 2003). Support appears to help bereaved people generally but does not buffer them against the grief (Stroebe et al., 2007). This suggests that for most people bereavement is a process they have to go to and, whilst support or intervention may be a comfort to them, it will not 'solve' their grief.

Summary

- Death is the ultimate crisis, when people are forced to confront and question their existence.
- Fear of death is common in terminal illness, especially in patients who are younger, have worse physical health, low life satisfaction, or anxiety or depression.
- Honest communication between terminally ill patients, family, friends, and health professionals may break down, and doctors may collude with patients to promote false optimism.
- The severity of grief and mourning will depend on how attached a person was to the deceased; the circumstances of death and situation of loss; and the extent of anticipatory mourning.
- Bereavement is associated with an increased risk of illness and mortality, particularly in older adults who lose their spouse.
- 15 per cent of people will develop chronic grief. This is more likely if the death was sudden, unexpected or a child; if there was high dependency in the relationship; if the person has a history of psychological problems, poor support, and additional stress.

6.4 DEATH AND MEDICAL PRACTICE

In the 1960s patients were usually not told they were dying but were instead heavily sedated and kept separate from other patients (Glaser and Strauss, 1966). Hospices today are founded on the idea that terminally ill patients should have compassionate care that addresses the medical, psychological, social, and spiritual aspects of dying (see Box 6.4). Palliative care focuses on relieving symptoms such as pain rather than curing disease. Painful or invasive treatments are usually discontinued. A greater emphasis is placed on the patient's psychological wellbeing. The patient is given as much control and choice as possible. Honest communication is emphasised and family are encouraged to be involved. Palliative care is increasingly provided to people in their own homes by specialist nurses or multidisciplinary teams. Dying at home or in a hospice is associated with better control of pain and symptoms and greater satisfaction on the part of the main carer (e.g. a spouse). However, the evidence is inconsistent over whether hospice care does result in a better quality of life (Finlay et al., 2002).

BOX 6.4   Aims of palliative care

1 Promote quality of life.
2 Manage the emotional and physical symptoms.
3 Support patients to live productively.
4 Empower patients to take control of life.

Working in palliative care puts considerable strain on staff, and burnout rates are high (see Chapter 3). A review of people working in oncology found that around 30 per cent had symptoms of burnout (Trufelli et al., 2008). The inability to cure patients and the fact that every patient dies can be unrewarding and frustrating. Healthcare professionals may detach or withdraw from patients to protect themselves emotionally. Others may focus their attention on patients who will benefit from medical intervention. Palliative care implicitly supports the idea of a 'good death' i.e. one where the patient is psychologically prepared, physically comfortable, and able to die in the best way possible. There has been extensive debate over the notion of a 'good death' and how far we should go to help patients achieve this.

CLINICAL NOTES 6.2

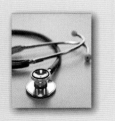

Working with terminally ill people

- Talk to patients about their illness and treatment.
- Involve them in decisions wherever possible.
- Try to address their fears and reduce anxiety.

- Be calm and mindful when with a terminally ill person – even if you don't feel like this.
- Empathise (e.g. 'That sounds…' 'I can imagine …') but do not say you 'know' or 'understand'.
- If they are angry do not take it personally – it is usually because of their illness.
- Help them make the most of the time they have left in the best way for them.
- Help them and their family work through anticipatory loss and grief.
- Help them die with dignity. If possible this should be where and how they wish.

Euthanasia and assisted suicide

Euthanasia comes from the Greek words for 'good death'. **Voluntary euthanasia** is when death is hastened at the dying person's request and with their consent. **Involuntary euthanasia** is killing a person who has not specifically requested assistance in dying. This occurs in situations such as brain-death or coma where family and/or doctors decide to withdraw life-support. The way in which euthanasia is done can be active or passive. **Active euthanasia** involves an active acceleration of death through the use of drugs or by other means. **Passive euthanasia** involves the withdrawal of treatment so that the patient dies. This is relatively common in critical care settings as it involves any situation where life support is removed. Passive euthanasia is therefore already practised in countries where active euthanasia is illegal.

BOX 6.5   Arguments for and against euthanasia

For	Against
<ul><li>People should have the right to decide when and how to die.</li><li>Euthanasia happens anyway.</li><li>It allows people to have a good quality of life when they are alive.</li><li>People will die in less pain and with dignity.</li><li>Passive euthanasia already occurs so is there any difference between passive and active euthanasia?</li><li>Most lay people (82%) are in favour of euthanasia.</li><li>The alternative is a protracted death with poor quality of life.</li></ul>	<ul><li>Sanctity of life.</li><li>Intentional killing is not allowed.</li><li>A cure may be found.</li><li>Voluntary euthanasia will lead to the involuntary euthanasia of people who do not want it but cannot express this.</li><li>People who chose euthanasia are depressed and/or not given adequate care.</li><li>Legalising killing leads to reduced respect for human life. This is potentially damaging for society.</li><li>Good palliative care means euthanasia is unnecessary.</li></ul>

(adapted from www.dignityindying.org.uk)

Assisted suicide is a form of active voluntary euthanasia where someone assists a terminally ill person to commit suicide in as painless and dignified a way as possible.

Some of the ethical arguments for and against euthanasia are given in Box 6.5. Euthanasia and assisted suicide are currently illegal in the UK, Australia, and most of the USA. Other countries have legalised euthanasia e.g. the Netherlands, Belgium, and Switzerland. Attitudes and laws on euthanasia are increasingly challenged by pressure groups such as Dignity in Dying, and terminally ill patients who fight for the right to take their own life. Medical opinion is also slowly changing, with many professional organisations changing their stance from explicitly opposing assisted suicide to being neutral.

ACTIVITY 6.4   Involuntary euthanasia

Consider the scenarios below and think about what you would do:

- In intensive care you have a 78 year old woman on life support with no hope of recovery. The family are unsure what to do. There is a 21 year old car accident victim who has just arrived and needs intensive care but you have no bed available. He will probably not survive the journey if you send him to the nearest alternative hospital.
- A terminally ill 67 year old man is in the advanced stages of cancer. He looks uncomfortable and is having trouble breathing. His relatives are very distressed. Should he be given a drug that will settle his breathing but will also mean he dies quicker?
- A 60 year old woman collapses in the Accident and Emergency department and is being actively resuscitated when the medical team find out she has advanced bowel cancer and has refused chemotherapy. Should they stop resuscitation?

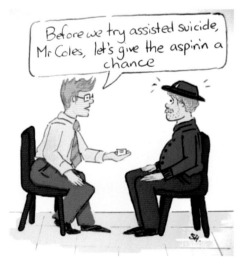

Research on healthcare professionals' experience of euthanasia is remarkably limited. One study in the USA carried out confidential interviews with ten nurses working in palliative or critical care settings (Schwarz, 2004). All of the nurses had been asked by patients to help them die. When patients asked for help the nurses reported (a) refusing assistance; (b) administering palliative drugs that might secondarily hasten dying; (c) ignoring and not interfering with the patient's or family's plans to hasten death; or (d) actively assisting the patient in dying. How nurses responded was influenced by the context and circumstances of each request. It was rare for nurses to consult with colleagues or the professional guidelines. Very few nurses immediately agreed or refused to help patients die; most struggled to find morally and legally acceptable ways to help them. Regardless of how they responded, nurses who had hastened death described feelings of guilt and distress.

This study illustrates a number of very important issues. First, medical professionals in critical and palliative care are exposed to patients asking for assistance to die. Second, the current legislation means staff will not be professionally supported when faced with these difficult ethical and moral decisions. Third, acting alone in these circumstances may have negative repercussions for emotional wellbeing. Consequently, some doctors are active campaigners for legal euthanasia (see Case Study 6.2).

In countries where euthanasia is legal, most guidelines insist that physicians are involved. For example, the guidelines in the Netherlands state that a doctor must ensure the request for terminating life is made voluntarily by the patient. They must also establish that the patient's situation means they are in unbearable suffering with no prospect of improvement. The procedure of euthanasia must include the consultation and agreement of two doctors; euthanasia can only be carried out on request and must be assisted by a doctor; and the death must be reported to the authorities as euthanasia or physician-assisted suicide.

CLINICAL NOTES 6.3

Dealing with death

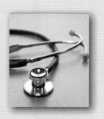

- When people are grief stricken the best thing you can do is calmly support them e.g. through touch or gentle words.
- If they are very distressed a useful technique is to get them to talk about something specific (but relevant). This will focus their mind and should reduce their immediate distress.
- Working with people who are dying is emotionally draining. It is OK to cry and feel upset.
- Make sure you look after yourself: use available support whether informal (e.g. peers, family) or formal (e.g. colleagues). Maintain activities that nourish you (e.g. exercise, music, being with friends).
- Be self-aware. If you start to feel overwhelmed or burnt out then get help straight away.

CASE STUDY 6.2   Helping people die

Retired doctor Michael Irwin is working to highlight the plight of people who are terminally ill and wish to commit suicide. His actions have increased the pressure on the UK Government to legalise assisted suicide.

At present, British people with chronic or terminal illnesses have to travel to a clinic in Switzerland if they wish to commit suicide. So far, approximately 140 people have done

(Cont'd)

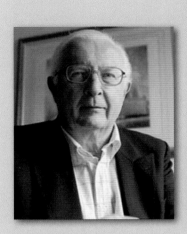

this and most friends or relatives that accompany them have not been prosecuted. However, a few people have been investigated or arrested.

One such case is the arrest of the partner of a man who killed himself at a Swiss clinic in 2007 with Dr Irwin's help. Dr Irwin helped pay for the trip and was there at the assisted suicide. Dr Irwin was also arrested and they were both held on bail for more than five months. Dr Irwin has been completely open about his involvement. He provided police with a diary of his trip that detailed how the suicide was carried out.

Dr Irwin has been investigated before for his involvement in assisted suicide. He spent two years under investigation after accompanying a woman with a severe degenerative disease to Switzerland to commit suicide. However, police did not have enough evidence to press charges. In 2003, he was held on bail for three months because he admitted helping a cancer sufferer die who was too ill to swallow the pills that Dr Irwin provided him with.

Dr Irwin has publicly stated that he intends to help other terminally ill patients to end their lives.

> I've done this before and I would do it again if someone is terminally ill. It's so wrong that people have to travel abroad to die when they could die here at home with dignity. I say to the police 'arrest me.

Reproduced courtesy of Dr Michael Irwin. All rights reserved.

Summary

- Palliative care is founded on providing terminally ill patients with compassionate care that addresses the medical, psychological, social, and spiritual aspects of dying.
- Palliative care implicitly supports the notion of a 'good death' but there is often tension between this and the ethical, moral, or legal opposition to euthanasia.
- Euthanasia can be voluntary (death hastened at the person's request) and involuntary (killing a person who has not requested it).
- Methods of euthanasia can be active (e.g. accelerated by drugs), or passive (e.g. the withdrawal of life-sustaining treatment).
- Assisted suicide is a form of active voluntary euthanasia which is legal in only a few countries.

- Research suggests that medical professionals in palliative care are asked by patients to assist death. Staff therefore face difficult ethical and moral decisions whilst being professionally unsupported.
- In countries where euthanasia is legal, most guidelines state that physicians must be involved in (a) establishing that assisted suicide is appropriate and (b) assisting death.

CONCLUSION

This chapter has addressed the challenges of chronic and terminal illness, including the significant impact these illnesses can have on the lives of patients and their family. In the final section we have also seen that these illnesses are a challenge for healthcare professionals – confronting us with difficult ethical and moral decisions as we watch patients die. In a medical system founded on saving life, it can be hard to accept that sometimes there is nothing to do except support a person's death. Yet it is this support they often most appreciate. As one doctor observed:

In my office adjacent to the medical intensive care unit, I have a growing file of letters from relatives of patients we have treated, thanking us for our care. But the majority of these letters are not from families of patients who survived. Rather, most come from people who have lost a loved one, from the bereaved survivors of patients who died in our intensive care unit. Yet they are deeply grateful for what we did. At first, I found these letters ironic and odd. I expected and basked in appreciation for lives saved. But the ones about lives we could not save – those I had trouble understanding. And I feel guilty. I read the letters over and over, wondering what the writers meant to me ... Saving deaths, I have come to realize, is as important and rewarding as saving lives. (Nelson, 1999)

📖 FURTHER READING

Ayers, S. et al. (eds) (2007) *Cambridge Handbook of Psychology, Health and Medicine*. Cambridge: Cambridge University Press. This handbook contains brief chapters on many topics in this chapter, including chronic illness, death and dying, quality of life, relaxation training, stress management, and the support interventions.

Fallon, M. & Hanks, G. (eds) (2006) *ABC of Palliative Care*. Oxford: Blackwell. This book covers both the medical and psychological aspects of palliative care and includes chapters on managing physical symptoms, communication, carers, and bereavement.

Martz, E. & Livneh, H. (eds) (2007) *Coping With Chronic Illness and Disability: Theoretical, Empirical, and Clinical Aspects*. New York: Springer. This is a comprehensive account of our psychological understanding of chronic illness. It also includes chapters on specific disorders, such as AIDS, arthritis, burns, cancer, diabetes, heart disease, and MS.

Murray Parkes, C., Relf, M. & Couldrick, A. (1996) *Counselling in Terminal Care and Bereavement*. Leicester: British Psychological Society. Though this is an older book than the others recommended here, it gives a good grounding in the issues that can arise for families and staff in palliative care, as well as useful counselling techniques for before and after bereavement.

? REVISION QUESTIONS

1 Outline the common emotional responses to chronic illness and discuss how these may affect health.

2 Describe one psychological intervention for people with chronic illness and discuss the evidence it is effective.

3 What is narrative-based medicine and how can it improve clinical care?

4 What challenges does terminal illness raise for individuals?

5 What are the reasons why doctors can find it difficult to 'diagnose' death and discuss this prognosis with terminally ill people?

6 Outline Kübler-Ross' stages of dying. Discuss how accurate and how useful these are in clinical practice.

7 Describe the processes of normal bereavement and pathological grief.

8 What are the common symptoms of bereavement?

9 What are the different types of euthanasia and what type of euthanasia is assisted suicide?

10 Describe some of the main ethical arguments for and against euthanasia.

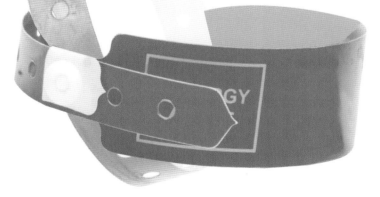

BASIC FOUNDATIONS OF PSYCHOLOGY

7 BRAIN AND BEHAVIOUR

CHAPTER CONTENTS

Figures

7.1   Organisation of the nervous system
7.2   Structure of a neuron
7.3   Anatomy of the brain
7.4   Divisions of the brain
7.5   The motor homunculus
7.6   Stages of sleep

Research boxes

7.1   Localisation of speech capacity
7.2   Sleep deprivation affects surgical skill

LEARNING OBJECTIVES

This chapter is designed to enable you to:

- Describe the functional organisation of the brain and nervous system.
- Describe how messages are communicated within neurons and from neurons to other cells.
- Describe how the nervous system controls involuntary and voluntary muscle movement.
- Outline explanations of the mechanisms of sleep, dreaming, and consciousness.

Medical professionals need to understand the normal functioning of the brain and nervous system. This chapter introduces: the structure and function of the nervous system, the control of movement, as well as sleep, consciousness, and biological clocks. Medical professionals also need to be able to recognise the physical and psychological aspects of abnormal brain functioning. Abnormal functioning will be covered in Chapter 16.

7.1 COMPONENTS AND ORGANISATION OF THE NERVOUS SYSTEM

7.1.1 ORGANISATION OF THE NERVOUS SYSTEM

There are two major divisions of the nervous system: the central nervous system and the peripheral nervous system (see Figure 7.1). The **central nervous system** (CNS) consists of nerves in the brain, brainstem, and spinal cord. Afferent nerves carry nerve impulses toward

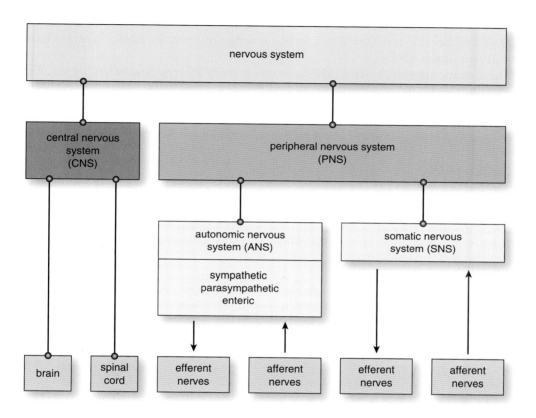

FIGURE 7.1   Organisation of the nervous system

the CNS; efferent nerves carry impulses away from the CNS. The structure and function of the CNS are described more fully later in this chapter.

The second major division is the **peripheral nervous system** (PNS). It consists of nerves that lie outside the CNS. The PNS can also be divided into different components: the automatic nervous system and the somatic nervous system. The **autonomic nervous system** (ANS) consists of nerves that innervate internal and glandular organs and regulate those processes that are not normally under voluntary control. The ANS comprises *sympathetic* and *parasympathetic nervous systems*. In general, the sympathetic nervous system prepares the body for action – e.g. opening airways, increasing the heart rate, inhibiting digestion, and stimulating the release of hormones from the adrenal glands. The parasympathetic nervous system tends to work in the opposite way to produce relaxation – e.g., slowing the heart rate, promoting digestion. The nerves of the sympathetic nervous system project from the thoracic and lumbar regions of the spinal cord. The nerves of the parasympathetic nervous system project from the brain and from the sacral region of the spinal cord. The *enteric nervous system* is part of the PNS which controls the gastrointestinal system. Because it receives considerable innervation from the ANS it is often considered as part of the ANS.

The **somatic nervous system** (SNS) receives sensory information (what we see, hear, smell, touch, and taste) and relays this to the CNS via afferent nerves. The CNS acts on this sensory information and sends motor signals (e.g. signals to pick and sniff a flower or to dodge a water bomb thrown at us) via efferent nerves to the skeletal muscles.

7.1.2 NEURONS

Humans have around 100 billion **neurons**. These are the functional units of the nervous system. Within neurons, messages are sent as electrical signals called action potentials. Between neurons, they are sent through the release of neurotransmitters into synapses, which are the small gaps between neurons. Neurons process and transmit information within the nervous system. Each neuron consists of:

- A cell body (or soma), which contains the nucleus and components vital for cell life.
- Dendrites that allow one neuron to receive messages from other cells.
- An axon, which carries messages from the cell body to the terminal buttons.
- Terminal buttons, which are important for passing messages from a neuron to other cells.

Neurons have a very high rate of metabolism. They cannot store their fuel and cannot extract energy in the absence of oxygen (unlike some other cells such as muscle cells). They therefore rely on a supply of glucose and oxygen from supporting cells. If blood

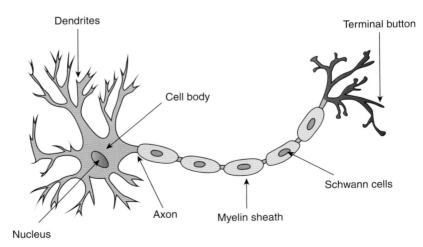

FIGURE 7.2   Structure of a neuron

flow to the brain is interrupted for as little as a few minutes, then permanent brain damage can occur.

Until recently, it was generally accepted that new neurons could not be produced in developed adult brains. However, recent research has identified neurogenesis in some areas of the adult brain (e.g. Bischofberger, 2007). Similarly, it was previously believed that the CNS was unable to repair itself. However, there is now evidence that there is the potential for some degree of neural regeneration and reorganisation within an adult CNS (e.g. Okano and Sawamoto, 2008). In the PNS, destruction of cell bodies leads to a permanent and irreversible loss of axons in the peripheral nerve. Severe damage to peripheral axons causes permanent impairment such as a loss of sensation and muscle bulk. If the damage is not severe, the nerve may be able to repair itself (Navarro et al., 2007). Some brain systems are able to be re-modelled in response to changes in input resulting from nerve damage (see for example Chen et al., 2002). The ability of neural circuits to undergo changes in organisation or function as a result of previous activity or damage is called neural plasticity.

Summary

- The two major divisions of the nervous system are the central nervous system (CNS) – the brain, brainstem, and spinal cord – and the peripheral nervous system (PNS) – nerves that carry information to and from the CNS.
- The PNS consists of three components: (a) the autonomic nervous system, which regulates bodily processes not normally under voluntary control; (b) the enteric nervous system, which controls the gastrointestinal system; and (c) the somatic nervous system, which processes sensory information.
- Neurons are the nervous system's functional units. Their dendrites receive information from outside the cell. Their axons transfer signals to other cells.

7.2 COMMUNICATION WITHIN AND BETWEEN NEURONS

7.2.1 ACTION POTENTIALS WITHIN NEURONS

An **action potential** is an electrical pulse used to send signals from a neuron to another cell. It is the result of changes in the balance of the concentrations of electrolytes inside and outside the neuron membrane. The neuron membrane has selective ions channels and ion pumps. Their action keeps the inside of the neuron slightly negatively charged relative to the outside (about -70 mV). An action potential is a burst of electrical activity that is of a fixed size and is an all-or-nothing response. A sequence of changes to the action of ion channels results in an action potential travelling along the axon toward the axon terminals.

7.2.2 SYNAPSES

When an action potential reaches the end of an axon it triggers the release of **neurotransmitters** from the terminal buttons into the synapse. Neurotransmitters are chemical messengers that bind to specialised receptors on the postsynaptic membrane of the target cell (which may be another neuron, a muscle cell, or a gland cell). The response may be the generation of an action potential in a neuron, the inhibition of neurotransmitter release, the contraction of a muscle, or the release of a hormone. Once a neurotransmitter has bound to its target cell receptor, it is broken down to prevent any further excitation or inhibition of the target cell. Many neurotransmitters are taken up and recycled by the pre-synaptic neuron to produce more of the neurotransmitter.

Whereas neurotransmitters within the central nervous system are involved in direct one-to-one neuron-to-neuron communication, neuromodulators secreted by some neurons diffuse through large areas of the nervous system and affect multiple neurons. Neuromodulators are not metabolised or re-absorbed by the pre-synaptic neuron. As a result, they influence the brain's overall levels of activity.

A number of different neurotransmitters and neuromodulators have been identified, some of which are briefly described in the remainder of this section.

Acetylcholine is released by neurons that stimulate the contraction of voluntary muscles. It also serves as a neurotransmitter in many regions of the brain and appears to be involved in the regulation of normal attention, memory, and sleep. Acetylcholine-releasing neurons die in people with Alzheimer's disease.

Monoamine neurotransmitters are divided into catecholamines and indolamines. The *Catecholamines* dopamine and norepinephrine are widely distributed in the brain and PNS. Within the brain, dopamine is present in three principal circuits:

- One circuit controls movement. Dopamine deficits in Parkinson's disease produce muscle tremours, rigidity, and difficulty in moving, but the dopamine precursor levodopa (L-Dopa) is an effective treatment.
- A second circuit is important for cognition and emotion and may be involved in psychosis.
- A third circuit regulates the endocrine system. In response to dopamine, the hypothalamus is stimulated to store or release hormones within the pituitary.

Norepinephrine appears to be involved in learning and memory. Deficiencies in norepinephrine occur in patients with Alzheimer's disease, Parkinson's disease and Korsakoff's syndrome – a cognitive disorder associated with chronic alcoholism. Depression is also often associated with low levels of norepinephrine.

The *indolamine* serotonin is implicated in sleep, mood, depression, and anxiety. Because serotonin appears to control various emotional states, much research has been directed toward developing serotonin analogs – chemicals with molecular structures similar to that of serotonin. Drugs that supplement or alter the action of serotonin can relieve the symptoms of depression and anxiety disorders.

Amino acids can act as neurotransmitters in the brain. Some inhibit the firing of other neurons e.g. glycine and gamma-aminobutyric acid (GABA), whereas other proteins have excitatory functions e.g. glutamate and aspartate.

Peptides are chains of amino acids linked together that are smaller than proteins. Opioid peptides have been the focus of much research. For example, endorphins act like opium or morphine to reduce pain and cause sleepiness.

Hormones are able to affect neural activity because hormone receptors are present on many neurons. In the brain, hormones can alter the structure and function of neurons. For example, stress hormones such as cortisol can affect learning. Severe and prolonged stress can cause permanent changes to the brain.

Thus far, the discussion of communication between neurons has focused on neurotransmitters acting at axon-dendrite synapses. However, the brain does contain axon-axon synapses in which the terminal buttons of one axon connect to a second axon and modulate (namely increase or inhibit) the release of neurotransmitters from the second axon. In addition, direct electrical transmission between neurons occurs at a small number of sites in the brain. These fast conducting gap junctions promote the rapid and widespread propagation of action potentials between neurons and may be important for synchronising complex brain activity.

Clearly, numerous events or processes could interfere with the transmission of action potentials within neurons and between neurons. Damage to the myelin sheath impairs the coordination of neuronal activity (see Multiple Sclerosis, Chapter 16). Disruptions or modifications to neurotransmitter or neuromodulator activity may impair memory and cognition and have been implicated in a range of psychiatric disorders (see Chapter 16). The normal effects of neurotransmitters on neurons become disrupted by addiction to alcohol or other drugs. The specific effects of different drugs vary, as do the neurotransmitters involved. Neurotransmitters involved in addiction include GABA, glutamate, opioid peptides, serotonin, and dopamine (Koob, 2006). Note that, although the physiological aspects of drug dependence are important, the biopsychosocial explanation of addiction highlights the importance of psychological and social aspects of addiction. The psychosocial aspects of addiction and its treatment are illustrated at various points in this book (see the Case studies in Chapter 5 on smoking cessation, and Case Study 2.2 in Chapter 2 on alcohol use).

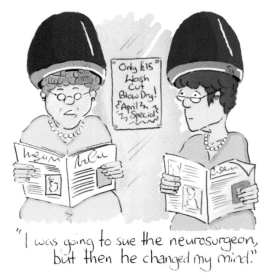

"I was going to sue the neurosurgeon, but then he changed my mind."

Summary

- Communication between a neuron and another cell (a neuron or muscle or gland cell) occurs across a synapse.
- When an action potential reaches the presynaptic neural membrane, it triggers the release of a chemical neurotransmitter which crosses the synapse and binds to the postsynaptic membrane of the target cell.
- The effect of a neurotransmitter on its target cell may be the excitation or inhibition of its function.
- Different neurotransmitters have specific roles within different regions of the CNS.

7.3 STRUCTURE OF THE BRAIN AND CENTRAL NERVOUS SYSTEM

7.3.1 SUPPORTING CELLS

Neurons rely on supporting cells to supply nutrients and oxygen and provide the optimal environment for neural functioning. The most important supporting cells are glia. There are several different kinds of glia – each with different functions. For example, oligodendrocytes provide physical support to CNS neurons and produce the myelin sheath. This appears as a string of beads along the axon and helps to insulate the axon and speed up the transmission of action potentials (see figure 7.2). In the PNS, Schwann cells perform the same functions as oligodendrocytes: they support axons and produce myelin.

The myelin sheaths of neural axons are vital for the efficient conduct of action potentials. Multiple Sclerosis (MS) is characterised by inflammation in the CNS and the destruction of the myelin sheaths of CNS axons (see Chapter 16). As a result, the myelin is completely or partially stripped from the nerves. There may also be damage to the underlying neurons. Damage to the myelin disrupts the passage of action potentials. Virtually all functions controlled by CNS innervation can be affected. The myelin produced by Schwann cells in the PNS has a different composition from the myelin produced by the oligodendrocytes in the CNS and it is not affected in MS.

7.3.2 MENINGES, CEREBROSPINAL FLUID, AND VENTRICLES

The whole of the nervous system – the brain, spinal cord, and nerves – is covered by tough connective tissue. The connective tissue that surrounds the brain and spinal cord is called the meninges and is arranged in three layers:

- The dura mater – the tough outer layer.
- The arachnoid membrane – the spongy web-like middle layer.
- The pia mater – the inner layer, which is closely attached to the brain.

The subarachnoid space between the arachnoid membrane and pia mater is filled with cerebrospinal fluid (CSF). Because the brain is completely immersed in liquid, pressure on the base of the brain is reduced. In the PNS there is no arachnoid matter or CSF and the dura and pia mater are fused to form a protective sheath.

The brain contains a number of spaces called ventricles which are filled with CSF. Besides providing physical support for the brain, the CSF performs a number of other functions: it protects against acute changes in arterial and venous blood pressure; is involved in intra-cerebral transport; helps maintain the ionic homeostasis of the CNS; and is a route for waste excretion.

7.3.3 BRAIN REGIONS

We now need to examine how neurons are organised in the brain (see Figures 7.3 and 7.4). The brain has three major divisions: the forebrain, midbrain, and hindbrain. The term 'brain stem' is often used to refer to the midbrain, pons, and medulla.

The **cerebral cortex** is the largest part of the human brain and is involved in 'higher' brain functions. This brain structure distinguishes mammals from other vertebrates: it is thought that the cortex is responsible for the evolution of intelligence. The cortex is the outer surface of the forebrain. It is highly wrinkled in order to increase the surface area of the brain and the number of neurons within it. The outer region of the cortex, which is grey in colour, contains neural cell bodies. Below this 'grey matter' is the 'white matter': this consists of axons which carry signals between cerebral neurons and other parts of the brain and body.

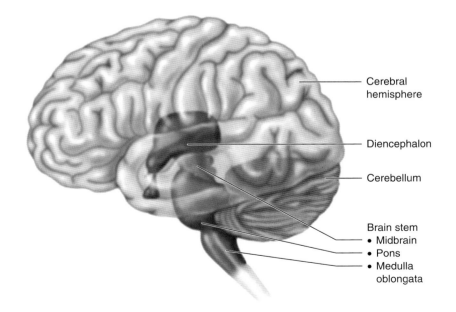

Cerebral hemisphere

Diencephalon

Cerebellum

Brain stem
• Midbrain
• Pons
• Medulla oblongata

FIGURE 7.3 Anatomy of the brain

major division	subdivision	principle structures
Forebrain	Telencephalon	Cerebral cortex
		Basal ganglia
		Limbic system
	Diencephalon	Thalamus
		Hypothalamus
Midbrain	Mesencephalon	Tectum
		Tegmentum
Hindbrain	Metencephalon	Cerebellum
		Pons
	Myelencephalon	Medulla oblongata

FIGURE 7.4 Divisions of the brain (adapted from Carlson, 2007)

The cerebrum is divided into the left and right hemispheres. Although the two hemispheres look mostly symmetrical, each side has slightly different functions. Sometimes the right hemisphere is associated with creativity and the left hemisphere is associated with logic. In each hemisphere, the cerebral cortex is divided into four sections, or 'lobes' – the frontal, parietal, occipital, and temporal. Each lobe has different functions, as described below. A bundle of millions of axons called the **corpus callosum** connects the right and left frontal lobe, right and left parietal lobe, right and left occipital lobe, and right and left temporal lobe.

The **frontal lobe** is involved in reasoning, planning, problem solving, aspects of speech, movement, and emotions. It contains the primary somatosensory cortex – which receives sensory input – and the primary motor cortex – which controls movement. The frontal lobe contains most of the dopamine-sensitive neurons in the cerebral cortex. As noted earlier, dopamine systems are involved in cognition and emotion. The frontal lobe is involved in more complicated or 'higher' mental functions. These include our capacity to: choose between different options; imagine the future consequences of our behaviour; and suppress socially unacceptable behaviour. The frontal lobe also plays an important part in our long-term memory of experiences by processing messages from the limbic system (see below).

The **parietal lobe** is important for integrating sensory information from various parts of the body and is also important for movement, orientation, recognition, perception of stimuli, and manipulation of objects.

The most important functional aspect of the **occipital lobe** is that it contains the primary visual cortex. Damage to specific areas of the occipital lobe leads to specific losses of visual capacity located in those areas.

The **temporal lobe** is the location of the primary auditory cortex. It is important for processing the meaning of both speech and vision. The temporal lobe also contains the hippocampus, which plays a key role in the formation of our long-term memory.

Wernicke's area – in the left temporal lobe – is particularly specialised for language comprehension. It is believed to have special connections to Broca's area in the frontal lobes. Although it has long been held that language comprehension and speech production are localised in Wernicke's and Broca's areas respectively, more recent research now suggests that these capacities may not be so clearly demarcated (see Research Box 7.1).

RESEARCH BOX 7.1   Localisation of speech capacity

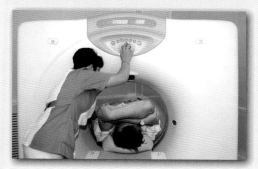

Background

Historically, our understanding of the brain's functional anatomy derived from post-mortem studies of brain-damaged patients. Later advances in neural imaging have led to dramatic changes in understanding how the brain works. It was traditionally thought that Broca's area was responsible for speech production, with speech comprehension localised in Wernicke's area.

Methods

The day after a surgical procedure, a 67 year old man referred to as MJE suddenly became unable to speak. He soon regained some speech capacity, but was only able to produce short phrases or say single words.

Results

Functional Magnetic Resonance Imaging (FMRI) revealed an infarction and a severe restriction of the blood supply in Broca's area. In addition to the expected impairments to language production, MJE also had impairments in some aspect of language comprehension. Restoration of normal blood flow to the affected area resulted in an immediate recovery of these functions.

Significance

Advances in imaging have improved our understanding of the brain's functional anatomy. This study shows that language comprehension and language generation may not be as separate as was originally thought. It is important however to note the limitations of this study. First, there was only a short time for observations before blood flow was restored to the affected area. Second, it may be difficult to generalise from case studies (a limitation common to many studies of brain abnormalities).

Photograph © Mikhail Malyshev/Fotolia

Davis, C. et al. (2008) Speech and language functions that require a functioning Broca's area, *Brain & Language, 105*: 50–58.

The **basal ganglia** consist of a cluster of neural nuclei connected with the cerebral cortex, thalamus, and brainstem. The basal ganglia are involved in a variety of functions including motor control, cognition, emotions, and learning. Disorders linked to the basal ganglia include cerebral palsy (basal ganglia damage during second and third trimester of pregnancy), Huntington's disease and Parkinson's disease.

The **limbic system** lies buried within the cerebrum, forming the inner border of the cortex. In evolutionary terms, this is an old structure which is present in the common ancestors of mammals and modern reptiles. This system contains the thalamus, hypothalamus, amygdala, and hippocampus. It is often referred to as the 'emotional brain' and is important for the formation of memories. It operates by influencing the endocrine system and the ANS. It is highly interconnected with the nucleus accumbens, which is the brain's pleasure centre.

The **thalamus** is a large mass of grey matter deep in the forebrain. Axons from every sensory system (except olfaction/smell) synapse here as the last relay site before the information reaches the cerebral cortex. However, it is not just a relay system: the thalamus also processes sensory information. The thalamus has sensory and motor functions. It plays an important part in regulating sleep, wakefulness, and consciousness (see section 7.5).

The **hypothalamus** is located just below the thalamus. It is mainly involved with homeostasis, including the regulation of thirst and hunger. It is also involved in the regulation of emotions and the control of the ANS and circadian rhythms (see section 7.5). Consequently, it receives input from a number of regions of the body and the brain. The hypothalamus sends messages to the rest of the body in two ways: via the ANS and via instructions sent to the pituitary gland (the 'master gland' of the endocrine system).

The **amygdala** are two almond-shaped masses of neurons located in each temporal lobe on either side of the thalamus. These neurons are involved in memory and emotion (especially aggression and fear). Damage to this area of the brain makes people indifferent to things that would normally invoke fear.

The **hippocampus** consists of two 'horns' of neurons projecting back from the amygdala. This part of the brain is important for converting our short-term memory into long-term memory, so it is important for learning (see Chapter 10). Damage to this brain region means that people may keep their old memories but will be unable to form new ones.

The term 'brain stem' is often used to refer to the midbrain, pons, and medulla. Collectively, these structures are responsible for basic vital functions such as breathing, heartbeat, and blood pressure. In evolutionary terms, these are old structures that were present in the ancestors of mammals and modern reptiles (indeed, the entire brains of some reptiles resemble the human brain stem). The midbrain lies at the 'top' of the brain stem and consists of the tectum and tegmentum. The anterior part of the midbrain contains the cerebral peduncle, which is a large bundle of axons involved in voluntary motor function which send messages from the cerebral cortex.

The **tectum** is involved in preliminary visual processing and in the control of eye movements. It is also involved in auditory processing. The **tegmentum** is a network of neurons that is involved in the control of motor functions, the regulation of awareness, and the regulation of many autonomic homeostatic and reflexive pathways.

Like the cerebrum, the **cerebellum** (literally the 'little brain') has a highly folded surface and is divided into two hemispheres. Although it makes up only 10 per cent of brain mass, it contains more than half of its neurons. Its functions include the regulation and coordination of movement, posture, and balance. In evolutionary terms, the cerebellum is an old structure.

The **pons** is involved in the regulation of consciousness, sleep, and sensory processing. Some structures within the pons are linked to the cerebellum and are therefore involved in movement and posture. The myelencephalon consists mainly of tracts carrying signals between the brain and the rest of the body. The **medulla oblongata** is responsible for maintaining vital body functions, such as breathing and heart rate.

Luria's functional model provides a useful summary: the brainstem regulates the arousal of the brain and muscle tone; the posterior areas of the cortex are involved in processing sensory information from the internal and external environments; and the frontal lobes and prefrontal lobes are involved in planning, executing, and monitoring behaviour (Zillmer et al., 2008).

Summary

- The brain is organised into different regions, each of which has different activities and functions. Major divisions of the brain are the forebrain, midbrain, and hindbrain. The forebrain is divided in two linked hemispheres.
- The frontal lobes are involved in reasoning, planning, problem solving, speech, movement, and emotions. They process sensory input and control voluntary movement. They also process information from other brain regions.
- The temporal, parietal, and occipital lobes all have specialised capacities for processing and integrating sensory information.
- The limbic system is the 'emotional brain'. It is also important for memory. It lies deep within the forebrain.
- The brain stem and the cerebellum are involved in regulating basic functions such as posture, movement, breathing, and heart rate.

Disruptions to normal functioning in different brain regions are related to different disorders and diseases. Disorders with primarily psychological symptoms are covered in Chapter 16. Other chapters discuss the regulation of emotions (see Chapter 2) and pain (see Chapter 4). The following sections will focus on control of movement and movement disorders. Later sections will address sleep and consciousness.

7.4 CONTROL OF MOVEMENT

All muscular activity is influenced by the nervous system. Although smooth muscle cells may contract spontaneously, their rate of contraction is influenced by motor neurons of the ANS. Although the contraction of the cardiac muscle is triggered by an internal pacemaker, the motor neurons of the ANS modulate the intrinsic rate and strength of the heartbeat.

Reflexive action in skeletal muscle is coordinated via the spinal cord without the involvement of the brain. Voluntary skeletal muscle activity is controlled by the CNS.

Motor neurons control muscle movement. We will examine first the innervation of skeletal muscles at the neuro-muscular junction (NMJ) and then the processes involved in reflexive and voluntary skeletal muscle activity. Skeletal muscles convert electrical action potentials from motor neurons into mechanical force by means of contraction. The presynaptic neuron membrane releases acetylcholine at the NMJ. The binding of acetylcholine to specific receptors on the muscle cell membrane causes muscle contraction. A single impulse from a neuron produces a single twitch in a muscle fibre. However, because muscle has a certain degree of elasticity, the duration of a muscle twitch is longer than the duration of the action potential. A rapid series of action potentials causes a muscle to produce a sustained contraction (rather than twitches). The overall strength of a muscle contraction depends on how many motor units fire and how rapidly they do so.

7.4.1 REFLEXES

If you touch something that is too hot, you will automatically move your hand away from it. This is not a conscious process: you do not think 'Oh, that pan is too hot, I should let go of it'. This type of movement is a **reflex** – an involuntary almost instantaneous movement in response to an external stimulus. Reflex actions can be made quickly because most sensory neurons do not pass directly into the brain. Instead they synapse with other motor neurons in the spinal cord. The stimulus could come in any sensory form (e.g. a heat or pain). This stimulus input is sent to the spinal column where it may directly synapse with a motor neuron, or an interneuron may relay the signal to an efferent motor neuron. The motor neuron then fires an action potential which causes the appropriate muscle movement (e.g. a withdrawal from heat). This arrangement of afferent and efferent neurons is referred to as a reflex arc. Although reflex arcs mean that the brain does not have to process sensory information before producing the appropriate response, the brain does receive sensory input while the reflex action occurs in order that we might become aware of our reflexive movements.

Spinal reflexes do not occur in isolation: rather, they involve control from the brain. In some cases the brain can inhibit the reflexive muscle action. The brain contains circuits which recognise that in some situations the reflex action may do more harm than good. For example, imagine you take a hot casserole out of the oven using a thin oven glove and begin to walk towards the kitchen table. After a few moments the heat will trigger a withdrawal reflex. However, your brain will recognise that dropping the casserole on the floor would be disastrous so it over-rides the reflex, allowing you to hold on until you get to the table.

7.4.2 VOLUNTARY CONTROL OF MOVEMENT

The nerves involved in generating the impulses for voluntary movement are located in the primary motor cortex. This is a band of neurons in the posterior frontal lobes which is organised like a map of the body. This 'motor homunculus' (see Figure 7.5) is not a scale model of the body. Instead, the size of each region indicates the level of innervation and reflects the degree of control of fine movements: the hands and fingers occupy more space than the rest

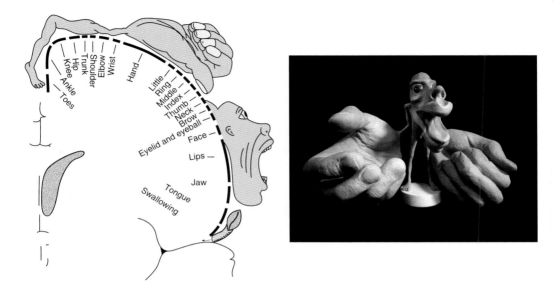

FIGURE 7.5 The motor homunculus
Photograph reproduced courtesy of the Natural History Museum

of the arm, and more space than the feet and toes. The image on the right of Figure 7.5 shows what we would look like if we were a scale model of the motor homunculus.

Each area of the primary motor cortex controls the movements of particular groups of muscles. It receives feedback from these muscles and the joints that they influence, via the somatosensory cortex. The term 'descending pathway' is used to refer to nerve pathways that go from the brain toward the spinal cord and allow the brain to control movement of the body below the head. In contrast, ascending pathways go upward from the spinal cord toward the brain. They carry sensory information from the body to the brain.

Electrical stimulation to the various areas of the motor homunculus produces muscle action in the relevant area of the body (but not other areas). Extensive damage to areas of the primary motor cortex may impair people's ability to move the corresponding body part independent of others (e.g. moving only one finger). However, voluntary movement is still possible because of the existence of pathways that descend directly from the secondary motor cortex without passing via the primary motor cortex.

The secondary motor cortices perform several functions. They are responsible for:

- Transforming visual information into motor commands (posterior parietal cortex).
- Guiding movement and controlling the proximal and trunk muscles (premotor cortex).
- Planning and coordinating complex actions such as those requiring two hands (supplementary motor area)

The secondary motor cortices may be involved in programming specific patterns of movement according to instructions received from the prefrontal cortex (which is involved in forming plans and strategies) and sending their output to the primary motor cortex.

In addition to these cortical areas, other brain regions are important for controlling motor function. Although skilled rapid movements are initiated in the frontal cortex, the control and timing of such movements require the involvement of the cerebellum. Extensive damage to the cerebellum results in a loss of ability to control movements, impairments in capacities to modify movements in changing conditions, and difficulty in maintaining posture. The basal ganglia also modulate movement. They do this via neural loops that receive input from a wide array of cortical areas and feed this back via the thalamus to the primary motor cortex, premotor cortex, and supplementary motor area. They also send outputs to the motor nuclei of the brain stem. Damage to the basal ganglia causes severe motor deficits such as Parkinson's and Huntington's Disease (see Chapter 16).

CASE STUDY 7.1   Parkinson's disease

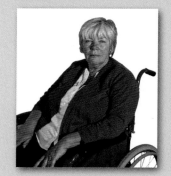

Beth is 62, and married with four adult children. When she was in her late thirties, she began to experience tremours in her arm, which were attributed to her response to the recent death of her son. However, the symptoms persisted and she was diagnosed with Parkinson's disease at age 44. Since then it has been treated with L-Dopa. Before she takes her medication and sometimes between daytime doses Beth often feels 'dull' and is often barely able to move and communicate properly:

> You can't think straight ... it's a horrible feeling, you feel as if, er, you you're not connecting, you know, that's all I can explain it, you're brain isn't telling your body what to do.

Overcoming her reduced capacity to control her movements requires purposeful effort: she talks herself through sequences of actions, such as walking or eating. Whereas she used to enjoy being active and 'never felt tired', Beth now feels fatigued and has difficulty doing things that used to be easy. Parkinson's disease has led to profound changes in how she sees herself and how others see her:

> They think that you're senile because you're moving like this and ... finding things hard to do like take a top off a bottle.

These changes to daily activities and quality of life are soul-destroying: Beth feels 'young at heart' but appears to others to be an 'old lady' who cannot manage. However, her efforts to conceal her muscle tremours so as to avoid negative evaluations from others usually only make the situation worse:

> I try and stop myself from moving. So I hold my arm or I put my arms to the back and clasp my fist ... but I look worse when I disguise it because I'm doing contortions.

To minimise such experiences, Beth adheres to her medication regimen. Although this lets her achieve daily activities at the right times, it limits her capacity to be spontaneous. She therefore feels empowered, but also disempowered by her medication.

(adapted from Bramley and Eatough, 2005

Summary

- All muscular activity is influenced by the nervous system.
- Spinal reflexes are muscular contractions made in response to sensory information that do not have to be processed by the CNS. However, the brain can over-ride reflexive muscle actions.
- Voluntary muscle movement is initiated in the primary motor cortex, a band of neurons in the posterior frontal lobe arranged as a motor homunculus. It also involves the secondary motor cortices, basal ganglia, and cerebellum.
- Damage to neurons in any of the areas involved in the control of movement can lead to severe motor impairments.

7.5 SLEEP, CONSCIOUSNESS, AND BIOLOGICAL CLOCKS

Sleep is an important topic: many people experience sleep difficulties (Groeger et al., 2004) and quality of sleep affects our wellbeing (see below). Given the high levels of neural and muscular activity described in the last section, one might think that sleep involves an absence of such activity. However, when we are asleep our brains are not simply at rest: important activities are going on.

Sleep research uses a range of devices to monitor the body's activity during sleep: electroencephalograms (EEG) record electrical activity in the brain; electromyograms (EMG) record muscle activity; and electrooculograms (EOG) record eye movement. Researchers may also monitor markers of arousal such as heart rate, breathing, and galvanic skin response (i.e. changes in the electrical resistance of the skin). The information gathered shows that rather than there being a single entity called 'sleep' there are various phases of sleep, each with specific patterns of bodily activity.

Sleep can be divided into five stages: **REM sleep** (so named because it is characterised by Rapid Eye Movement), and four stages of increasingly deep **non-REM sleep**. Typically, people will progress through Stages 1–4 of non-REM sleep before entering REM sleep, which is when dreaming occurs. This progression usually takes around 90 minutes. Normally, REM sleep must be preceded by slow-wave (Stage 3–4) sleep, and there is a refractory period after each bout of REM sleep when REM sleep cannot occur (see Figure 7.6).

The progression from stages 1 to 4 leads to 'deeper' sleep. People are easiest to wake during Stage 1 and hardest to wake during Stage 4 sleep. If people do wake from Stage 4 they are often groggy and confused. In Stages 3 and 4, EEGs show slow synchronised waves of neural activity. In contrast, EEGs during REM sleep show high frequency desynchronised activity more similar to those that can be seen when awake. During REM sleep the brain becomes activated: levels of neural firing, blood flow, and oxygen consumption increase to waking levels. REM sleep also differs from non-REM sleep stages because of the eponymous rapid eye movements that are observable through closed eye lids and via

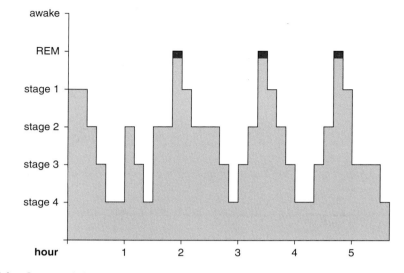

FIGURE 7.6 Stages of sleep

EOG. The EMG shows a marked loss of skeletal muscle tone compared to the moderate muscle tone in Stages 3 and 4.

Neural activity during REM sleep corresponds to the content of dreams. For example, talking and listening during dreams is associated with the increased neural activity in brain regions involved in talking and listening (Hong et al., 1996). However, physical movements made during sleep do not occur during dreams in REM sleep because of the loss of skeletal muscle tone. Sleepwalking and night terrors occur during slow-wave sleep – especially Stage 4. They do not occur during REM sleep and they also do not mean that a person is acting out a dream.

7.5.1 WHY DO WE DREAM?

There is no definitive explanation of why we dream. That there are specific patterns of brain activity during REM sleep absent from other stages of sleep suggests that it may have a distinct function. Studies of REM sleep deprivation show that the body tries to ensure a certain amount of REM sleep. In such studies, people will be allowed to sleep as much as they want, but will be woken each time they enter REM sleep. In response to REM deprivation, the body appears to enter REM sleep more rapidly than normal and on subsequent nights there is evidence of the body catching up on REM sleep.

Some research has indicated that REM sleep is important for consolidating learning and memory (Stickgold et al., 2001). However, there is also some evidence that deficits in total sleep or REM sleep do not affect learning and memory. For example, although REM sleep is significantly reduced by the three major classes of anti-depressant drugs, there are no corresponding disruptions to learning and memory (Vertes and Eastman, 2000). Although REM sleep appears to be important to the body, some studies have indicated that the body can do without it, at least in the short-term (Nykamp et al., 1998).

Just as there is disagreement about why we dream, there is also disagreement about what dreams mean. As you will probably know from your own experience, dreams will often relate to things you are preoccupied about. The content of dreams may have a literal interpretation. For example, if we are dehydrated we may dream about drinking water. However, objects and events within dreams may also have symbolic meanings. For instance, feeling thirsty but not being allowed to drink may symbolise some other frustration in our lives. When interpreting dreams, it is important to consider the individual items or events in dreams, their links to other objects/events in the dream, and the context of the dreamer's waking life.

Freud (1999 [1990]) believed that dreams are the 'royal road' to understanding our unconscious mental processes. In his psychoanalytic theory, he argued that subconscious urges and emotions appeared in a disguised form during dreams. An alternative to the psychoanalytic model is the activation-synthesis model, which proposes that dreams are simply the result of the brain trying to make sense of activation of neural circuits in the brain stem and parts of the limbic system during REM sleep (Hobson and McCarley, 1977). The brain's attempt to make sense of this neural activity is experienced as a dream.

7.5.2 WHY DO WE SLEEP?

Sleep deprivation appears to be a risk to human health through its effects on brain function. These include increased lapses of attention, deficits in cognition and memory, or involuntary sleep onsets (Dinges et al., 1997). Several lines of evidence indicate that sleep is linked to memory. Poor quality and/or quantity of sleep may impair the consolidation of memories and performance in learning tasks (Frank and Benington, 2006). Exposure to new environments or cognitive tasks can alter subsequent sleep. Research Box 7.2 highlights the consequences of sleep deprivation for surgeons. The findings of such studies have strengthened calls for legislation to limit doctors' working hours.

Sleep affects our physical health. People with reduced sleep have impaired immune function, a greater risk of diabetes and cardiovascular disease, and higher mortality rates (Alvarez and Ayas, 2004). A recent review focusing on cardiovascular disease revealed that sleep deprivation leads to changes in blood pressure, inflammation, autonomic tone and hormone activity that increase the risk of cardiovascular disease (Mullington et al., 2009).

Sleep seems to serve a restorative or recuperative function, allowing the body to repair and replenish itself following our daily activities. The 'deeper' sleep of stages 3 and 4 may have an important role here. Research indicates that Stage 3 and 4 sleep is protected: the sleep of people who are sleep deprived has a higher proportion of Stage 3 and 4 sleep, and may contain the same total amount of Stage 3 and 4 sleep as people with normal sleep (Reynolds et al., 1986).

RESEARCH BOX 7.2   Sleep deprivation affects surgical skill

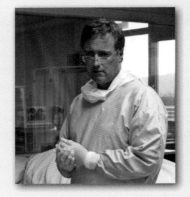

Background

Although it is known that sleep deprivation can lead to lapses in attention and impaired problem-solving capacities, less is known about how sleep deprivation affects the performance of resident physicians when spending 24 hours 'on call'.

Methods and results

The skills of 35 surgical residents were assessed using a laparoscopic surgery simulator. Participants were assessed at three time points – the morning of the day before going 'on call' (well-rested), the morning of the 'on call' period (well-rested), and the morning after being 'on call' (sleep-deprived).

Compared to the two 'rested' assessments, performance in the sleep-deprived state was poorer: residents took significantly longer to complete the task and made significantly more errors.

Significance

It is well-known that 'on call' schedules lead to acute sleep deprivation and fatigue. This study shows that such sleep deprivation and fatigue led to significant reductions in surgical performance. This may cause poorer clinical performance and patient outcomes.

Eastridge, B.J. et al. (2003) Effect of sleep deprivation on the performance of simulated laparoscopic surgical skill, *American Journal of Surgery, 186*: 169–174.

CLINICAL NOTES 7.1

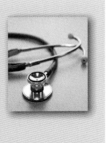

Sleep deprivation in medicine

- For your own sake, and for the safety of your patients, ensure that you get enough good quality sleep.
- Shift work can impair physical and psychological health, particularly if you are over 40 years of age.
- Be aware of how sleep deprivation impairs learning and memory.

- Be aware of the effects of sleep deprivation on your own performance.
- Shift patterns are better if they are forward rotating (i.e. move the biological clock forward with each shift) rather than backward rotating.
- These issues are important while you are a student, and will remain important throughout your working life.

7.5.3 WHY DO WE SLEEP WHEN WE DO?

Although sleep may have a restorative function, it is not simply the case that we sleep more when we have been more active, or sleep less when we have been inactive (e.g. Driver and Taylor, 2000; Ryback and Lewis, 1971). Rather than being responsive to activity levels, sleep patterns appear to be determined internally and to follow a circadian (literally 'about a day') rhythm (Lavie, 2001). The body also has circadian rhythms for body temperature and hormone secretion. These rhythms are determined by the body's internal pacemaker, the **suprachiasmatic nucleus** (**SCN**) in the hypothalamus. In the case of sleep, the SCN produces a circadian rhythm via the output of melatonin from the pineal gland. Increased melatonin output occurs during darkness and causes drowsiness.

The intrinsic rhythms provided by the SCN are around 24 hours long. They are kept in this pattern by the daily cycle of daylight and darkness. Jet lag occurs when there is a rapid desynchronisation of the endogenous rhythms of the SCN and external patterns of light and darkness. A similar desynchronisation happens among shift workers. In this case, the external patterns of light and darkness stay the same, but workers must adjust their sleep-wake cycles. Both people with jet lag and those working shifts tend to have disrupted sleep, feel more tired, and show impairments in cognitive function. Exposure to bright light at key times can make it easier for people to adjust to shift work or recover from jet lag (e.g. Burgess et al., 2002). Recent research has indicated that melatonin-analogue drugs can treat the range of symptoms associated with shift work and jet lag (Rajaratnam et al., 2009). A simple explanation is that they move the hands of the circadian clock.

Whereas the SCN regulates the periodicity of sleep, other brain regions are involved in the changes between stages of sleep. The reticular formation lies at the core of the brain-stem and runs through the mid-brain, pons, and medulla. Stimulation of this region ends sleep and may act as a 'wake up call' to the basal ganglia, thalamus, and forebrain. Serotonin activity within this region appears to be involved in sleep regulation. Activity in the pons appears to regulate REM sleep. Acetylcholine activity in the pons is involved in eye activity during REM sleep, whereas the inhibition of acetylcholine release in the forebrain causes slow-wave sleep. Increased norepinephrine release in the pons is linked to the change from sleep to wakefulness. Sleep-wake cycles can be disrupted in many disorders (including depression and seasonal affective disorder) and following brain injury. For example, 10–40 per cent of people with affective disorders report excessive sleep at night and napping during the day (Kaplan and Harvey, 2009).

CLINICAL NOTES 7.2

Self-treating insomnia

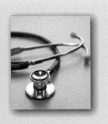

- Only go to bed when you are sleepy.
- Set your alarm for a normal waking hour and get up at the same time every day – regardless of how much you have slept.
- Do not sleep more than 10 hours a night and do not nap during the day.
- Paradoxically, if you wake up in the night it can sometimes help you get back to sleep if you try to force yourself to stay awake.
- Avoid alcohol, caffeine, or nicotine after 6 p.m. and do not eat a large meal late at night.
- Keep your bedroom for sleeping and sex - do not work in your bedroom.
- If you wake in the middle of the night for more than 20 minutes, get up and do something else. Only go back to bed when you feel sleepy.
- Do not worry about how much sleep you are getting or watch the clock – this may make it worse.

ACTIVITY 7.1   CONSCIOUSNESS

- Take a few seconds to write down everything that you are currently aware of – what you can see, hear, smell, feel, and taste.
- How much of your body's activities do you think you are consciously aware of?

7.5.4 WAKEFULNESS AND CONSCIOUSNESS

Sleep is not a single state and neither is wakefulness. **Consciousness** consists of the things that we are aware of – information, memories, or the rumblings in our stomach. Consciousness is the 'tip of the iceberg' of mental processes. There are other levels of mental activity which may or may not enter our conscious awareness. **Non-conscious** brain processes are those that we are never conscious of, such as the control of our heartbeat or digestion. The **pre-conscious** consists of information that is readily available to us should we need it, but of which we are not actively aware. For example, we may be able to tell someone what we ate for breakfast this morning, or where we were born, but that is not to say that we walk around all day consciously aware of this information just in case someone asks. The term **unconscious** is used to refer to information that we process but are never aware of knowing. In psychoanalytic thinking the unconscious contains primitive urges and repressed memories that are never available to consciousness. This psychoanalytic concept of the unconscious mind is controversial and less widely accepted than the concept of unconscious mental processes.

Levels of wakefulness and alertness are influenced by various neurotransmitters acting at different sites in the brain. Neurotransmitters with important influences on arousal are:

- Acetylcholine (released from neurons in the pons and the basal forebrain).
- Norepinephrine (released from neurons in the pons).
- Serotonin (released from neurons in the reticular formation).
- Histamine and hypocretin (both released from neurons in the hypothalamus).

The axons of these neurons branch to many important areas of the brain; some have direct effects on cortical arousal and others have indirect effects via the thalamus and hypothalamus.

7.5.5 DISORDERS OF CONSCIOUSNESS

Disorders of consciousness allow us insights into the physiology of consciousness. **Narcolepsy** is a neurological disorder characterised by brief bouts of sleep at inappropriate times. It appears to be caused by deficiencies in the production of hypocretin, a neurotransmitter involved in arousal and alertness (Nishino et al., 2000). Narcoleptic sleep attacks can occur at any time, but are most common in boring monotonous situations. People with narcolepsy may also experience cataplexy – a sudden muscular weakness caused by the inhibition of motor neurons in the spinal cord. This often leads to a collapse, followed by a period of immobility during which the person will remain fully conscious. Whereas narcoleptic sleep attacks are often preceded by boredom, cataplexy is usually precipitated by very strong emotions (see http://www.youtube.com/watch?v=3MBCeKn0Oeo).

Epilepsy is a serious neurological disorder, with a population prevalence of around 0.5 per cent. It is characterised by recurrent seizures – bursts of excess electrical activity in the brain which cause a temporary disruption to normal neural functioning. For around 70 per cent of people with epilepsy there is no known cause, but 30 per cent of cases can be linked to diseases or abnormalities such as imbalances in GABA-inhibition and the glutamate-excitation of neural activity. Partial seizures are localised and affect specific sites in one hemisphere (e.g. one temporal lobe). Simple partial seizures involve no impairment of consciousness, whereas complex partial seizures do. Partial seizures may be precursors to generalised seizures, which affect several areas of the brain and impair consciousness. These are also called tonic-clonic seizures: in the tonic phase the person briefly loses consciousness and their muscles tense up; in the clonic phase rapid contraction and relaxation of the muscles cause convulsions. Such seizures are usually followed by a period of sleep: upon waking people are often confused and may not remember events just prior to the seizure. Around two-thirds of patients cease having seizures within five years, usually as a result of anticonvulsant drug treatment. If such seizures have a localised origin and anticonvulsant medication proves ineffective, surgery may then be conducted.

Summary

- Sleep is not a period of rest for the brain: it consists of several phases, each characterised by specific patterns of neural activity.
- Dreaming occurs during Rapid Eye Movement (REM) sleep. The body tries to ensure a certain amount of REM sleep. This suggests that dreaming has important functions (e.g. the consolidation of memory). However, the functions of dreaming are not fully understood.
- Similarly, the functions of sleep are not fully understood. However, sleep does appear to have restorative functions, and sleep deprivation leads to impaired performance on cognitive tasks, and can lead to impaired health.
- The timing of sleep is determined by circadian rhythms in physiological systems controlled by the suprachiasmatic nucleus. These rhythms usually match natural patterns of daylight and darkness.
- Fluctuations in neurotransmitter levels affect levels of consciousness, and are involved in disorders of consciousness such as narcolepsy.

FURTHER READING

Carlson, N.R. (2007) *Physiology of Behavior* (9th edition). Boston, MA: Allyn & Bacon. A standard textbook for neuropsychology and biological psychology. It contains detailed descriptions and illustrations of brain structures and functions.

Pinel, J.P.J. (2007) *Biopsychology* (7th edition). Boston, MA: Pearson. Another standard textbook for neuropsychology and biological psychology. It also contains detailed descriptions and illustrations of brain structures and functions, along with descriptions of practical applications of concepts.

REVISION QUESTIONS

1   Describe the organisation of the nervous system (i.e. central, peripheral, autonomic, somatosensory) and the functions of each division.

2   How are action potentials conducted within and between neurons?

3   Outline the functions of the four lobes of the cerebral cortex.

4   Describe the action of the brain regions involved in the control of voluntary movement.

5 Discuss the accuracy of this statement: 'When you sleep your body and your brain are at rest'.

6 Why do we sleep? Why do we sleep when we do?

7 Describe the effects of sleep deprivation and dream deprivation.

8 Outline the key features of epilepsy and narcolepsy. Describe how neurotransmitters are involved in these disorders of consciousness.

8 PSYCHOSOCIAL DEVELOPMENT ACROSS THE LIFESPAN

Figures

Research boxes

LEARNING OBJECTIVES

This chapter is designed to enable you to:

- Describe the major psychosocial developmental changes that occur in childhood.
- Outline how language and thinking develop through childhood and adolescence.
- Describe the physical and psychological changes and challenges of adolescence.
- Discuss stability and change in physical and cognitive capacity during older adulthood.
- Appreciate how changes across the lifespan affect doctor-patient communication.

Psychosocial development occurs across the lifespan. At different ages, we will acquire different cognitive and social skills and enact different social roles (see Chapter 9). One way of thinking about these changes is by using Erikson's (1950) division of the lifespan into eight stages, each characterised by a particular developmental challenge that must be resolved for optimal psychosocial functioning (see Box 8.1).

Although these challenges are psychological in nature, health and illness can influence the extent to which people are able to resolve them. For example, physical disabilities may affect the development of autonomy in childhood. Similarly, people's health may be affected by their experience of each developmental conflict, such as adolescents engaging in risky behaviours as part of identity explorations. This model indicates that, although childhood is important, development and change in fact occur across the lifespan.

This chapter, therefore, outlines a lifespan approach to development. Medical professionals must be able to identify abnormal patterns of development and treat these appropriately to minimise disturbances to physical and psychological growth. We also need to be aware of people's capabilities at different ages to allow optimal doctor-patient communication.

BOX 8.1   Erikson's model of lifespan development

Age	Conflict	Outcomes
Infancy	Trust vs. Mistrust	Children develop a sense of trust in other people when their carers provide reliable care and affection.
Early childhood	Autonomy vs. Shame/Doubt	Children develop a sense of autonomy and independence derived from acquiring physical skills. Failure leads to shame and doubt.
Preschool	Initiative vs. Guilt	Children begin to assert control over their environment and develop a sense of purpose. Efforts to exert too much power result in disapproval and guilt.
School age	Industry vs. Inferiority	Children need to cope with new social and intellectual demands and develop feelings of competence.
Adolescence	Identity vs. Role Confusion	Adolescents need to develop a strong personal identity. Failure leads to role confusion and a weak sense of self.
Young adulthood	Intimacy vs. Isolation	Adults need to form strong intimate relationships. Failure leads to loneliness.
Middle adulthood	Generativity vs. Stagnation	Adults need to create and nurture things that will outlast them (e.g. children or social changes) to provide feelings of accomplishment and usefulness.
Maturity	Ego Integrity vs. Despair	Older adults need to feel fulfilled when they reflect on their lives. Failure leads to regret and despair.

8.1 CHILDHOOD

8.1.1 ATTACHMENT AND DEVELOPMENT

Attachment is a strong affectional tie felt for another. Children feel pleasure and joy when interacting with caregivers with whom they have a secure attachment, and comfort from being near them in times of stress. Unless infants have secure trusting attachments to their adult caregivers, normal cognitive, social, and emotional development may not occur.

Quality of attachment

Four different types of attachment have been identified by using a research technique known as the 'strange situation' (Ainsworth et al., 1978). This is a situation in which a mother brings her child to a room with toys in it, leaves the child for a short while, and then returns. By observing how much exploration and play the child engages in, and how they respond to their mother's departure and return, children's attachments may be divided into four types as shown in Box 8.2. The most common types of attachment are secure (around 70 per cent) and avoidant (around 20 per cent). Although there is some variation in the proportions found in each group, these general patterns have been observed in different cultures (van Ijzendoorn and Kroonenberg, 1988).

BOX 8.2   Attachment styles in the 'strange situation'

Attachment style	Child's behaviour when mother leaves	Mother's parenting style
Secure attachment	Child gets upset when mother leaves but calms down quickly when she returns and explores the environment when she is there.	Mother is quick to respond to physical and emotional needs of the child. Helps the child to cope with their stress.
Avoidant attachment	Child explores the environment and does not respond when mother leaves or returns.	Mother does not respond when child is upset. Tries to stop child crying and encourages independence and exploration.
Ambivalent attachment	Child gets upset when mother leaves but can be comforted by a stranger. When mother returns the child will act ambivalently and resist contact or appear angry.	Mother is inconsistent – varies between responding quickly and appropriately on some occasions and not responding on other occasions. Child is therefore preoccupied with whether mother is available before they can use her as a secure base.
Disorganised attachment	Can be secure, ambivalent, or avoidant but also shows some difficulty coping when the mother returns with behaviour such as rocking themselves or freezing.	Mother's behaviour can be negative, withdrawn, inappropriate, roles not clearly defined, sometimes child maltreatment.

The importance of secure attachment

Secure attachments to carers are important because they develop feelings in children that they are worthy of love and care and that others will be available to them in times of need. They establish children's 'internal working models' for all subsequent close relationships (Bowlby, 1973). The internal working models of children with less secure attachments do not include an expectation that they are worthy of love and care.

Secure attachment during childhood has broad and lasting influences on development. It promotes optimal development of the brain – especially the limbic system, which is crucially involved in emotional regulation (see Chapter 7). Insecure attachment resulting from neglect and a lack of stimulation can lead to serious underdevelopment in these brain regions (Gerhardt, 2004). Secure attachment also results in better social competence and peer relations, better emotional competence and self-reliance, better cognitive function, and better physical and psychological health (Ranson and Urichuk, 2008).

Given the importance of attachment, one might wonder whether all is lost if a secure attachment to parents does not develop or is not possible. Research has indicated that adopted children can develop secure attachments with their adoptive parents (van Londen et al., 2007). Most children will also have a degree of resilience which will allow them to recover to some extent from earlier neglect or abuse (see Research Box 8.1).

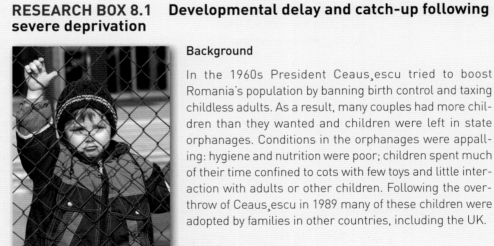

RESEARCH BOX 8.1   Developmental delay and catch-up following severe deprivation

Background

In the 1960s President Ceauşescu tried to boost Romania's population by banning birth control and taxing childless adults. As a result, many couples had more children than they wanted and children were left in state orphanages. Conditions in the orphanages were appalling: hygiene and nutrition were poor; children spent much of their time confined to cots with few toys and little interaction with adults or other children. Following the overthrow of Ceauşescu in 1989 many of these children were adopted by families in other countries, including the UK.

Methods and results

Longitudinal follow-up was conducted with 111 Romanian infants adopted by UK families and a comparison group of

British adopted children. When they arrived in the UK the orphans had severely impaired physical and cognitive development.

This study showed there was some 'catch-up' to normal levels of physical and cognitive development. This catch-up was nearly complete for children adopted in the UK before six months old. However, significant delays remained among those who were older when adopted.

Significance

For ethical reasons, it would never be possible to design an experiment in which children were subject to severe deprivation: the researchers took advantage of an unfortunate social experiment. Although all children displayed some resilience in being able to overcome early deprivation, severe prolonged deprivation produced significant deficits in physical and psychological development that were difficult to overcome fully.

Photograph © Forca/www.photoxpress.com

O'Connor, T.G. et al. (2000) The effects of global severe privation on cognitive competence, *Child Development, 71*: 376–390.

How does attachment develop?

Several different accounts for the development of secure attachments have been offered. Freud's **psychoanalytic theory** proposed that the mother becomes the primary love object in the baby's life because she satisfies the infant's need for food and oral pleasure. **Learning theory** argues that a positive perception of the mother is formed because the baby learns that breastfeeding satisfies hunger (and the mother learns that breastfeeding calms the baby).

Ethological theory argues that although breastfeeding is important for building the mother-baby relationship, attachment does not depend solely on the satisfaction of hunger and the provision of oral pleasure. Otherwise, how could we explain strong attachments between infants and their fathers? Bowlby (1969) argued that Freud's psychoanalytic perspective fails to acknowledge attachment as a psychological bond in its own right rather than an instinct derived from feeding or sexuality. Bowlby's view was supported by Harlow's (1958) research with monkeys separated from their mothers, which showed that attachment is formed on the basis of comfort rather than nourishment. In that research, baby monkeys separated from their mother were found to prefer a surrogate 'mother' covered in soft fabric to a wire 'mother' – even when the wire mother provided milk.

Bowlby argued that humans have a set of in-built attachment behaviours designed to maintain close contact with a particular person perceived to be better able to cope with the world. In babies, these include clinging to caregivers, crying for their attention, and smiling at their return. From a very young age, infants can engage in attachment behaviours such as imitating the facial expressions of parents (see Figure 8.1). From this early

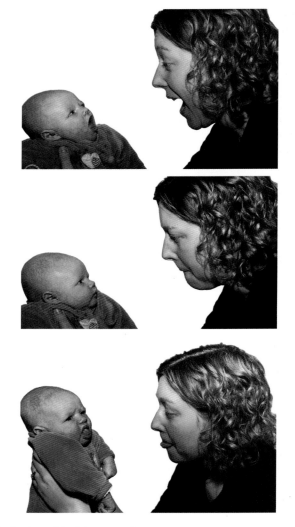

FIGURE 8.1   Infant imitation of facial expressions

unsophisticated (but amazing) behaviour, attachment develops in stages as infants develop greater skills for directing their attention and actions – the kinds of following and clinging behaviours assessed in the 'strange situation' with children aged 12 to 18 months.

Parent-infant bonding

For an attachment to parents to occur, infants must know who their parents are. The process of **bonding** to carers begins before birth. In the first few days of life, newborns use various senses to learn who their carers are. It is important, therefore, for parents to engage in behaviours which maximise this multisensory input for their children as follows:

- Physical contact: mothers should be encouraged to keep babies in contact with them as much as possible to provide sensory input in the form of touch, warmth, smell, sound, and sight.
- Smell: babies quickly learn to associate their mother's smell with comfort, pleasure, and nourishment.
- Sound: from an early age, babies can distinguish between their mother's voice and the voices of other people, and will prefer their mother's voice to similarly pitched female voices.
- Sight: even though their focal distance is only around 25cm, three-day old babies can visually distinguish between their mothers and others.

Although most of the research has focused on mothers, bonding with fathers is important and the principles described above also apply. Parent-infant bonding in the first days sets an important foundation for subsequent parent-child interaction. However, all is not lost if there is less contact during the early period. Strong parent-child bonds can be formed with children who must spend time in incubators, and between parents and adopted children.

8.1.2 BREASTFEEDING AND DEVELOPMENT

Breastfeeding is an important infant-mother interaction. The World Health Organisation advocates that infants be exclusively breastfed for the first six months of life (WHO, 2002). However, in developed countries most children are not exclusively breastfed for six months. For example, in the UK around 25 per cent of infants receive no breastfeeding and only 25 per cent are breastfed until six months (Bolling et al., 2007).

A number of prospective studies that followed infants into middle childhood or adulthood have found that those who were breastfed perform better on tests of intelligence (Clark et al., 2006; Kramer et al., 2008; Mortensen et al., 2002). The optimal duration for breastfeeding appears to be around 6–9 months, with lower test scores found for those not breastfed at all, breast fed for less than six months, or exclusively breastfed for more than nine months. Exclusive breastfeeding beyond nine months may produce nutritional deficiencies.

Several different factors may explain the links between breastfeeding and intelligence. First, nutrients in breast milk – especially long-chain fatty acids – may contribute to better neural development (Gustafsson et al., 2004). Second, physical and psychological attention during breastfeeding may foster greater intelligence. Third, factors related to both breastfeeding *and* children's intelligence may be important. Chief among these are characteristics of mothers who breastfeed, because better educated and more intelligent mothers are more likely to commence and continue breastfeeding (e.g. Coulibaly et al., 2006; Ladomenou et al., 2007).

Meta-analyses of studies designed to follow children over time show that exclusive breastfeeding during the first months of a child's life is associated with lower rates of childhood asthma, coeliac disease, and atopic dermatitis (Akobeng et al., 2006; Gdalevich et al., 2001a, 2001b). Some of the positive effects of breastfeeding may be due to immunomodulatory qualities of breast milk and/or the avoidance of allergens. Longer breastfeeding also appears to reduce the risk of subsequent obesity and diabetes.

8.1.3 LANGUAGE DEVELOPMENT

Learning to talk is one of the most important intellectual capacities a child will ever develop. As well as being essential for communication in its own right, language is important for many other learning skills: imagine what school would have been like if you were not able to understand your teacher or ask questions! Various theories have been developed and applied to explain how children progress from nonsensical babbling at six months of age to grammatically sophisticated speech just a few years later.

Some researchers have emphasised the importance of **operant conditioning** and **observational learning** (e.g. Skinner, 1957). Such perspectives argue that children develop their capacity for language in response to encouragement and correction from parents and other more mature people. They also argue that children's imitation of adult speech is important. Although children may learn the meanings of words in these ways, they cannot explain how children learn the complex rules of grammar – that is, rules about how words must be put together so as to make sense.

In contrast to behaviourism and social learning theories, **nativism** argues that children have an innate predisposition for language: i.e. they have in-built capacities for making sense of language. Chomsky (1965) argued that humans are unique in having an innate biologically based language acquisition device (LAD) which allows children who know a few words to generate grammatically correct utterances and understand what others say. The argument that the LAD is a *unique* human feature has received support from studies of language learning in primates. Such research indicates that although primates can learn to use sign language or symbols to communicate, they possess no understanding of grammar (Figure 8.2). Although Chomsky's ideas have been influential, they have some limitations. In particular, although there are specialised language areas in the human brain (see Chapter 7), there is no evidence that the LAD is located in a specific brain region.

Interactionism appears to offer a bridge between the opposing perspectives of Skinner and Chomsky. Interactionism argues that language learning is a combination of nature *and* nurture. Children learn language via the combination of an innate linguistic capacity, a strong desire to connect with others, a rich linguistic and social environment, and the reinforcement of their efforts.

Evidence for the interactionist perspective comes from the observation that adult-child communication is quite different from adult-adult communication. It involves closer physical proximity, more prolonged eye contact, exaggerated facial expressions and gestures, and the use of **motherese**. Motherese is an alternative name for adult-child speech, which is a simplified version of adult-adult speech. Box 8.3 shows that compared to adult-adult speech, motherese is shorter, less complicated, and much slower.

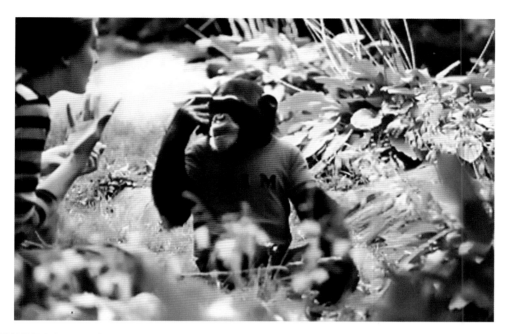

FIGURE 8.2 Nim Chimpsky using sign language
Photograph reprocuced courtesy of Susan Kuklin

BOX 8.3   Comparison of 'motherese' and adult-adult speech

	adult-child	adult-adult
Utterance length	4 words	8 words
Utterances with conjunctions (e.g., because)	20 per cent	70 per cent
Utterances with a pause at the end	75 per cent	51 per cent
Speed (words/min)	70/min	132/min

These differences are significant changes, not slight adjustments. Other features of motherese are that it is more likely to be in present tense; is more likely to use proper names rather than pronouns (e.g. 'Daddy's nose is bleeding' rather than 'My nose is bleeding'); has more repetition; and features exaggerated intonation. Young children appear to have a preference for motherese – the intonation and rhythm can attract and hold their attention. These features mean that children's natural predisposition for language learning is nurtured through interactions with others.

Stages of language development

Babies babble long before they speak their first real words. This is not a simple imitation of adult speech: it includes sounds that may not even be used in the language(s) spoken in a child's home. Babbling is a generalised system of vocalisations – nature provides infants with the sounds they may need, and nurture gradually moulds the use of sounds that are appropriate for their language. It is important that parents show interest in babbling because this indicates to the child that they are part of the social system. Parents' communication with babies at this stage can also help them to learn that vocal sounds have meanings (e.g. people's names).

The mean age of babies saying their first word is 12 months (but the range is 8–18 months). By this age, infants begin to use sounds to convey meaning. However, the meaning of these single word utterances is not always clear: when an infant says 'ear', this may mean 'This is my ear', or 'My ear hurts', or something else entirely. Parents can help their children learn words by giving a 'running commentary' of what they are doing and using expressions and gestures to provide clues to meaning.

From around the age of two, children begin to use 'telegraph speech' which contains mainly nouns and verbs. The sentences are similar to the sentences made by Nim Chimpsky (Figure 8.2). Words are used to express desires, e.g. 'Feel tired'. From age three there is a rapid progression to complete sentences. In addition to using more words per sentence, children begin to use possessive pronouns ('mine', 'Daddy's'); negatives (e.g. 'can't' rather than 'no'); and modifiers (adjectives like 'big' and adverbs like 'quickly'). Language begins to be used to express thoughts and emotions. Some of these changes can be linked to developments in cognitive capacity. By age five, children have vocabularies of thousands of words and can understand quite complex sentences.

Implications for doctor-child communication

As in all contexts, communication will be best when there is a match between the demands of the situation and the capacities of the people involved. Medical consultations with children are affected by:

- Children's language capacity: very young children may not possess the precise vocabulary used by medical professionals (e.g. what does 'I have a tummy ache' really mean?).
- Doctors' communication skills: health professionals should be sensitive to how a child's age may affect their ability to understand and should make appropriate adjustments to their manner of speech.
- Interaction between doctor and child: it is important to consider whether parents can be used as 'translators' for their children.

Medical professionals need to be aware of how language capacity develops with age and adjust their communication style as appropriate.

Summary

- All children have an innate capacity to learn language – the language acquisition device (LAD).
- The interactionist perspective argues that in addition to LAD, experience is important e.g. 'motherese' helps children to learn to use their innate capacity for language.
- Adults can help children develop their language capacity by encouraging them and providing feedback.
- Doctors should match their language to the capacities of child patients e.g. use elements of 'motherese' in consultations with young children.

8.1.4 INTELLECTUAL DEVELOPMENT

How does a child's mind grow? When and how do children begin to think symbolically, reason logically, and see things from another person's perspective? The following section attempts to provide answers to these questions and discuss the implications for medicine. It will commence with the influential theory of Piaget, followed by a discussion of some criticisms of Piaget's theory and the insights offered by Vygotsky.

Piaget's stage theory

Central to Piaget's (1954) influential theory was the idea that a child's mind is not a miniature version of an adult's mind waiting to be filled with information. The child's mind develops into an adult mind through four discrete stages (see Figure 8.3). Although each stage can be broken into sub-stages, development always proceeds in the same order and the order of

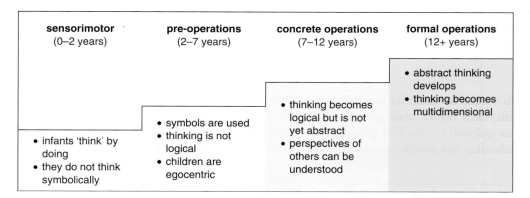

FIGURE 8.3 Piaget's stage model of intellectual development

stages is universal. The term 'operations' refers to the ways in which children work out problems. (Let's look more closely at each of the stages in Piaget's theory.)

- **Sensorimotor stage** – Babies experience the world through their senses. They cannot 'think' because they live in the moment with no abstract concepts. However, they can exhibit intelligent behaviour e.g. pulling a blanket to get a toy that is out of reach but resting on it. Before eight months, infants do not understand object permanence – the awareness that things which are out of sight still exist.
- **Pre-operations** – Language acquisition brings a fundamental change to intellectual development because language is symbolic: words are symbols used to refer to real things. Linked to this capacity for symbolic thought, a major change from the sensorimotor stage is the capacity to imagine things. This is reflected in play, where a stick can become a sword or a magic wand. In this stage, children are **egocentric**. They are unable to see things from another person's perspective or consider the point of view of others. For example, in hide-and-seek children may think that if they cannot see you, then you cannot see them.
- **Concrete operations** – Children begin to learn to use logical processes. They can manipulate real (concrete) objects to solve problems, such as using their fingers or blocks to do addition and subtraction. They also become able to classify things. Thus, carrots, oranges, apples, and peas could be sorted into vegetable/fruit or green/orange. In addition children can learn the principle of conservation i.e. that moving, spreading out, or re-arranging objects does not change them. In this stage, children develop the capacity to see things from another person's perspective.
- **Formal operations** – Children become able to reason not just on the basis of real physical objects, but also on the basis of hypotheses or propositions: e.g. '$x^2 + 4 = 13$, what is the value of x?' During this stage, thinking becomes multi-dimensional. Children become able to consider various possibilities rather than just the most obvious solution to a problem. Other important developments include the development of metacogniton – the capacity to think about thinking – and introspection – the capacity to think about emotions.

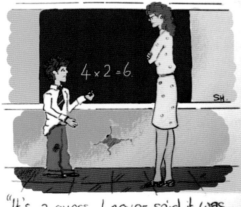

"It's a guess, I never said it was an educated guess."

Numerous studies have shown that development tends to follow Piaget's order. However, although Piaget's ideas have been highly influential they have been criticised (e.g. Amsel and Reninger, 1997). Development of intelligence is smoother and more gradual than Piaget's argument for step-like jumps between stages. Piaget seems to have under-estimated children's capacities and over-estimated adults' capacities (many adults fail to use formal operational reasoning). It has also been suggested that younger children's difficulty with reasoning tasks is also strongly influenced by their inability to understand complex adult language. Furthermore, recent research indicates that pre-operational children are able to consider others' perspectives.

Vygotsky's theory of social development

A fundamental principle of Vygotsky's theory of social development is that full cognitive development requires social interaction (Daniels, 1996). Vygotsky emphasised the importance of culture for learning. At a broad level, culture teaches children both *what* to think and *how* to think. At the individual level, children learn through problem solving that is shared with someone else (e.g. adult, peer). Compared with Piaget, Vygotsky gave greater emphasis to the importance of language in learning. Vygotsky argued that language is crucial for collaborative problem solving and that such collaborative problem solving is important for children's cognitive development.

Vygotsky also argued that learning occurs in the 'zone of proximal development', which is the gap between what a child can do without help and what they could do with appropriate guidance or collaboration. With such help from adults or peers, children can perform tasks they would be incapable of completing on their own. Furthermore, teaching and learning will be more effective if there is a continual adjustment of the level of help given so that children become more independent at solving problems.

Understanding others' perspectives

As noted earlier, young children are egocentric: they cannot take on the perspective of others. Young children also lack a **'theory of mind'**: they do not understand that other people have different thoughts, emotions, and perceptions. Children aged two or three use words like 'want' which reflect the development of knowledge of an inner self. Over time, this understanding is applied to other people and children come to understand that they can infer the mental states of other people. Thus, we may say that they possess a naïve theory of mind. Having a theory of mind allows us to empathise with others. However, it also allows us to deceive. For example, children who possess a theory of mind can understand what they need to do to feign illness to avoid school. Similarly, when poker players bluff they are applying their theory of mind.

Medical consultations with young children clearly need to take into account the issues of egocentrism and an absence of a theory of mind. Young children may assume others know what they are feeling and experiencing. Doctors therefore need to encourage young children to explain all of their symptoms and concerns, even if these appear obvious to the child.

Children's understanding of illness

Children's understanding of illness varies with age (see Box 8.4). An understanding of illness progresses from concrete, egocentric explanations to abstract multi-dimensional explanations.

Although Box 8.4 suggests a stage-like development of an understanding of illness, this is not strictly true: understanding illness is strongly influenced by experience. Thus young children with leukaemia may understand the disorder much more than other children of the same age. Such findings support Vygotsky's argument that children's understanding develops best if they receive appropriate help from sensitive adults. These findings also suggest that explanations of illness and disease should build on prior experience and not be based simply on chronological age.

BOX 8.4   Children's explanation of illness

age	explanation of illness
2–4	Phenomenism – particular objects are believed to cause illness but there is no sense of the mechanisms involved.
4–7	Contagion – illness is caused by proximity to ill people or to particular objects.
7–9	Contamination – illness is caused by physical contact with an ill person and may be viewed as punishment for misbehaviour.
9–11	Internalisation – illness is located within the body but may be caused by external factors e.g. people get colds from being cold.
11–16	Physiological – illness is caused by malfunctions in organs or systems which may be due to infections.
16+	Psychophysiological – psychological factors like stress and fatigue can affect physiological processes, rather than only being an outcome.

(Bibace and Walsh, 1980)

Children's understanding of illness can be enhanced by the use of developmentally appropriate interventions which break complex information into more easily digested pieces and present them in a child-friendly language like 'motherese' (see Research Box 8.2). Medical communication with young children – whether it is verbal consultations or information leaflets – should therefore avoid using abstract concepts. With all children, it is important to focus on their 'here and now' experiences and concerns.

RESEARCH BOX 8.2   Child-friendly interventions enhance understanding of illness

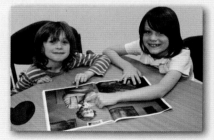

Background

Children's understanding of illness is limited, and is characterised by being incomplete and inaccurate. Research and theory suggest that interventions using materials and methods that are responsive to the cognitive capacities of children may lead to a better understanding of health and illness.

Method

Two groups of 30 children aged 4 and 30 children aged 7 were asked to explain three types of common ailments: chickenpox and a cold (contagious); asthma and cancer (non-contagious); and a scraped knee and broken arm (injury).

One week later, half the children in each age group took part in a small group session which involved learning age-appropriate information via the use of a storybook. The stories covered the cause, timing, and recovery for each type of ailment.

Results

Follow-up assessment revealed that the storybook intervention led to significant improvements in children's understanding of these three ailments.

Significance

Children's understanding of illness improves during early childhood. This improvement can be enhanced by providing age-appropriate factual information in an appropriate format.

Williams, J.M. and Binnie, L.M. (2002) Children's concepts of illness: An intervention to improve knowledge, *British Journal of Health Psychology*, 7: 129–147.

Summary

- Young children's thought processes are fundamentally different to adults'.
- Initial thought processes are based on real world objects and egocentric perspectives.
- Before developing a 'theory of mind' children will not know that others do not share their thoughts/feelings and may not disclose pain/symptoms.
- Young children cannot understand abstract or unobservable concepts like infection.
- Experience interacts with the developmental stage to produce an understanding of illness.
- Age-appropriate information increases children's understanding of illness and recovery.

CLINICAL NOTES 8.1

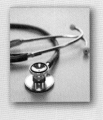

Communicating with children

- Adjust your consultation style to the capacities of children: pay attention to the language you use and the complexity of the ideas you are trying to convey.

- Younger children will not understand abstract concepts or internal bodily processes. However, be aware that some children can have very advanced knowledge of illnesses they have been exposed to.
- Explain things to children in age-appropriate ways e.g. use dolls or action figures to get their attention and help them to understand.
- Age-appropriate information booklets can increase children's understanding of illness, treatment, and recovery.
- Where applicable use parents or other adults to help you communicate with children.

8.2 ADOLESCENCE

Although adolescence is often equated with the physical changes of **puberty**, it is a biopsychosocial phenomenon that involves physical, cognitive, and social changes. The major psychological challenges of adolescence include adjusting to a changing body size and shape; coming to terms with sexuality; adjusting to new ways of thinking; and striving for emotional maturity and economic independence.

The average age of the onset of puberty is around 13 years, but there is a range of a few years around this average. Puberty begins one to two years earlier for girls than boys. Puberty is the most rapid growth period after prenatal development and early infancy. During a period of around four years, adolescents grow an average of 25cm/10 inches in height and gain 18kg/40lb in weight. There are also marked changes in hormone levels, especially testosterone and oestradiol. The end point is sexual maturation and an adult physique.

In developed countries, the age of onset of puberty has fallen by three to four years over the last few hundred years due to improved standards of living, including better health and better nutrition. These factors are important because puberty's onset is associated with girls reaching a critical body mass (~48kg/7.5 stone) and body fat proportion (~17%). These changes mean that it is now common to reach biological maturity at an age when cognitive and social maturity have not been reached.

8.2.1 PSYCHOLOGICAL ASPECTS OF PUBERTY

Responses to puberty are different for boys and girls and are tied to different body shape ideals. In terms of body shape, girls tend to be less satisfied than boys (Brooks-Gunn and Paikoff, 1992). This is influenced by the fact that the socially ideal body shape for women is often seen to be similar to that of pre- or early-adolescent girls (i.e. very thin), whereas the socially ideal body shape for men is adult (i.e. tall and muscular). However, it is important to note that during puberty both boys and girls feel worse about their bodies than before or after. There are also observed changes in mood. Boys tend to express more anger and irritability; girls tend to express more anger and depression. These alterations could be due to hormonal changes or responses to new life events and developmental challenges.

The timing of puberty will have different effects on boys and girls. For girls, early puberty tends to be associated with more difficulties than average or late puberty (Mendle et al., 2007). Because puberty onset is earlier for girls than boys, girls who mature early are the very first of their peers to mature. Early maturing girls tend to dislike the experience. They tend to be less sociable, engage in more risk behaviours, have a lower educational attainment, lower self-esteem, and poorer body image.

Boys tend to like maturing early because they are the first of their male peers to gain height and musculature. Early maturing boys tend to be more popular and likely to be leaders, good natured, and may have a cognitive advantage early on. However, they also tend to be more cautious, bound by rules and routines (Alsaker, 1992). Late maturing boys tend to be more dependent, insecure, aggressive, and more likely to rebel against their parents.

Many boys and girls express dissatisfaction with their body image during adolescence. For example, research indicates that although girls express more dissatisfaction with their bodies, the majority of adolescent boys and girls express a desire to change their body shape (Lawler and Nixon, 2010). Such studies also show that many girls and boys feel under pressure to conform to the ideal body shapes of modern consumer culture and that peer criticism of appearance is an unavoidable part of adolescent life for both boys and girls. Concerns about appearance do not only apply to body shape; they are also influenced by cultural ideals of clear, blemish-free skin (Kellett and Gilbert, 2001).

Relationships with parents and other adults

There are many explanations for the changes that occur in the parent-child relationship during adolescence. One explanation proposes that these occur because adolescents individuate from their parents, becoming more emotionally and behaviourally independent (Steinberg and Silverberg, 1986). An alternative view suggests changes in parent-child relationships can lead to psychological independence with continued connectedness. Studies of how adolescents spend their time show that although older adolescents spend diminishing amounts of time in family interactions, the time they spend one-to-one with parents does not change and the quality of such interactions often improves (Larson et al., 1996). The decline in time spent with family members appears to be due to pulls from external factors such as friends and work rather than pushes away from bad interactions with parents.

One important domain of adolescent-adult interaction is medical consultations. Research indicates that many adolescents are dissatisfied with their interactions with doctors. Some of this dissatisfaction stems from concerns about privacy and confidentiality; some arises from embarrassment arising from talking about sensitive issues such as body image, sexual behaviour, or illegal behaviours such as alcohol or drug use (Rutishauser et al., 2003; Towle et al., 2006). It is therefore important to be sensitive to these concerns and to remind patients that information exchanged in consultations will be private and confidential. It is also important to encourage adolescents to develop their capacity to discuss their health concerns during medical consultations (Towle et al., 2006).

We usually think of doctor-patient communication as a two-way interaction. However, it must be acknowledged that parents may have legal rights and responsibilities relating to medical consultations involving children below the age of consent. Older adolescents may feel uncomfortable or dissatisfied with three-way communications involving themselves, their doctor, and their parents. This may be more likely if they feel that they are being spoken about rather than spoken to. If parents insist on being involved in medical consultations involving their adolescent children, it may be helpful to ensure that at least part of the consultation involves seeing the adolescent patient alone (Rutishauser et al., 2003).

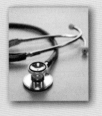

CLINICAL NOTES 8.2

Working with adolescents

- Adjust your consultation style to the capacities and experiences of adolescents: pay attention to the complexity of your explanation and check that they understand the terminology used.
- Be aware of adolescents' concerns about their appearance and body image.
- Be aware of patients' embarrassment when talking about their health concerns. Respond in a non-judgemental way and reassure them that information will be treated confidentially.
- You may need to be tactful when negotiating with adolescents and their parents about the role of parents in consultations and decision making.

8.2.2 COGNITION, RISK TAKING, AND IDENTITY

Piaget's (1954) stage theory argued that formal operational thought develops during adolescence. In this stage, adolescents become able to understand abstract principles and use propositional logic. Thinking also become multi-dimensional: a range of possible situations can be imagined.

The improved decision-making capacity of adolescents is supposed to make them better able to: identify alternative courses of action; identify the consequences of each alternative; evaluate the desirability of each consequence; assess the likelihood of each consequence; and logically combine all of this information to make the best decisions about their behaviour. This should reduce the likelihood that they will make bad decisions. However, adolescents seem to be good at making bad decisions! This is reflected, for example, in the fact that accidents are the leading cause of death among young people (Heron, 2007) and in the high rates of unplanned pregnancies (UNICEF, 2001) and unhealthy behaviours (e.g. de Visser et al., 2006).

Although the development of metacogniton (the capacity to think about thinking) and introspection (the capacity to think about emotions) should facilitate a better understanding of others, much of adolescents' thinking is directed toward themselves. Thus, adolescents may become self-absorbed and **egocentric**. However, this is different from the egocentrism characteristic of the pre-operational stage: pre-operational children cannot help their egocentrism whereas adolescents can. The combination of metacognition, introspection, and egocentrism can lead to feelings of there being an imaginary audience observing our actions. Adolescents tend to have a heightened sense of self-consciousness and may feel that their behaviour and appearance are the focus of everyone else's concern and attention. In this stage they may develop a 'personal fable' (Elkind, 1967). This is a belief that all of their experiences are novel and unique (e.g. 'Nobody has ever felt love this strong'). The personal fable may be dangerous when it is applied to health risk behaviour (e.g. 'I won't get pregnant' or 'I won't have a car crash').

Although young people may express unrealistic optimism about health risks, unrealistic optimism is not necessarily more common among adolescents than adults (Cohn et al., 1995). Higher rates of risky or unhealthy behaviour may, however, reflect differences in beliefs about the Subjective Expected Utility of different behaviours (Savage, 1954). Put another way, adolescents may not think the 'bad' outcomes of their behaviour are as likely or as bad as adults think they are.

A certain amount of risk taking is appropriate during the adolescent phase of development. For example, Erikson's developmental theory highlights the importance of 'trying out' different identities and related behaviours during adolescence (Erikson, 1968). Adolescents have increased access to a range of potentially risky behaviours – such as alcohol consumption, motor vehicle use, and sexual activity – and some of these behaviours are important aspects of their socialisation into adulthood. Furthermore, many health risk behaviours are gendered and adolescents may engage in risky behaviours as part of the development of their gender identities. Thus, many male adolescents seek to test or display their masculinity by engaging in risky or unhealthy behaviours (e.g. de Visser and Smith, 2007). Similarly, women's desire to conform to or resist traditional feminine roles influences whether they engage in risky or unhealthy behaviours (e.g. Lyons and Willott, 2008).

Summary

- Puberty onset is earlier today than 100 years ago – influenced by improved standard of living and better diet.
- Responses to the process and outcomes of puberty are different for boys and girls.
- Major developmental tasks include: adjusting to a new body size and shape; coming to terms with sexuality; using new cognitive capacities; developing maturity and independence.
- Adolescents begin to disengage from family activities but one-on-one quality interactions with parents may not alter.
- Adolescents' interactions with medical professionals can be affected by embarrassment when talking about sensitive issues, concerns about confidentiality, and the presence of parents during consultations. It is important to be responsive to these concerns.
- Although adolescents have an improved decision-making capacity, their egocentrism may distort risk perception.

8.3 ADULTHOOD

There is no clear line separating adolescence and adulthood. The differences between adolescence and adulthood have been blurred by the fact that in developed countries more young people are engaged in further education. They take longer than previous generations to gain their financial independence, establish their own households, form long-term relationships, and have children. It has therefore been suggested that the period from the late teens to the early twenties should be conceived of as 'emerging adulthood' (Arnett, 2004).

After rapid and profound changes in cognitive and psychological functioning during childhood and adolescence, adulthood is a time of relative calm. However, it is during adulthood that patterns of behaviour and psychological states linked to the major causes of morbidity and mortality become established. There are many examples of these throughout this book, but particularly in the chapters on body systems (see Section III).

Although adulthood is often thought of as a period of stability, there can be important changes. Many of these relate to changes in social roles and adjustment to major life events like having children, moving house, changing jobs, and experiencing the death of loved ones. As noted elsewhere, gaining, losing, or changing social roles can be stressful and may lead to depression (see 9.3.1, Chapter 9). Furthermore, prolonged stress can have serious negative consequences for immune and endocrine function (see Chapters 3 and 14). Although stressful life events and negative role changes tend to be linked to poorer physical and psychological wellbeing, the impact of such events will vary according to coping responses and social support. It is therefore important that adults develop and maintain effective individual coping skills and supportive social networks.

8.4 OLD AGE

Current life expectancy in the UK is 82 years for women and 77 years for men (ONS, 2008). The respective figures for the USA are 80 years for women and 75 years for men (NCHS, 2007). Life expectancy today is around 30 years longer than it was at the beginning of the twentieth century. While life expectancy has increased, birth rates have fallen (NCHS, 2007; ONS, 2008). As a result, the proportion of the population who are elderly is increasing. It is estimated that the proportion of the population aged over 65 will increase from around 15 per cent today to around 25 per cent by the middle of this century.

Control of infectious diseases means that there is a lower burden of disease among young people and a concentration of illness and death among the elderly. This **compression of morbidity** has occurred over the last century because the age of onset of chronic disease increased more rapidly than life expectancy i.e. people stay well for longer, but illness is compressed into the final phase of life (e.g. Fries et al., 1989). This, combined with changes in population composition, means a greater proportion of medical consultations and expenditure will be concentrated on older people.

8.4.1 HEALTH PROMOTION AMONG THE ELDERLY

It is generally accepted that ageing involves a reduced physical capacity. So should older people resign themselves to decline? The answer to this is a definite 'no'. Physical decline can be significantly reduced by encouraging older people to maintain or initiate healthy lifestyles. Research suggests that regular moderate physical activity among older men can lead to significant improvements in immune function (Smith et al., 2004). In addition,

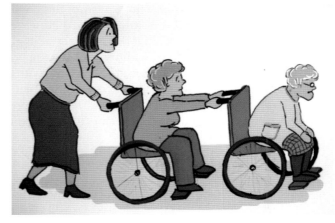

lung cancer and cardiovascular risk among smokers falls rapidly within a few years of quitting smoking (DHSS, 1990). Furthermore, even among people aged 65+ the likelihood of an earlier death is influenced by whether they continue or change unhealthy behaviours (Morey et al., 2002). However, behaviour change may be more difficult among older people than among younger people because their patterns of behaviour may have become more habitual.

ACTIVITY 8.1   BELIEFS ABOUT AGEING

- Stop for a moment and note the images that come to mind when you think about elderly people.
- Are the images that come to mind mostly positive or negative? Is there a mixture?

8.4.2 AGEING AND PSYCHOLOGICAL WELLBEING

Stereotypes of elderly people are often contradictory. On the one hand, elderly people are seen as 'sages' with a lifetime's knowledge and experience. On the other hand, they are seen as 'senile' or 'demented'. In general, our society has a negative view of ageing, which is seen as the loss of youth and a decline in physical, cognitive, and social functioning.

Dementia is present in around 3 per cent of people aged 70-74 and 25 per cent of people aged 85+ (Ferri et al., 2005). However, it is a myth that *all* old people suffer from fundamental intellectual decline (see Case Study 8.1). When discussing the intellectual capacities of the elderly, we must distinguish between 'crystalline intelligence', which reflects experience and long-term memory, and 'fluid intelligence', which reflects processing speed and short-term memory. Tests of fluid intelligence (e.g. IQ tests) suggest many older people are 'mentally disadvantaged'. However, their behaviour does not match this description. One reason for this is that crystalline intelligence may compensate for declines in fluid intelligence. In addition, IQ tests may not assess real-world skills. Age-related declines in fluid intelligence are associated with physical health and organic change in the central nervous system. Research suggests that enhancing physical fitness can therefore improve cognitive function in older adults, regardless of whether they have existing dementia or cognitive impairment (Angevaren et al., 2008; Heyn et al., 2004).

CASE STUDY 8.1   Successful ageing

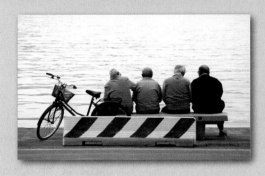

It is a myth that all old people suffer from a fundamental intellectual decline.

When Fred Hale Senior died in November 2004 at the age of 113 he was documented as the world's oldest man. Although few people achieve such old age, his experiences show that many elderly people maintain fully active lives:

- At 95 he tried boogie-boarding while visiting Hawaii.
- He participated in his last deer hunt at age 100.
- At 103 he was still living independently – shovelling the snow off his rooftop.
- His driving licence was renewed at age 104, but he gave up driving at 108 because slow drivers annoyed him.
- He maintained an active interest in sport and bee-keeping.

Although his longevity may have been influenced by genetic factors, his lifestyle was also important. He ate three full meals at the same time each day he never smoked, and he rarely drank alcohol. He ate at least a teaspoonful of honey and bee pollen every day.

Photograph © Bojan Stepanic/Fotolia

Depression in older age

The prevalence of depression tends to increase with age. Depression tends to be associated with declines or losses in other areas, including functional disability, cognitive impairment, and social deprivation (Djernes, 2006). As in earlier phases of life, depression is more common among elderly women than men. Reasons for increased rates of depression include role loss (see Chapter 9) – particularly among men for whom work was an important component of identity – and negative life events (Kraaij et al., 2002).

Bereavement has an important impact on rates of depression. Older people are more likely than younger people to experience the death of their spouse and friends. Given that average life expectancy is longer for women, in each age band there is a greater proportion of widows than widowers. This may help to explain higher rates of depression among older women than men.

CLINICAL NOTES 8.3

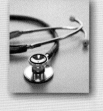

Working with elderly people

- Be aware of your own stereotypes and prejudices related to ageing and the elderly. Do not let these lead to poorer care for older people.
- Adjust your consultation style to the capacities of older patients.
- Do not assume elderly patients are frail or senile – difficulty with hearing or talking does not mean they are stupid!
- Encourage older patients to take regular exercise. Help them to understand that exercise can improve cardiovascular fitness, improve cognitive function, and extend their lives.

8.4.3 HEALTHCARE OF OLDER PEOPLE

As older people are an increasing proportion of the population, there are concerns that increased demands for health and social care will have to be met by a smaller proportion of tax payers of working age or an increased reliance on informal or voluntary care (Robine et al., 2007).

Negative stereotypes about ageing can lead to the stigmatisation of older people and a neglect of issues concerning them. It is often assumed that older people are physically frail, cognitively impaired, and have diminished social engagement. These stereotypes and prejudices then affect the quality of service provision: many elderly people are not treated with the respect and dignity to which all patients are entitled. Mistreatment of older patients in hospitals is not purely due to a lack of resources, but also reflects negative attitudes (Healthcare Commission, 2007).

Although some elderly people experience substantial declines in cognitive function with age, most do not. It is therefore important for doctors to check their patients' capacity and adjust their consultation skills accordingly. During consultations with older patients who have clear declines in fluid memory, allow more time for information to be considered before asking further questions. It is important not to fill any silences with more questions, as this can lead to a communication breakdown.

It is also important to consider patients' expectations of consultations. While younger patients may expect and appreciate a more patient-centred approach to consultations, older patients may be more comfortable with a patriarchal approach wherein the doctor is the expert who is expected to provide solutions and make decisions. As with patients of any age, it is important to tailor consultation styles to their capacities and preferences.

Summary

- Compression of morbidity means people stay healthier for longer, but have a concentration of illness and/or disability at the end of their lives.
- Even in old age, changes in health-related behaviour are beneficial to physical and psychological wellbeing.
- Ageing is linked to declines in fluid intelligence e.g. cognitive processing speed but not crystalline intelligence.
- Depression is common in old age, particularly in women.

FURTHER READING

Bee, H. & Boyd, D. (2009) *The Developing Child* (12th edition). Boston, MA: Allyn & Bacon. A standard text for development during childhood and adolescence, which is very reader-friendly with a range of illustrations of the major points. However, as this is a textbook for psychology students it gives a lot of detail, but little attention is given to medical applications.

Berk, L. (2008) *Child Development* (8th edition). Boston, MA: Allyn & Bacon. Also a standard text for child and adolescent development. It has reader-friendly images and text boxes to help with the understanding of key points. However, it is also a textbook for psychology students, so the focus is not on applications to medicine.

Durkin, K. (1998) *Developmental Social Psychology*. Oxford: Blackwell. This text has a more broad focus than the first two books, as it covers the whole lifespan. It does still give much attention to childhood development. However, this book is not as reader-friendly as those cited above.

REVISION QUESTIONS

1   Why is infant-adult attachment important for children's development?

2   Describe the link between breastfeeding and intelligence.

3   How does the interactionist approach to language learning differ from the nativist (LAD) approach?

4   What should doctors do to promote effective doctor-child communication?

5   Describe the central features of Piaget's theory of cognitive development.

6   How is 'Theory of Mind' important for medical consultations with young children?

7   Adolescents are supposed to have adult-like capacities for risk assessment, so why are they more likely to take risks?

8   What is meant by the compression of morbidity? How does this affect the number of medical consultations with older people?

9   Summarise the major changes in cognitive capacity observed in old age.

10 What factors need to be considered during consultations with older patients?

9 SOCIAL PSYCHOLOGY

Figure

9.1   Group behaviour and dress

Research boxes

9.1   Nurse-physician relationships
9.2   Doctors' attitudes to mental illness

LEARNING OBJECTIVES

This chapter is designed to enable you to:

- Discuss the links between attitudes and behaviour and the importance of attitude change in encouraging healthy behaviour.
- Describe how self-perceptions influence a range of health-related behaviours.
- Discuss the importance of group membership to individuals and how group membership can influence individual behaviour.
- Outline the different explanations of aggressive behaviour.
- Identify the factors that can increase the likelihood of pro-social behaviour.

Social psychology helps us to consider such issues as how we dress, our health behaviour, how a group makes decisions – and even whether we are able to challenge senior doctors if we believe they are wrong. For example, in 2003 one junior doctor was ordered by a registrar to administer a combination of two drugs to a man with leukaemia. The combination was lethal. The junior doctor asked the registrar twice if this was correct but was told to go ahead, with devastating consequences (Ferner and McDowell, 2006). Social psychology examines why we carry out such actions and which social forces contribute to them. In this chapter we shall consider, first, how people's attitudes and beliefs about themselves can influence their behaviour, including health-related behaviour, and then at the issues of conformity and aggression, and how individuals behave as members or leaders of groups.

9.1 ATTITUDES

In social psychology and health promotion a great deal of attention is given to attitudes. **Attitudes** can be defined as a measure of people's like or dislike of an object. The 'object' may be a real object, a person, or a behaviour like 'healthy eating'. The expectancy-value model suggests that attitudes are the product of expectancy about an object, and the value given to that object (see Chapter 5). For example, attitudes toward condom use will be shaped by expectancies (e.g. condoms reduce sexual pleasure) and the value of the expectancies (e.g. sexual pleasure is important). Thus, two people with the same expectancy may have different attitudes because they give different values to this expectancy.

Attitudes reflect what we think and feel about something and how we plan to behave (Eagley and Chaiken, 1993). Ideally, the thinking, feeling, and behaving components of attitudes will be consistent with each other. When we hold inconsistent beliefs or when our behaviour does not match our beliefs it leads to unpleasant **cognitive dissonance**, which we will be motivated to reduce (Festinger, 1957). People may seek to reduce cognitive dissonance by changing either their attitudes or their behaviour. Thus, an overweight person who knows this is unhealthy may either decide to lose weight or change their beliefs about their weight.

9.1.1 MEASUREMENT OF ATTITUDES

Attitudes cannot be observed. However, there are different ways to measure expressions of attitudes. Indirect measures of attitudes may use physiological measures (e.g. heart rate or galvanic skin response) or observations of behaviour (e.g. stopping to help a stranger) to infer people's attitudes. Direct measures of attitudes are more common.

A direct assessment of attitudes can be made in various ways. Likert scales are commonly used to collect people's responses to various statements of attitude. Ideally, assessments of attitudes using Likert scales will include a mixture of positively and negatively phrased statements which are then combined to give an overall assessment of attitudes. Likert scales are useful because they measure the direction of a person's attitude (i.e. positive or negative) and the intensity of the attitude (see Box 9.1).

BOX 9.1   Measuring attitudes: Likert scale

	strongly disagree	disagree	neither	agree	strongly agree
People should have the right to die if they are terminally ill and suffering	☐	☐	☐	☐	☐
No one should be allowed to decide to end a suffering person's life	☐	☐	☐	☐	☐

An alternative to Likert scales are semantic differential scales. These also measure the direction and intensity of attitudes. However, rather than being based on participants' agreement with statements, semantic differential scales assess individuals' position in relation to pairs of opposites. Each response is converted into a number, with higher summary scores indicating more positive attitudes toward the behaviours.

BOX 9.2   Measuring attitudes: semantic differential scale

		−2	−1	0	+1	+2	
Euthanasia is:	evil	☐	☐	☐	☐	☐	good
	cruel	☐	☐	☐	☐	☐	kind
	unacceptable	☐	☐	☐	☐	☐	acceptable

9.1.2 ATTITUDES AND BEHAVIOUR

Attitudes measured at one time can often be used to predict behaviour at a later time. Attitudes are therefore central to many models of health behaviour (see Chapter 5). However, it is important to note that other beliefs (e.g. normative beliefs) and social factors will influence whether attitudes are acted upon.

Changing attitudes and changing behaviour

Because attitudes predict subsequent behaviour, it is generally accepted that attitude change should be a productive way to change behaviour. The enormous sums of money spent on advertisements for soft drinks, cosmetics, and so on reflect the belief that people's purchasing behaviour will change if their attitudes toward products are changed. For example, in the last decade fast food chains have changed their advertising to counter concerns that their meals are unhealthy in an effort to retain their market share. Mass media health promotion campaigns also try to encourage behaviour changes by changing peoples' attitudes toward healthy and unhealthy behaviours.

These efforts are based on the hypothesis that there is generally agreement between people's behaviour and the affective, cognitive, and behavioural components of attitudes (Eagley and Chaiken, 1993). According to the theory of cognitive dissonance, if we change people's attitudes toward their current unhealthy behaviours, this will set up a dissonance between their new attitude and their established behaviours: they should then change their behaviour to reduce the dissonance between their attitudes and behaviour.

'Foot-in-the-door' techniques are an interesting illustration of how our desire to behave consistently with our attitudes can be manipulated (Burger, 1999). These techniques involve asking people to agree to a simple request which they are likely to comply with. Later the same person is asked to agree to a substantially more demanding request, which is the actual target behaviour. For example, one study found that women who had previously accepted a breast self-examination card were more likely than other women to agree to a request to schedule a gynaecological examination (Dolin and Booth-Butterfield, 1995). 'Foot-in-the-door' techniques produce better responses to requests for the target behaviour because once a person has agreed to the small initial request they have demonstrated to themselves and others that their attitudes toward the cause are favourable and that they are committed to the behaviour. Other techniques for encouraging behaviour change through attitude change are addressed below.

Persuasive messages

If we wish to change health-related behaviour by changing attitudes, then we must be sure about the most effective ways to do so. A message is most likely to change people's attitudes if it:

- Gets to its recipient – different approaches can be used, including discussion during consultations, leaflets, or the mass media.
- Is attention-grabbing.
- Is understood by the recipient – it must be couched in the appropriate language and 'pitched' at the appropriate level of complexity.
- Is seen by the recipient as relevant and important.
- Is remembered by the recipient, translated into an intention to change behaviour, and acted upon.

The characteristics of the sender of the message – be they individual doctors or organisations such as the Department of Health – will influence whether the message will be persuasive. We are more likely to be persuaded if the sender of the message is:

- Credible – the qualifications and occupational status of medical professionals may increase their persuasive power.
- Trustworthy – the perceived objectivity of medical professionals may increase their ability to encourage an attitude and behaviour change.
- Attractive – medical professionals must ensure that their personal presentation is attractive to patients.

Inducing a certain amount of fear may motivate people to change their behaviour, but fear campaigns can be counterproductive. If fear-based campaigns do not also include sufficient information about what people can do to avoid a feared outcome, people may simply avoid the issue rather than focusing on the issue and their behaviour (Witte and Allen, 2000).

CLINICAL NOTES 9.1

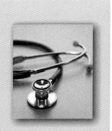

Persuading people to change their behaviour

If you wish to change patients' attitudes to their health-related behaviour:

- Make sure the message is clear, relevant to them, and easy to remember.
- Think of whether it is better to emphasise the gains or losses associated with current and desired behaviour.
- Pay attention to your own persuasive power based on your qualifications, occupational status, and credibility.
- Be aware of how your self-presentation can influence patients' perceptions of your status and credibility.

Framing effects are also important (Rothman and Salovey, 1997). They refer to whether a message emphasises the benefits of a certain behaviour or the losses associated with that behaviour. For example, a gain-framed message may be something like 'A regular saving plan will let you have your dream vacation' whereas a loss-framed message would be 'If you do not save regularly you will not be able to afford a vacation'. When we want people to take up behaviours aimed at detecting health problems or illness (e.g. breast self-examination or HIV testing), loss-framed messages may be more effective. When we want people to take up behaviours aimed at promoting prevention behaviours (e.g. using sunscreen or using condoms), gain-framed messages may be more effective.

ACTIVITY 9.1   FRAMING MESSAGES

Which of the two statements below will be most effective for breast self-examination?

1 If you do not undertake breast self-examination you may be more likely to die from cancer
2 If you undertake breast self-examination you may decrease the risk of dying from cancer.

Which of the two statements below will be most effective for promoting sunscreen use?

3 If you do not use SPF15 sunscreen, your skin will be damaged and you may die younger.
4 If you use SPF15 sunscreen, your skin will stay healthier and you may prolong your life.

*statements 1 and 4 will be the most effective

Ambivalence

For many attitudinal objects we do not have simple positive or negative attitudes. Instead, our feelings are often mixed. For example, we may have positive attitudes toward certain aspects of living in the countryside (fresh air, open space, less traffic, etc.) but negative attitudes toward other aspects of country life (social isolation, having to travel to town for movies and shopping, etc.). People are also ambivalent toward many health behaviours such as alcohol use, smoking, and condom use. This ambivalence can influence efforts to change health behaviours because ambivalent attitudes tend to be worse predictors of behaviour than homogeneous attitudes (Conner et al., 2003).

Summary

- People are motivated to keep their attitudes consistent with their behaviour. Thus, efforts to change health behaviour will often focus on changing attitudes.
- Attitude change messages should be tailored to maximise their persuasiveness. This means paying attention to the content of the message, the style of delivery, and the characteristics of the person delivering the message.

9.2 SELF PSYCHOLOGY

One important focus of our attitudes is ourselves. Here we shall examine why a person's self image is important for their health and wellbeing. We naïvely tend to assume that our selves are singular, continuous, and consistent: I think that when I wake up in the morning I am more or less exactly the same person I was the day before and will be when I wake up tomorrow. People with some psychiatric conditions may not always have this sense of unity (see Chapter 16).

Despite feeling that we have a singular self, it is possible to think of different definitions or different components of our selves. One important distinction is the difference between a personal self (how I perceive myself) and a social self (how others perceive me). These two selves may not always be in agreement. For example, I may be perceived as calm and confident when talking in public but will actually be a bundle of nerves. An important distinction can also be made between **personal identity**, which consists of everything that makes me a unique person, and **social identity**, which consists of the things I share with members of groups that are important to me (e.g. family resemblance, national identity, occupation). Processes of group affiliation and conformity will be addressed later in this chapter. For now we will focus on ideas of the self.

9.2.1 SELF-ESTEEM AND SELF IMAGE

Self-esteem has important links to behaviour and health. Self-esteem consists of feelings and evaluations about ourselves. It is generally acknowledged, that low self-esteem is undesirabled, but research suggests that this assumption is simplistic (Baumeister et al., 2003). For example, children and adolescents with high self-esteem may be more likely to experiment with smoking and using alcohol or sex rather than preventing such behaviour. One area in which there are clear links between low self-esteem and ill-health is in relation to eating disorders. One study of over 95,000 adolescents found that low self-esteem was a significant predictor of binge/purge eating practices and other weight loss behaviours (French et al., 2001). Self-esteem can also be lowered in certain illnesses, such as depression (see Chapter 16). Positive self-esteem is reflected in the promotion of a positive self image to oneself and other people.

Most of us put a lot of effort into developing and promoting a favourable self-image. An important part of self image is our appearance. Goffman (1959) used the analogy of acting in a play to explain how and why we modify our appearance and behaviour depending on where we are (the scene) and who we are with (our audience). For example, the clothes we wear and the amount of time we spend on our appearance will probably vary depending on whether we are at home studying, going to a party, or attending a formal meeting (see Activity 9.2). Appearance can also be an important marker of group membership (Figure 9.1).

ACTIVITY 9.2   SELF-PRESENTATION AND CLOTHING

Compare the following three settings:

1 The last time you were studying.
2 The last time you went out on a first date with someone.
3 The last time you had a formal interview.

In each of these situations:

- How much time did you spend planning what you would wear and getting ready?
- Did you do your hair/apply cosmetics/shave?
- If you need glasses, did you wear them, or contact lenses?
- How did the clothes you chose reflect the self image you were trying to project?

People also use appearance as a shorthand way of evaluating others. However, looks can be deceiving. In some cases this can have implications for health. For example, we often assume that if a person looks healthy they are healthy. This assumption can prove costly in the case of serious illnesses such as HIV/AIDS and cancer where there may be no visible signs of illness.

Hippocrates stated that physicians should be 'clean in person, well-dressed, and anointed with sweet-smelling unguents'. Research suggests that how physicians present themselves via clothing and accessories influences patients' trust and confidence in them (Lill and Wilkinson, 2005; Rehman et al., 2005). In general, patients feel less positive about medical professionals wearing casual clothes or jeans. However, preferences do vary between cultures: patients in the USA mostly prefer professional attire with a white coat, whereas those in New Zealand prefer semi-formal attire. In addition, older patients appear to prefer more formal attire.

How we behave in social situations is an important component of maintaining a positive self image. Most of us will try to obey social conventions about appropriate and inappropriate behaviour in order to be perceived favourably. It is important for our self-esteem

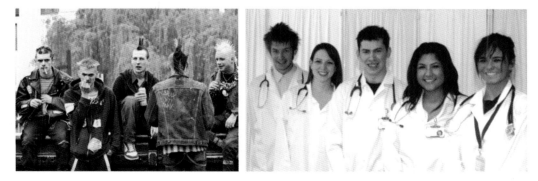

FIGURE 9.1   Group behaviour and dress
Photograph of punks reproduced courtesy of Jody Schofield

to affirm positive aspects of ourselves when we are criticised. This can be done in various ways. The example in Box 9.3 shows that when we are criticised we often try to publicly affirm positive aspects of our selves and/or denigrate the person who has criticised us.

BOX 9.3   Self-affirmation

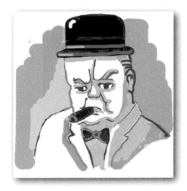

Quote copyright ©
Winston S. Churchill

The following exchange is reputed to have occurred between Labour MP Bessie Braddock and Conservative Prime Minister Winston Churchill:

Braddock: *Mr. Churchill, you are drunk.*
Churchill: *And you, madam, are ugly. But in the morning, I shall be sober.*

Churchill's response protected his self image and self-esteem by highlighting the fact that his undesirable behaviour was temporary (and therefore not a fundamental part of him), whereas his critic's undesirable appearance was permanent.

One way to boost our self image is to make downward **social comparisons** with people whose problems or situation are worse than our own. For example, a person who has had a leg amputated following a car accident may feel better off than someone who has been made quadriplegic in a car accident. Another example is the responses of some drug addicts to criticism of their behaviour: 'functional' heroin addicts may compare themselves favourably to 'junkies' who need to engage in crime or prostitution to support their drug use. In contrast, upward comparison occurs when people highlight the similarities between themselves and others who are deemed socially superior so as to make their self images more positive (Suls et al., 2002).

9.2.2 ATTRIBUTIONS

Our efforts to create and maintain a positive self image are also influenced by the attributions we assign to our own and others' behaviour. Internal attributions are based on the belief that a person's behaviour is internally motivated – that it is voluntary and reflects the person's attitudes. In contrast, external attributions are the belief that a person's behaviour is due to external factors such as luck, chance, or someone else demanding it.

In terms of our own behaviour, we tend to prefer internal attributions for our successes (e.g. 'I got an A for the exam because I studied really hard') and external attributions for our failures (e.g. 'I failed the exam because the lecturers set difficult questions'). In contrast, we tend to attribute others' behaviour to internal or dispositional causes rather than external or situational causes. This is known as the **fundamental attribution error** (Ross, 1977). This error means we are more likely to attribute negative facts about other people (e.g. being unwell, anxious or depressed) to their own behaviour or characteristics rather than to the broader social context. Examples of internal and external attributions for health are given in Box 9.4.

BOX 9.4   Attribution errors and illness

	Internal attribution	External attribution
Obesity	They are lazy, ignorant, greedy	There are not the right facilities or incentives to encourage activity and healthy eating
Depression	They are weak and unable to cope	They have experienced severely stressful life events

---

From this, it should be clear that attribution errors can have wide-ranging repercussions on clinical care through their impact on the doctor-patient relationship, understanding of the patient's illness, and therefore treatment. In healthcare practice, we must be aware of making this error and make sure we consider external and situational factors, such as life circumstances and competing priorities. As we will see below, in the section on conformity and obedience, situational factors can make us behave in unusual ways.

One application of attribution concepts within healthcare settings is the **health locus of control** (Wallston et al., 1978). An individual's locus of control reflects the extent to which they believe that they have control over their health. This can be divided into three components:

- Internal – the belief that what they do will affect their health. These people are more likely to seek information and to initiate and persist with changes in health behaviour.
- Powerful others – the belief that the most important influence on their health is other people such as medical professionals who possess important knowledge and skills. These people may be more likely to seek and follow professional advice but they are less likely to initiate changes in health behaviours.
- External – the belief that the maintenance of health and the onset of illness are due to fate, chance, or luck. These people are unlikely to take action to protect or promote their health.

An impressive example of the importance of attributions of control over health and illness comes from a longitudinal study which showed that children with a higher internal locus of control had a reduced risk of obesity, hypertension, and poor physical or psychological well-being during adulthood (Gale et al., 2008). Furthermore, a review of published research showed that a lower internal locus of control and a greater powerful other or external locus of control is associated with more symptoms of depression (Presson and Benassi, 1996).

9.2.3 IDEAL SELF AND ACTUAL SELF

To varying degrees most of us have biased appraisals of ourselves. Most of us probably think that we are more generous, helpful, and caring than others think we are. In most cases, this discrepancy between our own self image and how others see us is inconsequential. There may also be a discrepancy between our *actual* self (how we currently are) and our *ideal* self (how we would like to be) (Higgins, 1987). Perceived gaps between our ideal and actual selves can motivate a behaviour change. For example, a man may be motivated to take up regular exercise because when he looks in a mirror he does not see the ideal athletic physique he desires.

Sometimes, the discrepancy between the ideal self and actual self can be distorted, with important consequences for our physical and psychological wellbeing. This can often be observed among people with eating disorders such as anorexia and bulimia (Cash and Deagle, 1998). Influenced by cultural preferences and media images, many young women (and increasingly men) with eating disorders see themselves as having a substantially heavier physique than they actually do, and desire an ideal body image which is unrealistically thin and unhealthy (see Case Study 13.1). Men may also be affected in striving to attain an ideal which is unrealistically muscular (see Case Study 9.1).

CASE STUDY 9.1   Self image and body building

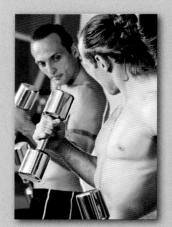

Sometimes, the discrepancy between the ideal self and actual self can be distorted, with important consequences for physical and psychological wellbeing. Muscle dysmorphia is a form of body dysmorphic disorder in which men who are already more muscular than most men become preoccupied with the desire to be more muscular than they are.

Tony initially became interested in weight training when he was in high school. He had always felt small and was impressed by a friend's change in physique after he started weight training. Tony quickly became 'hooked' on training. He began spending increasing amounts of time at the gym and less time with friends. He found himself constantly thinking about his body and comparing it to those of other men at the gym. Although he had developed an extremely muscular physique according to any objective standard, he felt ashamed of his lack of musculature, and when he was not at the gym he would wear baggy trousers and loose t-shirts to hide his body.

No matter how big I got, or how much bigger I was than other guys, it didn't matter – I had to be even bigger. I started using supplements, but I wasn't getting bigger fast enough ... so last year I started using steroids.

The steroids have produced some benefits, but they also have unwanted side effects. For someone so concerned about his appearance, the development of acne has been hard to bear. Tony's desire to be bigger has also led him to suffer in other ways:

I started pushing myself too hard and was getting all these injuries ... but that only made me want to train harder when I recovered to make up for the lost time. My shoulders and knees are shot from pushing weights that are too heavy.

Photograph © Sokolovsky/Fotolia

Summary

- Our beliefs about who we are and who we want to be can exert important influences on our behaviour.
- We tend to attribute our successes to our efforts and our failures to external factors.
- The fundamental attribution error is our tendency to attribute other people's poor health or lack of success to their disposition or character rather than to the broader social context.
- Our beliefs about what influences our health (our efforts, other people, or fate) can influence the likelihood of initiating and maintaining healthy behaviours.

9.3 INDIVIDUALS AND GROUPS

Humans have a basic need for the company of others to avoid loneliness, gain attention from other people, bolster our self image, and reduce anxiety. Some people do prefer to live in isolation, but these people are exceptions to a very strong social norm. Group membership and group identity are therefore important components of individual identity. Having a strong positive group identity can benefit our psychological and social wellbeing. In contrast, group membership may restrict our individual freedom due to pressures to conform to group norms, and membership of some groups may expose individuals to prejudice, stigmatisation, and victimisation.

When you finish your training and begin working you will acquire various identities from the broad group of 'health professionals' down to the specific group forming the department in which you work. **Social identity theory** (Tajfel and Turner, 1986) proposes that a sense of belonging to valued groups is an important component of maintaining a positive self image. Our membership of groups may be based on things we cannot change, including obvious physical characteristics such as ethnicity, sex, and age. However, our membership of other groups reflects the choices we make, such as our occupation, sporting team, or subcultural group (e.g. punks, Goths). Important markers of group identity include styles of dress and the kind of language use (vocabulary, accent, slang, etc.).

9.3.1 SOCIAL ROLES

Most everyday interactions run smoothly because of shared beliefs and assumptions about how people should behave. Many social interactions are quite complex, and most of us behave in ways that indicate our awareness of what is appropriate and inappropriate behaviour. It is usually only when someone 'breaks the rules' that we will become conscious of them.

Goffman's (1959) dramaturgical theory suggests that social interactions can be thought of as being like a play in which interactions between people inhabiting different social roles are guided by shared assumptions about normal or appropriate behaviour. **Social roles** can be ascribed or acquired. Ascribed roles are those given to us independent of what we do e.g. daughter/son. Acquired roles are those we attain through experience and social recognition e.g. doctor. Each social role entails certain rights and responsibilities. Different social roles also allow us to behave in certain ways. To be recognised as socially competent we must behave in ways that are appropriate to our social roles.

Changes in social roles can be stressful because of the links between social roles, identity, and social recognition. Gaining new roles can also be stressful because we need to learn new modes of behaviour and prove that we are competent (e.g. getting a job promotion, becoming a parent). Feelings of failure or incapacity in social roles can lead to depression. Role loss can also be stressful (e.g. someone who has retired after 45 years working for the same employer). Furthermore, role conflict can be stressful too (e.g. people trying to balance the new role of 'parent' with the established role of 'professional').

The concept of social roles is important in medicine and healthcare (Parsons, 1975). A person inhabiting the **sick role** has the right to relinquish other obligations – they can take time off work/school and avoid having to do the dishes or take out the rubbish. However, the sick role also entails obligations such as the obligation to strive to get better, follow advice, and not engage in activities that may hinder recovery. This may be difficult for people who possess other important or valued social roles. Another important aspect of the sick role (as an ascribed role) is that it must be formally acknowledged. Because medical professionals can certify sick leave they can be thought of as gatekeepers of the sick role. The social role of doctor bestows certain rights such as the right to ask personal questions and conduct physical examinations. However, it also entails certain responsibilities such as upholding professional standards and maintaining patient confidentiality.

9.3.2 CONFORMITY

People generally have strong tendencies for a **conformity** to the expectations of the groups to which they belong. The more we want to belong to a group, the more important it is for us to conform. Research has shown that people tend to go along with what others think – sometimes going against their own better judgement (Asch, 1956). When other group members have expressed a unanimous opinion, many people may find it hard to speak out against this.

ACTIVITY 9.3   CONFORMITY

Imagine you are a junior doctor on your first day. On ward rounds a senior consultant suggests a treatment you believe to be wrong. Several of the other group members seem to agree with the senior consultant.

- How easy would it be to say what you think rather than conforming to the group?
- What would you do?

An important reason to conform to group norms is to maintain distinctions between groups. One way to protect or improve our self image is to make favourable comparisons between the groups to which we belong (the ingroup) and other groups (outgroups). For example, if the team I support wins an important match, I will feel good about myself and happy to be part of my ingroup rather than the outgroup (i.e. not part of a losing team). However, making favourable comparisons often means relying on and reinforcing prejudices and stereotypes about outgroups.

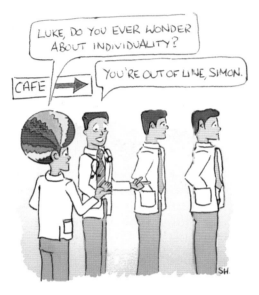

Groups can also have powerful effects on decision making. With group decision making it is not always the case that 'the whole is greater than the sum of its parts' (Mesmer-Magnus and DeChurch, 2009). This seems to be because the urge to conform can sometimes stifle creative thinking. This may be particularly so for new members of groups. For example, junior doctors or medical students may have fresh insights, but find it difficult to question the professional opinions of other members of the team.

Group decisions are often more narrow than the decisions of individual group members. The phenomenon of polarisation means that through group discussion, agreement within a group tends to intensify so that each individual's attitude becomes stronger. For example, imagine we have six individuals who have moderately positive attitudes toward euthanasia. Following a group discussion there will tend to be a concentration and polarisation of attitudes. The group will become more positive toward euthanasia. If individuals were moderately opposed to euthanasia before the group discussion, the group attitude would be more extremely opposed following group discussion. Three explanations have been given for why this polarisation occurs (Hogg and Vaughan, 2008):

- Persuasive arguments: people in groups of like-minded people will hear arguments that they already agree with as well new arguments supporting their original beliefs. These will galvanise the initial attitude. In addition, making public commitments to our own beliefs via statements to other people may strengthen our initial attitudes.
- Social comparison: to prove they really belong to the group and seek approval, individuals will make more intense statements of their initial belief.
- Self-categorisation: people will develop stereotypes of group members and be aware of what distinguishes the ingroup prototype from stereotypical outgroup members. Therefore for individual and group identity reasons people's opinions will move toward the ingroup prototype.

Another example of how group decision making may be worse than individual decision making is called **groupthink** (Janis and Mann, 1977). Groupthink occurs when the desire for group unanimity overrides rational decisions. It is more likely to happen when a group is already homogeneous and cohesive. However, groupthink also depends on the characteristics of the situation, such as if a decision has to be made in stressful or rushed situations or when the group is isolated from external sources of information. Thus, groupthink may be most likely to occur when cohesive groups are placed in stressful situations. Given the urgency of many medical situations, it is therefore vitally important that health teams are aware of how groupthink can lead to erroneous or poor decision making.

9.3.3 OBEDIENCE, POWER, AND LEADERSHIP

The processes of conformity just described refer to situations in which people think or behave in certain ways because of a perceived pressure to do so. Of course, there are many situations in which we behave in certain ways because of a need to be obedient to people who have power or authority.

Obedience

The powerful effects of obedience to authority have been observed in many settings, including those directly relevant to the practice of medicine. The study described in Research Box 9.1 shows how an unquestioning obedience to authority may have disastrous consequences.

RESEARCH BOX 9.1   Nurse-physician relationships

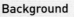

Background

The professional status of nurses is sometimes challenged by doctors' behaviour – one example being when nurses are directed by doctors to behave in ways that go against their professional standards or established procedures.

Methods and findings

22 nurses were observed in their normal work environments. The researchers placed a bottle of a fictional drug 'Astroten' in the ward drug cabinet. The label on the bottle clearly stated 'Maximum daily dose 10mg'. A researcher posing as 'Dr Smith' – someone unknown to the nurse – telephoned each nurse and asked her to administer 20mg of Astroten to a patient, stating that he would sign for it when he arrived at the hospital.

Nurses had four good reasons not to administer the drug:

1   The requested dosage was double the safe daily dose stated on the bottle.

2 Hospital procedures stated that they should only take instructions from doctors they know.

3 Hospital procedures also stated that nurses should not take telephone instructions.

4 Astroten was not on the approved medication list and had not been signed for.

Nevertheless, 21 of the 22 nurses complied with the request to give an overdose of the drug. They were intercepted by the researchers after they prepared the dose.

Significance

Power differentials in the status of doctors and nurses can affect nurses' behaviour. No nurses involved in this study expressed concern about the excessive dose – indeed, many repeated and clarified the dosage without questioning it. Such conformity has consequences for the professional and personal esteem of nurses and the health of patients.

Hofling, C.K. et al. (1966) An experimental study of nurse-physician relationships, *Journal of Nervous and Mental Disease, 143*: 171–180.

In a classic study of obedience, study participants were told by a researcher in a white coat to give increasingly strong electric shocks to people who made mistakes in a word memory task (Milgram, 1974). No shocks were actually given, but the 'voltage generator' included descriptions of increasing voltage levels – 375v was labelled 'Danger: Severe Shock', and 435v was labelled 'XXX'. At different levels of shock, the learner (actually a co-researcher) gave standard responses: after 150v they asked to leave the study; after 250v they screamed in agony; after 300v they lapsed into silence. If participants hesitated or asked to stop the researcher urged them to go on, informing them to treat silence or non-responses as errors and to administer another shock. Although it was predicted that fewer than 10 per cent of participants would administer shocks greater than 195v (labelled 'Very Strong Shock'), all of the participants went beyond this. In fact, 63 per cent went all the way to 450v.

Leadership and influence

Effective leadership involves the appropriate use of authority and influence to ensure the efficient management of people and resources to achieve group aims. Good leadership involves more than simply 'getting the job done'. Good leaders will aim to develop and maintain good team relationships and provide appropriate opportunities for individual input.

Leadership styles can be grouped into three broad categories. Autocratic leaders assume total responsibility for making all decisions, and managing team members. This style characterises dictators who do not tolerate the views and decisions of ingroup or outgroup members. Democratic leaders are consultative, allowing group members to be involved in decision making, planning, and the monitoring of performance if they possess the appropriate knowledge and skills. Laissez-faire leaders do not impose their leadership, but allow group members to decide on goals and strategies. In most professional settings it is rare to find purely autocratic or laissez-faire leaders. However, democratic leaders may tend more toward autocratic or laissez-faire styles: the context may determine the extent to which they do so.

Leaders often vary in terms of how they try to encourage or enforce compliance with their decisions (Raven, 1965). One common strategy is to apply the principles of operant conditioning (see Chapter 10). According to this approach, good performance may be recognised via bonuses or other material rewards. One example is performance-related pay for general practices in the UK. In contrast, coercive leadership is based on a leader threatening to remove privileges if their instructions are not obeyed.

It is also possible to identify different sources of authority or reasons for leadership. One basis for power is recognised hierarchies of power. These are often based on the leader possessing superior knowledge, experience, or expertise. Thus a consultant is in a superior position relative to a junior doctor. However, this is not always the case. For example, in the military a newly commissioned officer has a higher leadership position than a senior non-commissioned officer with forty years of experience. It is also important to note that people sometimes become leaders not because of their expertise or experience but because of their charisma, charm, or connections to powerful people.

CLINICAL NOTES 9.2

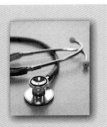

Hierarchy and leadership in medicine

- Being a doctor entails certain rights and responsibilities. Your reputation will be damaged if you disregard these responsibilities or abuse these rights.
- Pay attention to the different leadership skills people use. Use good leaders as role models and avoid following the examples set by bad leaders.
- Be aware of your own tendency to conform to authority. Ask yourself whether it is always in patients' best interests to do what your superiors suggest.
- Be brave enough to challenge your superiors if you think they have made a decision that will not lead to the best care for patients.

9.3.4 STEREOTYPES AND PREJUDICE

An important aspect of the study of individuals and groups is stereotypes and prejudice. **Stereotypes** can be defined as generalisations that we make about specific social groups and members of those groups. Stereotypes are 'rules of thumb' which are broadly correct, but may sometimes be erroneous (Tversky and Kahneman, 1974). The social groups for which people have stereotypes are various and include nationality, occupation, and religion. However, they can be more specific. Stereotypes form the basis of many jokes in which a dominant ingroup denigrates an outgroup that is perceived as being inferior. For example, Australians make jokes about New Zealanders. You may also be aware of jokes based on stereotypes of different medical specialisations (e.g. orthopaedic surgeons, psychiatrists).

Although many of these jokes may appear harmless, it is important to note that incorrect or inaccurate stereotypes can lead to undesirable social behaviour. **Prejudice** towards particular social groups is commonly based on inaccurate stereotypes. Taken literally, prejudice means to judge prior to having relevant facts. History is replete with clashes between groups based on erroneous assumptions about differences due to sex, sexuality, nationality, ethnicity, or religion.

ACTIVITY 9.4   STEREOTYPES OF PATIENTS

- Take two minutes to write down quickly words that describe people with AIDS, people with chronic fatigue syndrome (ME), and people with cancer.
- How did you acquire these beliefs?
- How have your interactions with people with these conditions been shaped by your initial beliefs?
- How have your initial beliefs been changed by your interactions with people with these conditions?

Stereotypes and prejudice can also affect medical care. The example in Research Box 9.2 shows that prejudices about mental illness can result in poorer care for some patients (Lawrie et al., 1998). It is notable that many medical students also express prejudices about patients with mental illnesses (Dixon et al., 2008). Stereotypes and prejudices about people with certain health conditions, ethnic minorities, or the elderly (see Case Study 8.1) are important because of the known links between attitudes and behaviour noted earlier. Indeed, some research has highlighted how prejudice and stereotyping can lead to increased ethnic disparities in health (Balsa and McGuire, 2003).

Stereotyping in healthcare is not restricted to medical professionals. Patients' stereotyped beliefs about medical professionals are also important. One study found that patients who expressed more negative stereotypes about physicians were less likely to seek medical care when they became ill, were less satisfied with the medical care that they did obtain, and were less likely to be adherent to the treatment prescribed by their physician (Bogart et al., 2004). Identifying the reasons for patients' negative stereotypes in an attempt to change these may help to improve the health of the population. It may also be important for doctors to try to change their behaviour so that they do not reinforce unhelpful stereotypes.

RESEARCH BOX 9.2   Doctors' attitudes to mental illness

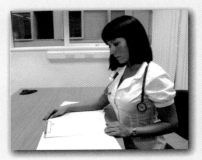

Background

Many members of the general population possess negative stereotypes and prejudices about people with mental illness. Previous research has indicated that many people with mental illnesses report unfair treatment from their own general practitioners.

Methods and findings

166 GPs were randomly allocated to receive a letter from a 30 year old married housewife with a 5 year old child who wishes to be registered at the GP practice because since moving to the area two months previous she has been troubled by insomnia, fatigue, and nausea. The letter was altered to say that she either had (1) no previous major illnesses, or a past history of (2) schizophrenia, (3) depression, or (4) diabetes. For options 2 – 4 it was made clear that the illness was well controlled by the appropriate medication.

In spite of the clear statement that the mental illnesses were well controlled, GPs were significantly less happy to register a patient with schizophrenia than the three other patient types. GPs who received the letter with a history of schizophrenia were significantly more concerned about the risk of violence and the child's welfare, and were more likely to say that they would personally contact the patient's previous GP.

Significance

Schizophrenia arouses concerns in GPs that are not simply due to the fact that patients have a mental illness. Patients with schizophrenia may have difficulty finding a GP prepared to register them, and this can hamper the likelihood they will receive the integrated community-based healthcare they need. These findings also suggest a need to educate GPs about the care of patients with schizophrenia.

Lawrie, S.M. et al. (1998) General practitioners' attitudes to psychiatric and medical illness, *Psychological Medicine, 28:* 1463–1467.

Summary

- Group membership is an important part of individual identity.
- Different social roles entail different rights and obligations. In medicine social roles influence the behaviour of doctors and patients (e.g. the sick role).
- People tend to conform to the expectations of the groups to which they belong.

- People often conform to people in leadership positions without questioning – sometimes even when what they are being asked to do is harmful to others.
- Group decision making can be impaired by the tendency toward conformity and because alternative positions are not considered.
- Effective leadership involves the appropriate use of authority and the best use of the skills and capacities of group members.
- Stereotypes are cognitive short-cuts which are a core aspect of prejudices. They can exert important influences on health-related behaviour.

CLINICAL NOTES 9.3

Avoiding racism and careless assumptions in medicine

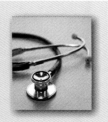

- Be aware of your attitudes toward different groups of people – whether they are ethnic groups, particular types of patients, or particular professions in healthcare.
- Ensure that your attitudes do not affect your treatment of different patients.
- The fundamental attribution error means we are prone to assume that peoples' behaviour is due to them and not their circumstances.
- Remember that people's behaviour is often due to their history or current social circumstances – do not assume people are intrinsically difficult or badly motivated.

9.4 ANTI-SOCIAL AND PRO-SOCIAL BEHAVIOUR

9.4.1 AGGRESSION

Aggression involves behaviours that are enacted to cause physical or psychological harm or pain to another person. Aggression can be actual (e.g. physical attacks) or symbolic (e.g. burning flags). Different explanations to explain aggression are outlined below. Strategies for dealing with angry or aggressive patients are covered in Chapter 18.

The **frustration-aggression** hypothesis (Berkowitz, 1989) argues that when we are prevented from achieving our goals we become frustrated and this can lead to aggression. Although frustration may be important in the lead-up to aggression, it cannot be the sole answer. For example, if someone is frustrated because a library book they want has not been returned they do not automatically become violent, because they know that the library is not an appropriate place for aggressive behaviour. The **cue-arousal** theory of aggression therefore argues that frustration is more likely to lead to aggression if there are situational cues that aggression is appropriate (Geen and O'Neal, 1969). In medical contexts, such situational cues may include rude or aggressive behaviour that is exhibited by other patients or medical professionals. Other important situational factors include the effects of alcohol and other drugs, which may impair cognition or reduce inhibitions against violent behaviour.

A recent review revealed that patient aggression and violence are prominent occupational hazards for medical professionals: half of all healthcare professionals working in general hospitals have experienced verbal assaults, and one-quarter have experienced physical assaults (Hahn et al., 2008). The reviewers suggested that the likelihood of aggressive behaviour is influenced by organisational procedures, such as prolonged waiting times, which will increase patient frustration, and by medical procedures that induce pain or anxiety. It has been suggested that patients who are anxious or in pain pay more attention to threatening stimuli and that aggression may be a response to increased feelings of threat (Winstanley, 2005).

Patients with certain conditions may be more likely to become aggressive – this could be particularly likely in dementia or psychiatric conditions characterised by cognitive impairments, delusions, or disinhibition (see Chapter 16). However, situational factors are important because not all patients with such conditions will become aggressive or violent. Reflecting the fundamental attribution error referred to earlier, it is interesting to note that healthcare professionals tend to attribute aggressive behaviour among psychiatric patients to internal characteristics such as delusional thoughts or stress, whereas patients tend to attribute their aggressive behaviour to external or situational factors such as being provoked, teased, or 'bugged' by staff (Nolan et al., 2009).

Summary

- Several different theories of aggression have been put forward. Although there is support for most theories, no single theory explains all acts of aggression.
- Aggressive behaviour appears to be a combination of individual tendencies toward aggression, the psychological state of the individual at a particular time, and situational cues or stressors.

9.4.2. PRO-SOCIAL BEHAVIOUR

Although social psychology often focuses on why people engage in undesirable behaviours like aggression and prejudice, many researchers focus on positive social behaviours such as helping and altruism. Such **pro-social behaviours** include the activities of medical professionals and other healthcare workers (although people may not engage in such behaviours for purely altruistic reasons).

Altruistic behaviours are pro-social behaviours that we engage in without expecting to be rewarded – although the feeling of 'doing good' that arises from altruistic behaviours may be a form of reward in itself. Some people would argue that our capacity for empathy explains why we do help others: we can imagine what it would be like to be in their position, so we try to help them (Batson et al., 1981). Others would argue that we choose to help others to relieve our own distress at seeing someone in need of help (Cialdini et al., 1987). It is also possible that people engage in seemingly altruistic behaviours because they expect a reward or recognition in the future (e.g. we may do voluntary work because we think it will look good on our CV). Consenting to donate one's organs for transplantation after death could be seen to be purely altruistic because there is no possibility of a reward for such behaviour. However, it is also possible that the knowledge that we will be helping others after we die would be construed as a reward.

In more mundane everyday circumstances, the likelihood that we will help others is influenced by our perceptions of the costs and benefits of helping. We are more likely to help others if we perceive that doing so will not be too taxing for us in terms of time, effort, and emotion (Piliavin et al., 1969). For example, we are less likely to help someone get their cat out of a tree if we are rushing to a job interview. This principle helps to explain mobile blood donation services. Such services eliminate some of the time and money costs associated with donation, thereby increasing the attractiveness of this behaviour.

In addition to being influenced by perceived personal costs and benefits, the likelihood of helping others is influenced by our perceptions of whether other people are helping. Social learning and modelling concepts (see Chapter 10) suggest that we are more likely to help if we can see others doing so, and less likely to help if we see others not getting involved. In situations where nobody helps this can be because of a diffusion of responsibility. Each individual assumes that somebody else will take responsibility for helping, with the net result that nobody does so (Latané and Darley, 1970). This can be illustrated by the fact that people are more likely to help when they are not in groups. For example, if a person has an epileptic seizure people are more likely to help if they are the only bystander, but the likelihood of helping will decrease as the number of inactive bystanders increases.

Social cues to helping can be used to encourage pro-social behaviour (just as social cues may encourage aggression). Examples include the coloured badges, ribbons, and wristbands worn to demonstrate support for various charities. These are in some part symbolic of a material exchange e.g. you donate money so you get a reward. They are also a public demonstration of commitment and a signal to others that they should also support the cause.

Summary

- Altruistic behaviours are helping or pro-social behaviours that people do for others with no expectation of a personal reward.
- The likelihood of helping appears to be influenced by the personal costs and benefits of helping.
- The behaviour of others is also a cue for helping behaviour. We are more likely to help if we can see others helping, or if there are no other people available to offer help.

📖 FURTHER READING

Hogg, M.A. & Vaughan, G.M. (2008) *Social Psychology* (5th edition). Harlow: Pearson Prentice Hall. A good introduction to a wide range of social psychology topics. However, this book is designed for psychology students, so it lacks a specific focus on medical applications of key concepts.

Stroebe, W. (2000) *Social Psychology and Health* (2nd edition). Buckingham: Open University Press. This book discusses health from a social psychological perspective but is less reader-friendly than mainstream social psychology textbooks.

❓ REVISION QUESTIONS

1. What is meant by the term 'cognitive dissonance'? How can it be used to encourage healthy behaviour?

2. Outline the characteristics of messages and messengers that will increase the likelihood that people will respond to them in positive ways.

3. How does the clothing doctors wear affect patients' perceptions of them? Why is this the case?

4. How can perceived discrepancies between people's actual and ideal selves prompt behaviour change? Give one healthy example and one unhealthy example.

5. What is meant by the 'fundamental attribution error'? Give two health-related examples of this phenomenon.

6. What is meant by the term 'sick role'? What does it mean to say that doctors are 'gatekeepers' of the sick role?

7. How well does the proverb 'Many hands make light work' apply to medical decision making? Discuss with reference to the concepts of conformity and groupthink.

8. What is a stereotype? What is the link between stereotypes and prejudice?

9. Why is the cue-arousal theory likely to be a better explanation of aggression than the frustration-aggression hypothesis?

10. Describe the characteristics of situations that make it more likely that people will help others.

10 LEARNING, PERCEPTION, AND MEMORY

LEARNING OBJECTIVES

This chapter is designed to enable you to:

- Describe perceptual processes and give examples of how these are relevant to medical settings.
- Understand the processes of attention and how they contribute to medical errors.
- Describe classical and operant conditioning and discuss how these can be used in clinical practice.
- Understand the characteristics of (a) short-term and (b) long-term memory.
- Use this information to to help devise effective ways to revise for exams.

Learning to be a doctor involves the accumulation of knowledge, clinical, and surgical skills – all of which are driven by cognitive processes of perception, attention, learning, and memory. Understanding how these processes work can help us in a wide variety of ways. We can find better ways to learn; be more alert to the conditions under which medical errors might occur; and help patients to change behaviours such as helping children with eczema to stop scratching. In this chapter we shall look at perception, attention, learning, and memory, with examples of how these are relevant to medicine.

10.1 PERCEPTION

Perception involves the way information from our environment is transformed via our senses (hearing, touch, smell, taste, and sight) into experience. It is helpful to clarify the difference between perception and attention, which we shall look at in the next section. **Attention** is broader and involves those aspects of our environment we focus on and process.

Let us focus on visual perception because, on the surface at least, this appears quite straightforward. Light from the environment is projected onto our retina and transformed into electrical impulses by the rods, cones, and ganglion cells of the retina. These impulses are transmitted via the optic nerve to the visual cortex where we 'see' the image. However, the mind has a strong influence on how we interpret stimuli. Activity 10.1 is an example of this. Many people will get this wrong because we tend to process small and frequently used words, such as 'the' and 'of', as single units. This makes it much harder to 'see' the individual letters in these words.

ACTIVITY 10.1

How many F and T letters are there in this sentence?
'INFERTILITY TREATMENT IS THE RESULT OF YEARS OF SCIENTIFIC STUDY COMBINED WITH THE EXPERTISE OF CLINICIANS'

Visual perception is therefore a combination of visual stimuli (bottom-up processing) and our existing knowledge (top-down processing). Other examples of top-down processing are **size and shape constancy** and **depth perception**. In size and shape constancy, an object is perceived as remaining the same despite the fact that it appears larger as we move towards it and changes shape depending on the angle we see it from. Our mind knows that most objects do not change shape so therefore concludes that we are moving and seeing it from different perspectives.

This knowledge is used in the perception of depth. For example, we know that people are approximately similar in size. In Figure 10.1 we can therefore see that the person in the background is further away from the camera. In this instance, our previous knowledge gives us clues about depth. Our interpretation of it happens very rapidly at a subconscious level. This effect is so strong it can even override our conscious perceptual processes. Compare the size of the image of the person in the background with the image of the person in the foreground. How much smaller would you say the person in the background is, compared to the person in the foreground? Now look at Figure 10.2 on page 223 in which the image is actually brought forward in the picture. You probably would not have judged the image to be this small because size constancy and depth perception will automatically bias your judgement.

The study of perception has established that not only are we unable to realise the extent of some true differences (such as the difference in size between the two people in Figure 10.2), but that we are also actually quite selective and biased in what we perceive. The underlying concept here is that of **perceptual sets**, where the influence of attention, previous experience, and motivation is combined so we perceive information that is relevant to us,

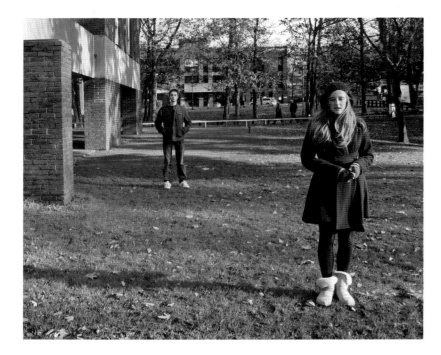

FIGURE 10.1   Size constancy and depth perception

both as humans and individuals. A perceptual set is influenced by the factors summarised in Box 10.1. **Threshold for perception** is where one stimulus has a lower or higher threshold for perception than others. If someone shouts 'Fire' it is more likely to get your attention than if they shout 'Air'. Similarly, in a noisy environment where lots of people are talking, you might suddenly become aware that someone across the room has said your name. This is because you will naturally have a lower threshold for 'hearing' your name.

BOX 10.1   Factors that influence perceptual sets

- Threshold for perception.
- Past experience.
- Current drive state.
- Emotions.
- Individual values.
- Environment.
- Cultural background and experience.

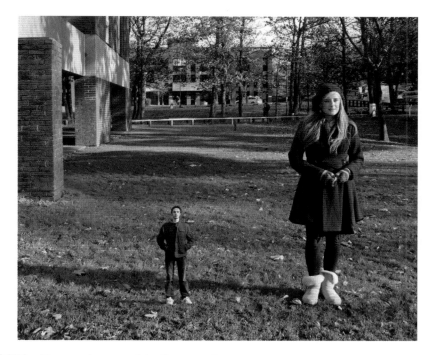

FIGURE 10.2   Size constancy and depth perception

The influence of **past experience** is evident through the effects of size constancy and depth perception. Past experience, **expectations** and **individual values** will combine to influence perception in more subtle ways as well. For example, experiments of symptom perception show that just telling people a stimulus might be painful makes them more likely to report pain in response to it (Colloca et al., 2008). The placebo and nocebo effects provide classic examples of the role of expectations and learning in the perception of symptoms (see Chapter 4). Poor children and adults will overestimate the size of coins compared to more affluent people (Ashley et al., 1951).

Current drive state affects what we perceive in different ways. First our level of arousal determines how much attention we will pay to our environment. When we are sleeping we do not consciously perceive much, if anything, of our external environment unless there is a large change, such as a loud noise or a change in temperature. The processes through which people perceive stimuli when in a low level of consciousness are important in anaesthesia. Anaesthesia aims to remove conscious awareness, yet approximately 1 per cent of people report some perception during surgery (see Research Box 10.1). Second, our motivational state will also determine what we pay attention to in our environment. For example, when we are hungry we are more likely to notice food-related stimuli (Seibt et al., 2007).

RESEARCH BOX 10.1   Awareness and memory during anaesthesia

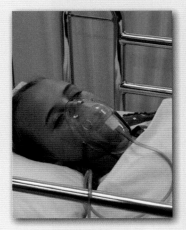

Background

Epidemiological research has shown that awareness during anaesthesia is more likely during some types of surgery, in people who have a history of awareness, are obese, use central nervous system depressant drugs, and who are younger – particularly children. This study looked at awareness and memory in children during surgery.

Methods

184 children aged 5 –18 were tested for awareness and memory during surgery via various means:

1 During surgery children were told to squeeze their hand if they could hear (awareness).
2 During surgery words were played 20 times then children were tested after surgery for their increased recognition of these words (implicit memory).
3 After surgery children were asked if they remembered anything from the surgery (explicit memory).

Results

Children could not explicitly recall the events of surgery or recognise the words played during surgery. However, two children (1 per cent) showed awareness during surgery by responding to the command to squeeze their hand. These two children were similar to the rest of the sample in terms of type of surgery, anaesthetic technique, and previous history.

Significance

This study added to existing evidence by using in-surgery techniques to measure awareness and memory in children. The 1 per cent of children who showed awareness during surgery is similar to that reported by adults. However, it is interesting that these children had no implicit or explicit memory for surgical events.

Andrade et al. (2008) Awareness and memory function during paediatric anaesthesia, *British Journal of Anaesthesia, 100(3)*: 389–396.

Emotions will also affect what we attend to and perceive. It has been well established that anxiety results in an increased perception of threat and a narrowing of attention onto threatening stimuli (Ouimet et al., 2009). Perceptual changes can also be seen for positive emotions. Classic studies of young children's perception of Santa Claus found that before Christmas children's drawings of Santa Claus were much larger and more elaborate than after Christmas – suggesting children's emotional state influenced their perception and representation of Santa Claus (Sechrest and Wallis, 1964).

The **environment** provides the external stimuli that we interpret into experience. Despite top-down influences and our perceptual set, most of us are remarkably accurate in what we see. This is partly due to our previous experiences of the environment which can help us interpret what is happening. However, sometimes our knowledge of the environment can override what we see and result in a distorted perception. A classic example of this is the Ames room – a specially constructed room where the walls, window, and floor are faked to look like a square room when the back wall is in fact on the diagonal. This means that if a person in the room walks from one corner to the other they appear to shrink or grow. In reality this is because they are walking further away. However, to a viewer, the perceptual cues that the room is square can override this so they 'see' the impossible i.e. that the person shrinks or grows as they walk (there are many examples of the Ames illusion on www.youtube.com).

Cultural factors influence perception less than might be expected. Many aspects of visual perception are consistent across cultures. One of the strongest effects of culture on perception is that we are quicker and better at recognising people of our own ethnic group compared to people of another ethnic group (Meissner and Brigham, 2001). This can influence how healthcare professionals interact with patients of different ethnicity. A review of cultural influences on doctor-patient communication found that with patients from ethnic minorities, consultations involve less emotional expression by the doctor and patient and less verbal expression by patients. The authors concluded perceptual biases contributed to culture-related communication difficulties in medical consultations (Schouten and Meeuwesen, 2006).

So far we have discussed the influence of perceptual sets on normal visual perception. However, we also need to understand abnormal perceptual processes. These are relevant to many disorders, including autism and schizophrenia. For example, people with autism and antisocial characteristics both have poor perception of facial expressions of emotion (Marsh and Blair, 2008). Schizophrenia and other psychotic experiences are particularly interesting because they involve the perception of illusory events as real. Research in this area is relatively new but suggests psychotic-type thinking is more likely when people with schizotypal characteristics are put in situations of perceptual ambiguity and overload (Tsakanikos, 2006). This type of research could eventually help us understand more about the conditions that trigger psychotic symptoms, which in turn could inform the treatment and management of schizophrenia.

Summary

- Perception is the way information from our environment is transformed and inter-preted into experience.
- Perception is the combination of environmental stimuli (bottom-up processing) and existing knowledge (top-down processing).
- A perceptual set is where attention, previous experience, and motivation determine the information each person perceives.
- Perceptual sets can be influenced by thresholds for perception, past experience, individual values, current drive state, emotions, environment and culture.

10.2 ATTENTION

Attention is the ability to select information in the environment to attend to and process. Attention is therefore an important part of perception, learning, and performance – particu-larly in situations where we need to multitask (i.e. divide our attention between different tasks). What we attend to and how much attention we pay to it will be influenced by our physical arousal, motivation, and emotion. Attention can also be biased by these factors. Knowledge of how attention works can therefore help us understand errors in medicine, such as giving wrong drug dosages or surgical errors.

Attention involves many different mental processes and it would be wrong to think in terms of a single attentional system. For example, studies of people with brain damage show they often have problems with some aspects of attention but not all (Posner and Petersen, 1990). Attention can be voluntary, such as when we concentrate on learning or doing a task, or involuntary, such as when a loud noise or sudden movement grabs our attention. Attention has been likened to a spotlight or filter that can have either a broad or narrow focus. When attention is focused, central information is processed in detail but peripheral information may be ignored or lost. At a basic level, we can distinguish between being able to:

- Focus our attention on a particular stimulus.
- Remove or disengage our attention from a stimulus.
- Shift attention between one stimulus and another.

Attention is intertwined with cognitive processes of perception and memory (see Figure 10.3). **Sensory buffers** are short-term stores of incoming information that can be used to select which information to attend to consciously. Auditory sensory buffers register all incoming sounds for a few seconds so this information is potentially recoverable during this time. A good example of this is when we 'tune out' of a conversation for a few seconds but can then replay what was just said in our head. This is especially useful if we are accused of not listening to something someone has just said!

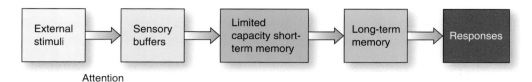

FIGURE 10.3 Cognitive processes

Many theories of attention propose that we have a **limited capacity processor** that restricts the amount of information we can consciously attend to. Research has broadly confirmed this, although capacity is not as fixed as this implies. There is evidence that we can still unconsciously perceive information not attended to and that our capacity to process information or multitask increases as tasks become more practised or automatic and hence demand less conscious attention. For example, neuroimaging research indicates that even when we do not consciously attend to stimuli there is similar but weaker neuro-logical activation in the same parts of the brain that are activated during conscious atten-tion (Vuilleumier, 2005).

10.2.1 ATTENTION AND CLINICAL SKILLS

Clinical skills are essential for medical practice and so during training you will learn skills such as clinical interviewing, physical examinations, and surgery. **Skill acquisition** draws on the processes illustrated in Figure 10.3. Learning a new skill demands our concentrated attention, short-term memory, cognitive motor processes, and effortful responses. Initially, attention is needed for both perception and response stages. As we learn and practise a skill it gradually becomes easier and requires less of our attention or concentration. There are three broad stages in skill acquisition (Adams, 1971):

1 *Cognitive stage* – development of a mental representation of the skill and how to perform it. At this stage learning usually relies on explicit instruction through teaching from an expert, demonstra-tion, and self-observation e.g. relying on a driving instructor to tell you what to do.
2 *Associative stage* – an effective motor programme has been developed so the person is able to carry out the broad skill but lacks the ability to perform finer subtasks with fluency. Development is guided by knowledge or feedback e.g. able to drive but consciously aware of actions such as turn-ing the wheel and changing gear.
3 *Autonomous stage* – the skill is largely automatic and relies on implicit knowledge and motor co-ordination, rather than explicit instruction e.g. able to drive automatically without conscious effort.

Studies of skill acquisition show that practice is more important than aptitude. For example, hours of practice are the strongest predictor of musical ability – more so than musical aptitude, parents' musical ability, and social class (Sloboda et al., 1994). If learn-ing or practice is spaced out over time it also improves learning (see 'Memory', p. 238).

Multitasking is easiest when the skills are automatic and the tasks are not too similar or complex. You might write an essay whilst listening to music or talk to someone whilst driving a car. However, even under easy conditions multitasking leads to competing processes which will influence how each task is carried out. For example, using a phone while driving results in slower response times, a reduced ability to notice when the car in front slows down, and less attention to sensory inputs. This effect on driving appears to occur regardless of whether the phone is hands-free (Esgate and Groome, 2005). Studies of attention have shown that incorrect actions or mistakes are most likely:

- When the correct response is not the strongest or most habitual.
- When our full attention is not given to the task.
- Under conditions of stress and anxiety.

The advantage of developing a skill to the autonomous stage is that it frees up our attention for multitasking (although other tasks will still impinge on the automatic one). The disadvantage is that automatic behaviour is no longer consciously controlled so it is possible to make mistakes. This is particularly relevant to medicine: it is estimated that in the USA alone nearly 100,000 patients die every year from preventable mistakes (Ferner and McDowell, 2006). Studies of British manslaughter cases against doctors over the last century have shown that the majority of cases arise from errors in administering or prescribing medication. Other types of errors are wrong treatment or diagnosis and surgical errors (see Research Box 10.2).

RESEARCH BOX 10.2   Medical mistakes and manslaughter

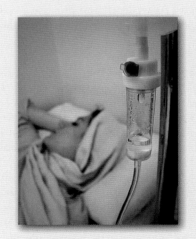

Methods

UK newspapers and journal archives were searched to identify legal cases where doctors were charged with manslaughter to examine the causes of death.

Results

85 doctors were charged with manslaughter between 1795 and 2005, with a large increase in prosecutions since 1990. The majority of doctors were acquitted: only 29 per cent were convicted or pleaded guilty. The main causes of manslaughter were:

Mistakes (44%) – errors in planning

For example, a 20-year-old man with muscular dystrophy died after circumcision. The surgeon guessed the patient's weight and inadvertently gave three times the recommended dose of lidocaine. He was charged with manslaughter but acquitted.

Slips (20%) – errors due to distraction or a failure of concentration

For example, a 6-week-old boy died after cardiac arrest during surgery for pyloric stenosis. The anaesthetist injected air into the bloodstream instead of the nasogastric tube. The anaesthetist was charged with manslaughter but acquitted.

Violations (19%) – deliberate violation of medical practice

For example, a 2-year-old boy died from hypoxia that occurred during a hernia operation. The anaesthetist had deliberately inhaled anaesthetic before and during the operation. He was charged with manslaughter and found guilty.

Technical errors (4%) – failure to carry out an action successfully even though the plan of action and technique were appropriate

For example, a 16-year-old girl being treated for leukaemia died after an attempt to insert a Hickman line (central venous catheter) caused cardiac rupture. The surgeon was charged with manslaughter but acquitted.

Significance

Over half of patient deaths brought to prosecution are due to unconscious errors (mistakes or slips) that could be a direct consequence of automatic behaviour. The authors argue that the prosecution of individual doctors would not improve patient safety as much as changing healthcare systems to incorporate checks that reduce such errors.

Photograph © Hamed Saber, http://flickr.com/hamed

Ferner, R.E. and McDowell, S.E. (2006) Doctors charged with manslaughter in the course of medical practice, 1795–2005: a literature review, *Journal of the Royal Society of Medicine, 99*: 309–314.

Skilled surgeons will carry out surgery relatively automatically at the same time as doing other things such as listening to music (which is quite common). Although music can be quite calming emotionally and physically, research into attention suggests that if something goes wrong and quick decisions or actions are required music will interfere with our ability to focus attention on the emergency situation and responses. Research suggests this is particularly the case for novice surgeons. Miskovic et al. (2008) examined surgical skill in junior doctors who carried out simulated (virtual reality) laparoscopies with no music, calming music, or lively music. Junior doctors who did not listen to music were almost three times better at the simulated laparoscopy than those listening to music. This difference was less obvious once junior doctors had had more practice, illustrating the effect of

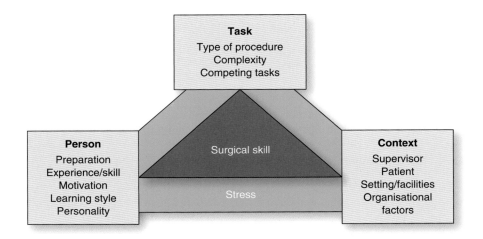

FIGURE 10.4 Influences on surgical skill (adapted from Schout et al., 2010)

practice and automaticity. Other research into surgical skill showed that student and junior doctors' performance was strongly affected by the context and that adverse events were usually preceded by individual errors, often in response to contextual factors as summarised in Figure 10.4.

10.2.2 BIASED ATTENTION

As with perception, attention is biased towards certain stimuli. Normal and abnormal biases have been found. Normal biases include being more likely to attend to faces and emotional stimuli. Infants will spend more time looking at faces or face-shaped stimuli than other shapes (Dannemiller and Stephens, 1988). Studies of reaction times to different objects have shown we are quicker to pay attention to emotional items and take longer to disengage from them. Neuropsychological research shows emotional stimuli will produce stronger neurological responses than neutral stimuli regardless of whether they are visual or auditory. In other words, if we see emotional expressions or hear emotional voices, we will have stronger neurological responses than we do to neutral expressions or voices (Vuilleumier and Huang, 2009).

Attention is also biased in some psychological disorders. People with eating disorders are more likely to attend to stimuli that are food, body, or weight related (Faunce, 2002). Anxious people are more likely to attend to threat-related stimuli and may be hypervigilant for particular stimuli. This is the case in generalised anxiety disorder, obsessive-compulsive disorder, post-traumatic stress disorder (PTSD), and phobias. For example, a person with a blood phobia will continually scan the environment for signs of blood, which takes up cognitive processing and attentional resources. In other psychological disorders, normal biases may be disrupted. For example, Pearson et al. (2009) found that most pregnant women found it harder to disengage their attention from pictures of distressed infants compared to adults or neutral infant faces (as measured by reaction times). However, this bias was not observed in women who were depressed during pregnancy.

Emotions are also important in how attention is directed and focused. Positive emotions are associated with a broadening of attention and negative emotions with a narrowing of attention onto particular stimuli (Vuilleumier and Huang, 2009). This can have various repercussions. On the one hand, narrowing our attention in emergency situations is useful because it helps us focus on the problem and what actions are needed to resolve it. On the other hand, this narrow focus means subsidiary or peripheral information is potentially ignored or less likely to be picked up. There are many examples of accidents that have occurred because vital information has been missed and mistakes made (Esgate and Groome, 2005). Knowledge of attention processes shows that, to a certain extent, slips and mistakes are inevitable parts of being human. It is therefore important to recognise the role of systems and organisations in such circumstances. If adequate systems of checking and monitoring are in place then individual errors are more likely to be caught and corrected before they have severe consequences.

Summary

- Attention concerns the ability to select information in the environment to attend to and process.
- Attention influences the way in which we perceive, process, and respond to stimuli.
- Learning new skills involves concentrated attention, short-term memory, cognitive motor processes, and effortful responses.
- There are three stages involved in learning skills: cognitive, associative, and autonomous.
- When autonomous, skilled behaviour can be carried out without conscious or effortful control.
- Multitasking requires divided attention and is easiest when one or both tasks are practised and automatic.
- Mistakes are most likely when the correct response is not strongest or habitual, when our full attention is not given to the task, and in conditions of stress or anxiety.
- Attentional biases include a bias towards emotional expressions and voices and the influence of emotions on the breadth of attentional focus.
- Abnormal biases are found in some psychological disorders where people show a bias towards stimuli that are relevant to that disorder.

10.3 LEARNING

Associative learning is how we learn the relationship between two events that occur together. For example, if one event occurs at the same time as another it indicates a temporal relationship; if one event always follows another it indicates a causal relationship. Different learning processes have a range of implications for medicine, both in terms of your own learning and helping patients recover and change their behaviour. Key learning processes include classical conditioning, operant conditioning, modelling, and imitation. Conditioning processes are particularly useful when working with young children or people with cognitive impairments who are less likely to change their behaviour in response to verbal reasoning.

10.3.1 CLASSICAL CONDITIONING

Classical conditioning is best known and illustrated by the work of Pavlov and his dogs. Dogs have a normal reflex to salivate when food is presented. Food is therefore an **unconditioned stimulus** and salivation is an **unconditioned response** because it occurs naturally without learning. Pavlov noticed that his dogs began to salivate at other times, such as when he entered the room, because they had learned that he was associated with being fed. Pavlov formally demonstrated classical conditioning by ringing a bell just before feeding the dogs. The bell was initially a **neutral stimulus** because it was not associated with food and did not produce salivation. However, after a short while the dogs began to salivate when they heard the bell. The bell had therefore become a **conditioned stimulus** and salivation to the bell a **conditioned response** because the dogs had learned the association between the bell and food.

Many other characteristics of classical conditioning have been identified. For example, the *nature of the stimulus* is important, as some stimuli are more easily conditioned than others. Novel food or drinks are more readily associated with physical symptoms such as nausea. This is probably due to biological mechanisms that encourage learning in situations that may be dangerous – in this case to prevent us eating poisonous foods. Therefore, if a novel food is associated with illness or vomiting most of us will develop an aversion to that food.

ACTIVITY 10.2

- Is there a food that you particularly dislike and will not eat? What learning processes do you think this might be due to?

The *order and timing of the stimulus* will also determine whether conditioning takes place. The neutral stimulus (e.g. a bell) must be presented very shortly (e.g. half a second) before the unconditioned stimulus (e.g. the food) for conditioning to occur. If it is presented afterwards very little or no conditioning will take place.

Finally, conditioning can be blocked or unlearned. Once classical conditioning has occurred then attempts to condition a third stimulus can be blocked. In other words, once dogs learn that the bell predicts food they will not always respond if a third stimulus is introduced, such as a flashing light, but may continue to rely on the bell. Conditioning can be *extinguished* or undone by presenting the conditioned stimulus repeatedly without the unconditioned stimulus.

Classical conditioning and physical symptoms

Many physical responses can be classically conditioned, including immune and neuroendocrine responses (Figure 10.5), allergy symptoms, and nausea. Classical conditioning is therefore highly relevant to medicine and occurs in many clinical situations, especially where illness or treatment involves pain or other adverse symptoms. The sights, sounds, or smells associated with hospitals may induce physical and emotional responses such as anxiety, or nausea. A good example of classical conditioning involves chemotherapy because cytotoxic drugs can often have strong side effects such as nausea and vomiting. After the first one or two sessions, up to 30 per cent of chemotherapy patients will experience anticipatory nausea and vomiting when they return for subsequent sessions (Stockhorst et al., 2006). This is because some aspect of the hospital environment has become associated with symptoms of nausea and vomiting. Thus when patients are re-exposed to the hospital stimulus associated with chemotherapy they will feel nauseous or vomit.

Our understanding of classical conditioning can be used to reduce symptoms or induce positive physical responses. For example, we know that physical symptoms are more easily conditioned in response to novel food or liquid. We also know that once conditioning has occurred it can block a third stimulus becoming conditioned. Research has confirmed that giving chemotherapy patients a novel drink before each chemotherapy infusion prevents anticipatory nausea and even shortens the time that nausea is experienced during chemotherapy because they associate nausea with the drink and not the hospital context (Stockhorst et al., 1998). This has also been demonstrated with allergy symptoms. If people are given a novel drink just before taking antihistamine drugs for five days, the drink alone will start to trigger the same drop in basophil activity and improvement in symptoms as the antihistamine drug (Goebel et al., 2008). Classical conditioning therefore plays an important role in placebo effects (see Chapter 4) and may underpin many of the effects of alternative therapies.

Classical conditioning and psychological problems

Classical conditioning can be involved in the development of psychological problems such as phobias. A traumatic experience can lead to a particular object becoming associated with severe anxiety and fear. Subsequent exposure to this object can then trigger severe anxiety and, if the person then avoids the object, a phobia may develop. An example of this is needle phobia which usually develops following a negative experience of an injection or blood test. To treat phobias we need to extinguish the learned association by exposing the person to the

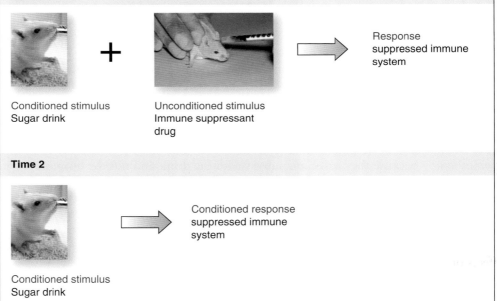

Decreasing and enhancing the immune function using classical conditioning

The immune system can be conditioned using classical conditioning to decrease or improve the immune function with a previously neutral stimulus. Studies typically pair a drug that suppresses or enhances the immune system with a new taste, such as saccharin, then re-administer the saccharin at a later date without the immune altering drug, to see if the immune function is affected.

The immune system can be suppressed or enhanced in this way through classical conditioning, although the effects are small (Ader, 2003). Research in humans has shown a similar conditioning of symptoms, such as anticipatory nausea before chemotherapy.

Time 1

Conditioned stimulus
Sugar drink

+

Unconditioned stimulus
Immune suppressant drug

→ Response
suppressed immune system

Time 2

Conditioned stimulus
Sugar drink

→ Conditioned response
suppressed immune system

FIGURE 10.5 Classical conditioning and placebo

Photograph of mouse drinking reproduced courtesy of © Edstrom. Photograph of mouse being injected reproduced courtesy of the Comparative Biology Centre, Newcastle University object whilst reducing or minimising the conditioned response. This is usually done through flooding or systematic desensitisation, which are based on the fact that strong anxiety responses cannot be sustained indefinitely. **Flooding** therefore involves exposing a person to the feared stimulus for a long enough time so that their anxiety reduces and the association between the stimulus and anxiety is extinguished. However, this is very hard for people with phobias to accomplish because it is an extreme way to face their fear.

Systematic desensitisation is a more gradual procedure where people are taught relaxation techniques and gradually exposed to stronger versions of the feared object or situation. For example, a person with a needle phobia might be asked to imagine a needle whilst relaxing. Once they are relaxed in this situation they might repeat it whilst looking at a picture of a needle, then a real needle, then perhaps a nurse giving someone else an injection. Thus they can learn to relax when exposed to the feared stimulus and the association is gradually extinguished. Research shows both flooding and systematic desensitisation are highly effective treatments for phobias (Wolitzky-Taylor et al., 2008). Advances in technology also mean virtual reality programmes can be used for simulated exposure treatments.

10.3.2 OPERANT CONDITIONING

Operant conditioning is learning from the consequences of our behaviour and reinforcement. In operant conditioning, behaviour is shaped by whether it results in positive reinforcement (e.g. a reward) or negative reinforcement (e.g. a punishment). In particular, behaviour is very quickly learned if it is followed by **positive reinforcement** such as food or praise. **Primary reinforcers** are those needed for survival, such as water, food, sleep, and sex. **Secondary reinforcers** are those that acquire value through experience, such as money, praise, and attention. People's behaviour can therefore be 'shaped' by reinforcement. Different patterns of reinforcement are given in Box 10.2 and vary in effectiveness. Variable ratio patterns of reinforcement usually lead to the strongest responses and are hardest to extinguish. This may explain why gamblers often find it hard to stop. It also has repercussions for drug abuse treatment. For example, methadone blocks the positive effects of heroin, but if it is used intermittently and the drug user gets occasional highs from heroin they are on a variable ratio pattern of reinforcement and may find it even harder to stop.

BOX 10.2   Patterns of reinforcement

- Fixed ratio: behaviour is always rewarded after a fixed number of times (e.g. bonuses when you reach a target).
- Variable ratio: behaviour is usually rewarded after an average number of times but this varies (e.g. gambling).
- Fixed interval: behaviour is rewarded after a fixed time interval (e.g. once a week).
- Variable interval: behaviour is rewarded but at varying time intervals.

In contrast to positive reinforcement, **negative reinforcement** reduces or extinguishes behaviours. Negative reinforcement can occur in two ways. The first is if the behaviour results in the removal of an aversive stimulus. For example, taking drugs that relieve pain will reinforce the use of painkillers. This kind of reinforcement is highly relevant to avoidance or escape behaviours where people learn to avoid situations that hurt or make them anxious. The second form of negative reinforcement is **punishment** where the behaviour results in aversive consequences. Research has shown that punishment is much weaker than positive reinforcers and any effect of punishment is short-lived. In fact, it has been argued that punishment only suppresses a response, rather than leading to new learning. This may explain why a hangover is not enough to stop people drinking again! Given this knowledge, it is ironic that our society places so much emphasis on punishment, from disciplining children to our penal system (Eysenck, 2000).

Operant conditioning and medicine

Operant conditioning shows that to learn and improve at any task, including medicine, we need feedback on our performance – preferably immediately – and this feedback is most powerful if it is positive. Operant conditioning can be used by healthcare professionals to encourage adaptive behaviours and is particularly useful with children or people with cognitive impairments (see Case Study 10.1). Research with people with severe learning disabilities shows that behaviours such as destructive outbursts or refusing to eat can be changed very effectively by positively reinforcing an alternative behaviour (Petscher et al., 2009). Operant conditioning can also be useful for families caring for ill relatives. For example, chronic pain behaviours can be reinforced if families are overly sympathetic, or urge the patient to lie down or rest and do everything for them. Although the family may believe they are doing the right thing, in the long term it will lead to more pain behaviour. Hence, families need to learn to ignore pain behaviour and respond positively to non-pain behaviour.

10.3.3 MODELLING AND IMITATION

Social learning theory has shown that we also learn by observing and imitating others. In a series of famous experiments, Bandura showed that when children observed an adult being aggressive towards a life size doll they were more likely to do the same when playing with the doll (Bandura et al., 1961). Similarly, recent research has shown children who play violent video games have more aggressive behaviour, thoughts, emotions, cardiovascular arousal, and less helping behaviour (Anderson, 2004). However, social learning cannot account for all of our behaviour, because we do not imitate the behaviour of everyone we encounter. Social learning is more likely to take place if the person is seen to be rewarded, is high status (e.g. a teacher, a medical consultant), is similar to us (e.g. colleagues, family), or friendly (e.g. friends).

Modelling and imitation is an integral part of medical education where students will learn from observing and (selectively) imitating the behaviour of senior staff. Positive role models can be used in other settings to promote positive behaviours, such as national health promotion campaigns, patient support groups, and helping people prepare for surgery. The importance in health promotion of using models that are perceived as similar or relevant is illustrated by the anti-smoking campaign in Chapter 19 (see Figure 19.3).

CASE STUDY 10.1   Conditioning and paediatric pain

How could you use conditioning to help?

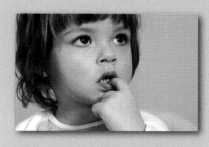

Jessica is a 3 year old girl who has third degree burns to her legs. She needs physiotherapy and must wear uncomfortable splints on her legs. Treatment is not progressing because Jessica gets increasingly upset until therapy is stopped. Her mother tries to comfort her but finds it very difficult and is starting to question whether therapy is really necessary.

The physiotherapist sometimes tries offering Jessica sweets to pacify her but she seems to be getting worse rather than better. When Jessica is put into bed she struggles until she has removed the splints. If she can't get them off her crying intensifies to the point of screaming and she remains sobbing well into her sleeping time until she falls asleep or staff come and distract her.

Jessica has learned that the more she cries and struggles the more likely it is that:

- Her mum will cuddle her.
- She will be offered sweets.
- The splints will be removed.
- The physiotherapy will stop.
- Staff will come and distract her.

Some of these reinforcements are occasional so these may be a variable ratio pattern of reinforcement which leads to the strongest responses and is hard to extinguish.

To help Jessica we need to stop reinforcing the negative behaviour and positively reinforce the behaviour that helps her recover. This could include:

- Star charts, praise, and treats to reward her when she keeps her splint on for a period of time, does physiotherapy exercises, etc.
- Preventing distress by using distraction and encouragement at critical times (e.g. the beginning of physiotherapy and bedtime) can also help.
- Teaching her ways to relax or cope during physiotherapy or when in bed that may reduce the pain felt.
- Ignoring the distress as much as possible and using a decreasing schedule of contact. For example, when she first cries in bed a staff member might check her and with minimal words or contact tell her it is OK and she must keep the splint on. Jessica could then be left for increasingly longer intervals with minimal or decreasing interaction at each point. The splints must be put back on if she removes them.
- Physiotherapy should not be ended because of Jessica's distress. However, this needs to be managed sensitively. It might help to reduce the length of physiotherapy initially to help Jessica to cope with this, then gradually increase it.

Photograph © Renata Osinska/ www.photxpress.com

Summary

- Associative learning occurs when we learn the relationship between two events that happen together.
- Classical conditioning occurs where a neutral stimulus (e.g. a bell) is paired with an unconditioned stimulus (e.g. food) to produce a conditioned response (e.g. salivation to the bell).
- Physical responses can be classically conditioned – including immune and neuroendocrine responses, allergy symptoms, and nausea.
- Classical conditioning can be used to create placebo effects and may underpin the effects of alternative therapies.
- Phobias can be a result of classical conditioning and are treated using extinguishing methods i.e. flooding or systematic desensitisation.
- Operant conditioning occurs when we learn through the consequences of our behaviour – namely positive or negative reinforcement.
- Positive reinforcement is an effective way to encourage adaptive behaviour in patients.
- Modelling and imitation can also influence behaviour, but people are selective in whose and what behaviour they imitate.

10.4 MEMORY

How and why we remember things affects every aspect of our lives from day-to-day functioning to exam performance. The importance of memory is most apparent in the devastating impact of disorders such as dementia and amnesia. Understanding memory processes can help us improve our own memory and also the way we give information to patients so they are more likely to remember it. Research suggests patients will immediately forget around 50 per cent of information they are told by their doctors (Kessels, 2003). In this section we shall look at the basic organisation and characteristics of memory and the relevance of this to medicine – namely effective revision techniques and clinical applications.

10.4.1 ORGANISATION AND CHARACTERISTICS OF MEMORY

Learning and memory involve three stages of encoding, storage and retrieval. **Encoding** takes place when the stimuli are presented and memory traces are created. **Storage** involves memory stores where information is organised and stored. **Retrieval** involves how we access and recall stored information. Memory problems can occur at any of these stages – information can be encoded wrongly (or not at all), storage may be partial or retrieval may fail.

Memory is thought to be broadly structured as shown in Figure 10.3. Initially, information is held in sensory buffers. Some of this information is then processed by our short-term memory and the relevant or learned information will go on to be stored in our long-term memory.

The **short-term** or **working memory** is used to manipulate and temporarily hold incoming information. Examples of using our working memory are when first learning a patient's history, making a diagnosis, or calculating drug dosages. The working memory has visual and auditory components, both with a limited capacity. For example, the auditory loop will usually only hold as many words as we can read aloud in two seconds. This is consistent with early research that established the average short-term memory span is 7±2 pieces of information (Miller, 1956). However, if the information has meaning or is chunked together our memory span can be significantly increased. An everyday example of this is chunking telephone numbers. It is much easier to remember 0800-234-145 than 0-8-0-0-2-3-4-1-4-5.

Other characteristics of working memory are primacy and recency effects. The **recency effect** means people are most likely to remember information that has been most recently presented, such as the last few words on a list. This is probably because this information is most accessible in our working memory. The **primacy effect** means people are more likely to remember items at the beginning of a list compared to the middle. This is probably because of the extra time they have had to rehearse these items. Thus, when giving information to patients we need to present the most important information first and last and chunk information so more is remembered.

The **long-term memory** holds information for future retrieval and is dependent upon the formation of associations between nodes when information is active in our working memory. Different types of long-term memory are shown in Figure 10.6 and many theories have been put forward about how long-term memory stores work. The known characteristics of our long-term memory are shown in Box 10.3.

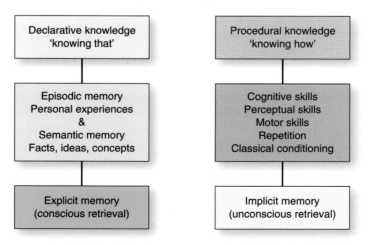

FIGURE 10.6 Long-term memory stores (adapted from Eysenck, 2000)

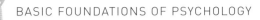

BOX 10.3   Characteristics of memory

- Distinctiveness: distinctive or unique information is more likely to be remembered.
- Elaboration and processing: if information is elaborated in terms of meaning it will be processed more deeply and remembered better.
- Categorisation: information is stored in semantic categories e.g. animals, food, people, which influences how quickly new information is processed and recognised.
- Spacing and chunking: chunking information increases the amount that can be learned and spacing out learning over time improves memory and retrieval.
- Construction of memories: memories are actively constructed and can be influenced by subsequent events e.g. eyewitnesses' memory is notoriously subject to distortion.
- Context dependent: memories are associated with the context in which they were encoded – this includes environment and mood. Retrieval is therefore better in the context it was first encoded in.
- Power of retrieval: the more information is retrieved the better it is remembered – probably because the neural trace is strengthened.

10.4.2 MEMORY AND STUDYING MEDICINE

It is peculiar, given what we know about memory, that many students do not revise effectively. With a few rare exceptions, studies of people with an outstanding memory have shown it is down to practice and using strategies, such as mnemonics, rather than being innately gifted. Memory is improved through:

- Meaningful encoding – e.g. relating information to knowledge you already have.
- Structured retrieval – e.g. adding as many different cues as possible to the information to help retrieval.
- Practice – to make memory processing quick and automatic (Chase and Ericsson, 1982).

Successful encoding of information involves concentrating on understanding the meaning rather than learning things by rote. Elaborating and organising information means it is processed more deeply and integrated into existing knowledge. Effective revision strategies include summarising your notes and reorganising the information into different categories, thinking about connections between new information and the things you already know, finding personal relevance or a connection, adding visual images or drawing diagrams or mind maps. Encoding is better if it is spaced out rather than crammed into one long session. Research clearly shows that spacing learning over time results in better memory and retrieval (Esgate and Groome, 2005). The most effective strategy is to gradually increase the time between each session.

Using visual imagery can increase our learning because it means both the auditory and visual aspects of our working memory are being used; and it adds further associations in the long-term memory. Visual imagery has been shown to increase memory performance, particularly if objects are pictured together (Esgate and Groome, 2005). For example, if you have to remember to get a suture kit, a sandwich and patient records for Mr Smith you might visualise Mr Smith with a sandwich that has been sutured up balancing on his head. This is a visual mnemonic. **Mnemonics** are strategies that can help you remember lists of information that have little connection or meaning. Mnemonics are effective at increasing memory and are widely used in medical education for things like the cranial nerves or how to perform examinations for pain (see Clinical Notes 10.1).

CLINICAL NOTES 10.1

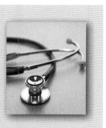

SOCRATES examination for pain

- Site – where is the pain?
- Onset – when did the pain start; was the onset sudden or gradual?
- Character – what is the pain like?
- Radiation – does the pain radiate anywhere else?
- Associations – any other signs or symptoms associated with the pain?
- Time course – does the pain have a pattern over time?
- Exacerbating/relieving factors – does anything help the pain? Make it worse?
- Severity – how bad is the pain?

Research has shown that medical students who use strategies like these to improve their revision and memory do better in exams (Lahtinen et al., 1997). In particular, summarising notes and drawing mind maps are very effective. If you want to find out more about how to improve your revision technique see the Further Reading at the end of this chapter.

Retrieval in exams can be improved using the characteristics of memory previously outlined (see Box 10.3). First, the more times you retrieve a piece of information the more you will remember it. Therefore doing practice exams, testing yourself and others, or talking about topics are all good strategies to help remember information better. Second, memory is context-dependent. In other words, you are more likely to remember information if the context in which you learned it and then recall it remains the same. Therefore, try to revise under exam conditions. If you get writers' block in an exam, try imagining yourself in the lecture theatre or the place where you revised. Focus on cues such as what was around you, the PowerPoint slides, the paper you wrote on, books, etc. This can help retrieve the information you need.

CLINICAL NOTES 10.2

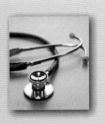

How to revise effectively for exams

- Summarise lecture notes and draw diagrams or mind maps.
- Concentrate on the meaning of the information rather than rote learning.
- Elaborate information as much as possible – how does it fit with what you already know? How does it relate to your personal experience? How could you use it clinically?
- Chunk information into meaningful groups or categories.
- Use mnemonics to remember lists – distinctive mnemonics are more easily remembered.
- Space out your learning – do not cram revision into one long session.
- Recall the information regularly through testing yourself and doing mock exam papers.
- Work with other people in revision groups where you can explain or discuss different topics.
- If you are stuck in exams, think back to the context in which you learned the information.
- Useful websites include www.medicalmnemonics.com and www.medicalfinals.co.uk

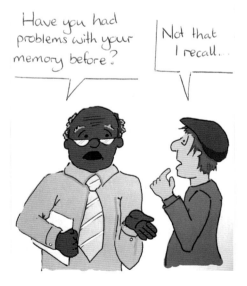

Clinical applications

There are many clinical applications of understanding memory, not least in trying to treat memory disorders such as Alzheimer's disease, or understanding why most of us have amnesia for the first two to three years of our life. Particularly vivid memories are commonly reported by people after shocking or extreme events, such as traumatic events, car accidents, and a myocardial infarction (Tedstone and Tarrier, 2003). These 'flashbulb' memories will usually occur in response to events that involve strong emotion. Re-experiencing these memories through flashbacks can be a symptom of PTSD. Research has shown that in situations of strong emotion people tend to remember emotions at the expense of facts. For example, if a doctor appears worried patients may well think the situation is more severe, become more anxious themselves, and remember fewer facts from the consultation (Shapiro et al., 1992).

The most common clinical situation where memory is important is giving information to patients. From our understanding of memory and other cognitive processes in this chapter there are a number of things we can do to improve the likelihood a patient will remember what we tell them (see Clinical Notes 10.3). It also helps to avoid distractions, use written and visual information aids, ask patients to say in their own words what they have been told, correct any inaccuracies, and to be aware of the impact of emotions on the consultation (Watson and McKinstry, 2009).

CLINICAL NOTES 10.3

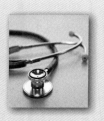

Giving information to patients

- Put important information first and last.
- Emphasise the information that is important.
- Chunk information into meaningful groups or categories.
- Make the categorisation explicit e.g. 'Now I am going to tell you: what is wrong with you, what tests are needed, and what you must do'.
- Use repetition.
- Make the information salient to the person.
- Use simple words and short sentences.
- Be specific.
- Avoid overloading people by giving them too much information (Ley, 1997).

Summary

- Learning and memory involve three stages of encoding, storage, and retrieval.
- Memory involves sensory buffers, the short-term or working memory, and long-term memory stores.
- The short-term or working memory manipulates and temporarily holds incoming information.
- The long-term memory stores hold information for future retrieval.
- Memory is improved through meaningful encoding, structured retrieval, and practice.
- The characteristics of memory can be used to improve revision techniques and memory performance.
- Memory is context dependent – this includes the physical and emotional context.
- We should use our understanding of memory to give information to patients in ways that make it more likely they will remember it.

📖 FURTHER READING

Ayers, S. et al. (eds) (2007) *Cambridge Handbook of Psychology, Health and Medicine* (2nd edition). Cambridge: Cambridge University Press. Includes short chapters on cognitive dysfunction in specific disorders including dyslexia, dementias, amnesia, aphasia, head injury, and stroke.

Esgate, A. & Groome, D. (2005) *An Introduction to Applied Cognitive Psychology*. Hove: Psychology Press. An introduction to how cognitive theory and evidence relate to things like everyday memory, biological cycles, performance, and decision making.

Herrmann, D., Raybeck, D. & Gruneberg, M. (2002) *Improving Memory and Study Skills: Advances in Theory and Practice*. Ashland, OH: Hogrefe & Huber. A book on study skills based on memory research and evidence.

❓ REVISION QUESTIONS

1   What is a perceptual set? Discuss the evidence for three factors that influence our perceptual set.

2   How do we learn skills? Outline the three stages involved in learning skills.

3   Discuss the conditions under which people can multitask. What are the implications of these for clinical practice?

4   Discuss two biases of attention and their implications for clinical practice.

5   What is classical conditioning? How can it be used to create a placebo effect?

6   Describe operant conditioning. What are the most effective forms of reinforcement?

7   Describe modelling and imitation and the three characteristics that make it more likely children will imitate someone's behaviour.

8   What are (a) short-term and (b) long-term memory? What characteristics do they possess?

9   Discuss five techniques from our understanding of memory that should be used when giving information to patients.

10   How can our understanding of memory help improve revision techniques and memory performance?

11 IMMUNITY AND PROTECTION

LEARNING OBJECTIVES

This chapter is designed to enable you to:

- Understand the effect of stress and emotion on the immune system.
- Describe the role of psychological factors in immune disorders.
- Describe aspects of psycho-dermatology.
- Outline the psychosocial risk factors for cancer.
- Explain how psychological factors might affect the progression of cancer.

Do you get sick around exam time? Your greater susceptibility to infections at such times may be related to inadequate sleep, a lack of exercise, a poor diet, and may also be affected by stress. Links between emotions and health have long formed a part of medical thinking. Pre-modern medical thought, for example, was based on the beliefs that optimal health depended on a balance of the four humours (blood, yellow bile, black bile, phlegm) and that imbalances influenced disease and behaviour. For example, the depressive melancholic personality is named after the Latin words for black bile.

Our understanding of disease is now very different but modern medicine continues to find evidence of intricate links between psychological and physical wellbeing. In a classic early study, Ishigami (1919) found decreased phagocyte function among people with tuberculosis when they were emotionally agitated. Since then, our understanding of the links between psychological states and immune function has increased. Over the same period, there has been increasing evidence of pathogenic involvement in diseases previously not thought to involve the immune system (e.g. *Helicobacter pylori* infection is often implicated in peptic ulcers and myocardial infarctions) (see Chapters 12 and 13).

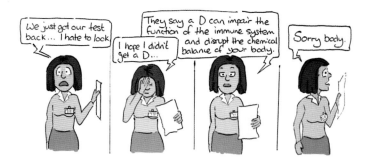

Psychoneuroimmunology (**PNI**) examines how psychological states affect our immune function. Although most PNI research has focused on negative psychological states such as stress and depression, recent research has examined the beneficial effects of positive moods. In this chapter we shall first look at the effect of psychological factors on the immune system and immune disorders. The next section looks at our main protective organ – the skin. Finally, the large body of knowledge on psychosocial factors and cancer is examined as an illustration of how immune impairment can ultimately lead to disease.

11.1 INFECTION, INFLAMMATION, AND IMMUNITY

The presence of protein molecules called antigens on the surface of each cell allows the immune system to distinguish body cells from potentially harmful foreign cells.

There are two broad types of barriers to infection – non-specific and specific. The non-specific barriers include mucous membranes, which destroy many foreign microorganisms and phagocytes, which consume and destroy foreign microorganisms and debris.

The specific immune barriers involve the action of specialised white blood cells called lymphocytes. There are two components to this type of immune response. The **cell-mediated immune response** begins when a macrophage ingests a foreign microorganism and then displays the mircoorganism's antigens on its surface. T lymphocytes with a receptor for the foreign antigen bind to the macrophage and create more T lymphocytes with the specific receptor. These T lymphocytes then bind to and destroy all foreign microorganisms with the specific antigen and all the cells that have been infected by it.

The **antibody-mediated immune response** begins when a B lymphocyte binds to foreign microorganisms for which it has the appropriate antigen receptor. This binding causes the B lymphocyte to multiply and produce copies of its receptor molecules called antibodies, which then bind to cells with foreign antigens and destroy or deactivate them.

11.1.1 STRESS AND IMMUNE FUNCTION

Stress has measurable effects on our immune function, susceptibility to infections, severity of infections, response to vaccinations, and wound healing (Glaser and Kiecolt-Glaser, 2005; Segerstrom and Miller, 2004; Zorrilla et al., 2001). Whether these effects are beneficial or detrimental is determined by the duration of stress.

Acute stress produces improvements in the immune function – particularly non-specific barriers – with this reverting to normal levels fairly quickly after the stressor ends (Bachen et al., 2007). Thus, stressful events such as public speaking or an athletic competition may temporarily enhance our immune function. If threats are brief stressors that invoke the fight-or-flight response, there is evidence of the body preparing adaptively to deal with potential infection and/or injury arising from that threat. The immune response to stress is affected by activation of the sympathetic nervous system and hypothalamic-pituitary-adrenal axis (see Chapter 3). There is a complex interplay between the nervous, endocrine, and immune systems so it is difficult to determine which factors are more or less important. The sympathetic nervous system increases immune system activity, particularly large granular lymphocyte activity such as natural killer cells. However, the HPA axis suppresses some immune activity through the production of cortisol, which has an anti-inflammatory effect and reduces both the number of white blood cells and the release of cytokines.

Chronic stress tends to impair our immune function. Chronic stress can arise from various causes e.g. work, unemployment, difficult relationships, caring for sick relatives. More severe and longer lasting stressors are associated with more global immunosuppression – initially in our cell-mediated immunity and then across the spectrum of immune

functions. Immune down-regulation associated with prolonged stress can lead to impaired wound healing, poorer responses to infectious diseases, autoimmune diseases, and the progression of cancer (Kiecolt-Glaser et al., 2002a).

A different pattern can be seen in people who have been exposed to traumatic events, such as natural disasters, war or terrorism, particularly those who also develop symptoms of post-traumatic stress disorder (PTSD). In these instances, exposure to a severely traumatic event is associated with increased immune measures such as antibodies, lymphocytes, interleukins, and natural killer cell activity which may persist many years after the traumatic event. Thus it appears that trauma and PTSD are associated with a long-term enhanced immunity. This is an intriguing contrast to the effect of chronic stress and other negative affects (e.g. depression): it may be explained by the observation that PTSD leads to a dysregulation of the HPA axis and reduced cortisol responses (Bachen et al., 2007). Paradoxically, despite an enhanced immune function, people with PTSD report increased symptoms of illness and greater use of medical services (Ramchand et al., 2008).

Substantial evidence of the effect of stress on the immune system has led to interest in whether interventions that alleviate stress can counter the stress-related suppression of immune function. There is some evidence that emotional disclosure (e.g. writing about negative emotions and experiences), hypnosis, and conditioning are effective at producing positive changes in our immune function (Miller and Cohen, 2000). The evidence for the efficacy of stress-management or relaxation programmes, however, is less convincing. It should be noted that many studies involve small samples from specific groups of people. Therefore, in addition to developing more effective approaches to stress management, there is a need to conduct trials which will allow for valid statistical conclusions and generalisations to be made.

11.1.2 EMOTIONS AND IMMUNE FUNCTION

Negative emotions

Negative emotions like depression are associated with impaired immune function (Herbert and Cohen, 1993; Kiecolt-Glaser and Glaser, 2002b). The effect of negative emotions on the immune system may be the common pathway between negative emotions and illnesses such as cardiovascular disease, rheumatoid arthritis, Type 1 diabetes, and some cancers. There is substantial evidence that negative emotions are associated with a dysregulation of the immune system, an increased susceptibility to infections, and slower wound healing.

Depression is associated with several changes in the immune function (see Box 11.1) as well as changes in clinical outcomes. For example, depressive symptoms have been linked with the more rapid progression of disease among people with HIV/AIDS (Leserman, 2008), cancer (Speigel and Giese-Davis, 2003), and heart disease (Chapter 12). However, not all studies find the same results. It must also be acknowledged that the links between depression and impaired immune function may be influenced by unhealthy behaviours among depressed people, including poorer adherence to treatment (DiMatteo et al., 2000).

ACTIVITY 11.1

- The last time you were ill, what was the relationship between your physical symptoms and emotions?
- Do you think one caused the other, that they influenced each other, or that they were separate?

BOX 11.1 Changes in immune function related to depression

- Lower total numbers of lymphocytes.
- Reduced proliferation of lymphocytes in response to mitogens that usually promote lymphocyte production.
- Reductions in the numbers and functioning of natural killer cells.
- Increased CD4/CD8 ratios.
- Changes in pro-inflammatory cytokines.
- Increases in interleukin-6 (an important mediator of fever and inflammation).

Given the association between depression and immune function, it is not surprising that psychotherapy for depression can also affect the course of immune disorders. Moreover, interventions that improve psychological wellbeing can lead to improvements in endocrine function and immune status (Antoni et al., 2006; Carrico and Antoni, 2008).

Positive emotions

There is emerging evidence that positive moods and personalities are associated with enhanced immune function (Barak, 2006). For example, optimism, emotional expressiveness, and extraversion are associated with greater numbers of helper T lymphocytes and greater natural killer cell cytotoxicity (Segerstrom et al., 1998). Such results suggest our mood may be an important moderator of the links between stress and immune function. Whereas some studies have examined optimism as a dispositional characteristic of individuals, other studies have examined the effect of positive psychological experiences. For example, watching humorous films produces significant improvements in several parameters of immune function (Berk et al., 2001). Some of these effects may last for several hours.

Whereas hundreds of studies have examined the effects on our immune function of negative psychological states (allowing for the publication of meta-analyses), fewer studies have examined the links between positive emotions and immune function. It is therefore more difficult to be sure about the immune benefits of positive moods and positive experiences. More research is required to determine the causal mechanisms through which positive moods might affect immunity. However, some studies have made interesting comparisons of the effects of positive and negative moods (see Research Box 11.1).

RESEARCH BOX 11.1   Positive and negative emotions and immune function

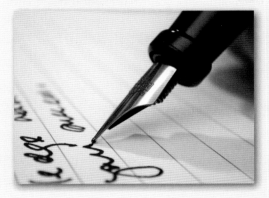

Background

The aim of this study was to examine how day-to-day changes in psychological states could affect our immune function.

Methods and results

96 healthy married men completed a diary of daily events and emotions for three months. On each day, participants indicated their experience of various emotions provided on a checklist (e.g. determined, distressed, inspired, irritable, nervous, upset).

They also indicated their daily experience of a range of positive and negative events in various domains (e.g. work, friends, household, activities, finances). The men's reports were corroborated with those of their wives. Responses to an orally ingested pathogen were recorded via an analysis of daily-collected saliva samples.

Production of antibodies to the orally ingested antigen was higher on days when men reported more positive moods and lower on days when they reported more negative moods. The strongest positive immune effects were found for experiences of desirable leisure and household events. The strongest negative effects were found for undesirable work events. There was some evidence that positive experiences and moods had longer-lasting effects than negative experiences.

Significance

This study demonstrates that positive and negative experiences and emotions have opposite effects on immune function. The study shows that daily variations in affect have observable effects on the single immune parameter that was assessed. In the years since this study, more evidence has accrued to support these findings, although more research is required to provide a fuller understanding of the mechanisms involved.

Photograph © Lim Jerry/Fotolia

Stone, A.A. et al. (1994) Daily events are associated with a secretory immune response to an oral antigen in men, *Health Psychology*, *13*: 440–446.

11.1.3 IMMUNISATIONS

Immunisations are an important part of tackling disease and promoting health in our society. Immunisations prime the immune system to respond to a disease by giving a small,

usually disabled, form of the virus or bacteria. The ability of vaccines to protect against the disease depends on the strength of the immune response to the vaccine. Given the relationship between stress and immune functioning, it is perhaps not surprising that people who are stressed, upset, or anxious will have weaker, delayed, or less lasting responses to vaccines (Glaser and Kiecolt-Glaser, 2005).

In recent years there has been some controversy over vaccines for young children, and this has led to reduced uptake: for example, the uptake of measles/mumps/rubella (MMR) immunisation has fallen to below 70 per cent in some areas. Whether parents decide to immunise their child is determined by beliefs about the perceived risks associated with the disease and with vaccination. Parents are less likely to immunise children if they perceive dangers associated with the vaccine, have doubts the vaccine will be effective, believe they can protect their children from exposure, or think their children are unlikely to catch the disease (Sturm et al., 2005).

Vaccinations and other medical procedures involving needles can cause substantial anxiety and distress in children, adolescents, and some adults. Many children and parents consider needle-procedures to be one of the most traumatic experiences of hospitalisation (Cordoni and Cordoni, 2001). Needle-related distress and anxiety has adverse short- and long-term psychological effects, including anticipatory nausea, insomnia, eating problems, PTSD, and avoidance behaviour (Kennedy et al., 2008; Young, 2005). Furthermore, needle-related distress can escalate with successive procedures. Effective management of needle distress in children is therefore critical. Pharmacological management involves analgesics during or after the injection, which can be topical (applied to the skin) or oral. However, the use of such methods by healthcare professionals is variable.

Parents and healthcare professionals have a strong influence on children's distress during needle procedures. Perhaps counter-intuitively, being empathic, reassuring, or critical is associated with increased distress in children. Conversely, using humour, talking about other things, and instructing the child to cope by using distraction or other adaptive means are associated with decreased distress (Mahoney et al., 2010).

11.2 PSYCHOLOGICAL ASPECTS OF IMMUNE DISORDERS

So far we have focused on how psychological states can affect immune function. Of course, the reverse is also true: changes in immune function can lead to changes in psychological wellbeing. We all know that when we have a cold our mood can also be affected. In the case of more serious and/or chronic infections, the psychological consequences can be more severe. Research indicates that rates of depression are higher among adults and children with chronic illnesses (Bennett, 1994; Dickens et al., 2002). In general, self-reported quality of life also tends to be lower among people with chronic autoimmune diseases (e.g., Cohen, 2002). Such experiences of depression, stress, and anxiety resulting from disease may in turn impair the immune function.

Autoimmune diseases occur when the body's immune system mistakenly identifies self-cells as foreign cells and mounts an immune response against initially healthy tissues.

Some examples of autoimmune diseases are given below. Others include coeliac disease and lupus erythematosus. The mechanisms involved in many immune diseases are not fully understood. Thus, patients may have no hope of a cure, and must adjust physically and psychologically to the long-term management of symptoms (see Chapter 6).

Rheumatoid arthritis is a chronic systemic inflammatory autoimmune disorder which can affect many tissues and organs, but principally attacks the synovial lining of joints. There is no known cure for rheumatoid arthritis, but different treatments may be used to alleviate symptoms including pain, and/or to try to prevent future joint destruction. People with rheumatoid arthritis are more likely than healthy controls to report anxiety and depression (Pincus et al., 1996). Longitudinal research indicates that greater anxiety and depression lead to increased perceptions of pain, and higher levels of pain and/or disability in turn predict higher levels of distress. These findings suggest a reciprocal relationship between psychological wellbeing and experiences of pain or disability (Odegård et al., 2007).

There is a paradox in the role of stress in inflammatory diseases like rheumatoid arthritis. Physical responses to stress involving the HPA axis and autonomic nervous system can play a vital role in inflammation. As we have seen, the release of cortisol via the HPA axis should reduce inflammation. Thus, in theory, stress should improve the symptoms of rheumatoid arthritis. However, stress actually results in worse immunological markers, physical symptoms, and disability (Geenen et al., 2006). This seems to be due to a physical hyporesponsiveness to stress: people with rheumatoid arthritis have consistently reduced autonomic nervous system responses to stressful events. HPA responses to stress will also appear blunted and out of proportion to corresponding immune activity. It is not clear whether these altered stress responses predate the onset of rheumatoid arthritis, or are due to a past experience of stress or the physical deconditioning accompanying disease (Capellino and Straub, 2008; Geenen et al., 2006).

Type 1 diabetes mellitus (also called insulin-dependent diabetes mellitus; **IDDM**) is an autoimmune disease in which the insulin-producing cells of the pancreas are destroyed by an inappropriate immune response. As a result, the body is unable to regulate blood sugar levels. There is no known cure for IDDM, and patients must use insulin replacement therapy to avoid potentially fatal diabetic ketoacidosis. Among people with diabetes, hyperglycaemia resulting from poor glycaemic control is linked to depression, however neither the direction of causation nor causal mechanisms linking depression and hyperglycaemia are known (Lustman et al., 2000). A synthesis of published research has revealed that experience of diabetes-related complications, including retinopathy, neuropathy, renal disease, coronary artery disease and sexual dysfunction, is associated with depressive symptoms (de Groot et al., 2001). It is important to address the psychological wellbeing of people with diabetes because those with more depressive symptoms have a poorer compliance with medication regimens, poorer diets, and greater functional impairment (Ciechanowski et al., 2000).

Unlike the autoimmune diseases discussed above, **HIV/AIDS** is an acquired immune deficiency. There is increasing evidence that the course and development of HIV/AIDS is affected by psychosocial factors such as stress, emotions, and support. Animal studies show that social stress can lead to quicker disease progression and death (e.g. Capitanio et al., 1998). Longitudinal studies of humans show that a faster progression to AIDS

occurs among men with higher stress levels and less support (Leserman et al., 1999). Depression is more common among people with HIV/AIDS than among the general population, probably because of the widespread impacts of the virus on patients' health and social lives (Ciesla and Roberts, 2001). HIV has profound and long-lasting impacts on health, work, finances, and sexual relationships (e.g. Dray-Spira et al., 2003; Ezzy et al., 1999). This affects how people experience their current health and wellbeing, and how they plan for the future (see Case Study 11.1). The net effect is that people with HIV/AIDS will tend to have a lower quality of life. However, it is important to note that interventions designed to treat depression among people with HIV/AIDS also result in better immune function, as indicated by a lower viral load (Antoni et al., 2006).

CASE STUDY 11.1   Living with HIV (adapted from Ezzy, 2000)

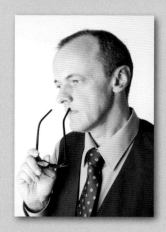

The following comes from an interview with Andrew, a 42 year old bisexual man who was diagnosed with HIV seven years before the interview.

HIV had had a marked influence on Andrew's plans for the future and the prospect of death affected every aspect of his life – especially his emotional wellbeing.

Before I found out I was HIV positive, I was determined to live forever – and live life accordingly. I had great expectations of making a bloody fortune with the company I was running.

As far as I was concerned the diagnosis meant I was dying. The drug choices were limited or none and I had no control over it.

It screwed up my emotional life, it screwed up my marriage, it screwed my work up because I was spending so much time dealing with the virus, I was facing death. I hadn't really thought about it before. I told my doctor at the time, so much for our wonderful technology when I've got a disease and I depend on you to deal with it and you can't.

Now I just live day to day because these drugs I'm on are not the answer. Resistance can develop, if I don't take these drugs strictly in accordance 100%, resistance develops fairly rapidly and I don't have too many options at this point in time.

I'm a person obviously living with a disease that our medical science can't deal with. And there's no prospect of them dealing with it in the foreseeable future in terms – even in fact as long as I live. However, long or short that may be. I've become very self-centered. I get angry very easily. I have a short fuse about just about anything.

Photograph © Coka / Fotolia

Summary

- Acute stress leads to enhanced immune responses, but chronic stress impairs immune functioning.
- Negative emotions, such as depression, are associated with reduced immune functioning.
- Conversely, positive emotions appear to have a positive effect on immune function.
- Immune disorders are associated with a reduced quality of life, increased anxiety, and increased depression.
- There is a reciprocal relationship between negative mood, pain, and disability.
- Some psychological interventions, such as disclosure and conditioning interventions, may result in improved immune function in disorders such as HIV/AIDS.

11.3 SKIN

The skin is a key protective organ that is made up of many layers of epithelial tissues. It protects the body against pathogens, insulates the body, prevents dehydration, and protects the internal organs, muscles, etc. against damage from external sources. The impact of psychological factors on skin has mainly been examined in relation to wound healing and skin disorders.

11.3.1 WOUND HEALING

Wound healing research typically carries out punch biopsies or suction blisters on volunteers and monitors immune activity and healing over time. It has consistently shown that stressed people heal 20–40 per cent slower than people who are not stressed, apparently because of an interaction between glucocorticoids (e.g. cortisol) and proinflammatory cytokines (Christian et al., 2007). For example, Marucha et al. (1998) made small punch biopsy wounds in students' oral hard palates: once during the summer vacation and once just before exams. In the exam period, students took 40 per cent longer for their wounds to heal and had 68 per cent less interleukin 1ß messenger RNA than during the vacation.

Wound healing is slower when we experience difficult circumstances, such as caring for chronically ill people or having relationship difficulties. However, wound healing is not only affected by stress. Wounds also heal slower in people who are depressed, anxious, or have poor anger control (Gouin et al., 2008). Positive factors that speed up wound healing include emotional disclosure, close personal relationships, and exercise (Emery et al., 2005). Psychological interventions such as writing about stressful or traumatic events can also lead to faster wound healing (see Chapter 6 and Research Box 2.1).

The prospective experimental design of wound healing studies makes it possible to establish a causal link between stress and healing. This is relevant to many areas of

medicine, but particularly surgery. There is substantial evidence that negative emotions such as fear and anxiety are associated with worse outcomes after surgery, including more post-operative distress, pain, use of analgesia, a longer hospital stay, and a slower return to normal functioning. Similarly, research shows that preparing people for surgery by providing more information, coping skills or relaxation techniques reduces distress and improves all the aspects of recovery mentioned above, in addition to other clinical and physical markers of recovery such as post-operative complications (Johnston and Vogele, 1993). This is therefore an area of medicine where psychological preparation has the potential to make a big difference to clinical outcomes.

CLINICAL NOTES 11.1

Immunity, vaccinations, and surgery

- Negative emotions are associated with a poorer immune function. This is especially important for people who have serious health conditions.
- It is therefore important to address negative emotions via appropriate psychosocial interventions.
- You can have a strong influence on children's distress during invasive procedures – use distraction, humour, and give them strategies to help them cope.
- Empathy, reassurance, and criticism are more likely to increase children's distress during invasive procedures.
- Wound healing is slower when people are stressed.
- Surgical outcomes are better if patients feel prepared for surgery and are relaxed. Anxiety and distress lead to worse outcomes.
- Give surgical patients as much information as they want, help them develop coping skills, and encourage them to use relaxation techniques.

11.3.2 SKIN DISORDERS

Psychological factors can affect the course of dermatological disorders in several ways. First, stress is associated with increased symptoms in disorders such as psoriasis, atopic dermatitis, alopecia areata, and urticaria (Picardi and Abeni, 2001). This is likely to be due to physiological mechanisms such as those detailed above and changes in behaviour that are also associated with stress, such as scratching and increased tobacco or alcohol use. Scratching can exacerbate symptoms and cause further skin damage and is usually a conditioned response (see Chapter 10). Early research showed that people with skin conditions such as eczema develop conditioned scratching responses more quickly. They are also slower to unlearn them than people without skin disorders (Robertson et al., 1975).

ACTIVITY 11.2

If scratching is a conditioned response, how might you go about reducing scratching behaviour in someone with eczema?

Second, people with various skin disorders have increased anxiety, depression, and dysfunctional coping strategies like avoidance. Approximately 30 per cent of dermatological outpatients report some form of impaired mental health (Picardi et al., 2000; Stangier and Ehlers, 2000). However, there is little prospective research into the causal relationship between negative emotions and symptoms of skin disorders. It is therefore difficult to know whether negative emotions make physical symptoms worse or whether physical symptoms cause people to become more anxious or depressed. The severity of skin disorders is not associated with the level of distress a person feels. Instead, distress and quality of life are more closely related to physical appearance, disfigurement, a fear of negative evaluation, and social stigma (O'Leary, 2007).

Psychological interventions can be very effective in the clinical management of skin disorders (Ehlers et al., 1995). Interventions draw on a variety of techniques such as education, relaxation training, biofeedback, cognitive restructuring, and social skills training to manage stigma (see section 6.2 and Chapter 19). The most important part of these interventions appears to be improving self control of scratching through habit-reversal training. This involves helping patients to:

- Recognise scratching cues or triggers.
- Interrupt and prevent the automatic scratching response.
- Use a competing response, such as relaxation, to reduce the itching sensation.

Providing relaxation techniques helps reduce stress and is a good substitute for scratching. Relaxation techniques include progressive muscle relaxation and using calming or healing imagery. Research shows that improving the self control of scratching and using relaxation techniques are both effective for reducing the symptoms of skin disorders (Stangier, 2007).

Summary

- Stress and negative emotions are associated with slower wound healing.
- Distress and anxiety are associated with poorer psychological and physical recovery from surgery.
- Stress is also associated with increased symptoms of skin disorders.
- Up to 30 per cent of dermatological outpatients report psychiatric symptoms, which are less influenced by the severity of the skin disorder than physical appearance, disfigurement, the fear of a negative evaluation, and social stigma.
- Psychological interventions add significantly to the effectiveness of clinical management of skin disorders, resulting in less psychiatric and physical symptoms.

BODY SYSTEMS

11.4 CANCER

There are over 100 different types of cancer and around one-third of us will have cancer at some point in our lives (Cancer Research UK, 2008). The development of cancerous tumours is a complex process dependent upon a cascade of events that is a bit like cellular anarchy. At least three different types of gene damage or mutation are necessary for cancer to develop. Cancer cells have to avoid the process of programmed death (apoptosis) that usually protects against the proliferation of abnormal cells. Normal cells have a fixed capacity of division and growth, but cancer cells manage to divide indefinitely. As the tumour grows, it requires nourishment and the removal of waste products, so it has to encourage blood vessel growth around it. The tumour also has to be able to invade other areas of the body. This requires the inactivation of a whole series of factors that will usually restrict cells to a specific site. In the later stages of the disease, cancer cells break off (metastasise) and migrate to other areas of the body.

Psycho-oncology examines (a) psychosocial risk factors that influence the development of cancer, (b) responses to cancer and (c) interventions for people with cancer. These are looked at in turn.

11.4.1 PSYCHOSOCIAL RISK FACTORS FOR CANCER

Cancers are often caused by the interplay between environmental factors such as toxins, viruses, and lifestyle, and internal factors such as genetic vulnerability and hormones. Psychosocial factors that influence cancer onset include:

- Demographic factors.
- Lifestyle and health behaviour.
- Social support.
- Coping and adjustment (see Section 11.2).

Demographic factors that influence cancer include ethnicity, country of residence, and socioeconomic status. For example, malignant melanoma (skin cancer) is more common in white people; breast cancer is common in Northern European and white American women but relatively rare in Asians; Japanese people are up to ten times more likely to get stomach cancer than white Americans or Europeans. Figure 11.1 shows the most common cancers for men and women living in different countries. For many cancers, people who have poor socio-economic status are more at risk, although this is not true for all cancers. For example, in England low socio-economic groups have higher rates of lung cancer and cervical cancer, but lower rates of melanoma or breast cancer (Shack et al., 2008).

The role of ethnicity, socio-economic status, and country of residence in cancer risk is often due to differences in lifestyle. For example, higher rates of stomach cancer in Japan are associated with the high salt content of the Japanese diet. If Japanese people move to the USA, their risk of stomach cancer decreases compared to people who remain in Japan but their risk of breast cancer increases (Keegan et al., 2007; Tsugane, 2005). Similarly, higher rates of melanoma in people from higher socio-economic groups may reflect the fact that they can afford holidays to sunny locations but do not properly protect their skin.

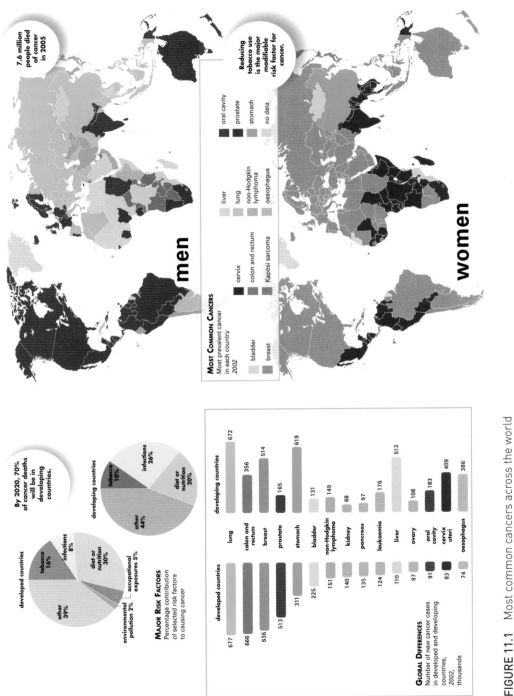

FIGURE 11.1 Most common cancers across the world

Reproduced from *The Atlas of Health*, by Diarmuid O'Donovan, "Most common cancers", pp. 44–45, Earthscan 2008. Copyright © 2008 Myriad Editions Ltd/ www.MyriadEditions.com

Lifestyle factors include *health behaviours* such as smoking, diet, exercise, and alcohol use. They also include *exposure to toxins or infections* such as asbestos (lung cancer), *Helicobacter pylori* (stomach cancer) and human papiloma virus (cervical cancer). As shown in Figure 11.1, tobacco, diet, and infections alone are thought to be responsible for 54 per cent of cancers in developed countries. Changing people's behaviour so that they live healthier lifestyles could prevent up to 60 per cent of cancer deaths, particularly smoking-related and gastro-intestinal cancers (Institute of Medicine, 2005). Risk factors vary for different cancers and many cancers have multiple risk factors. For example, risk factors for breast cancer include genetic vulnerability, greater age, the early onset of periods, being childless or not having children until over 30, using hormone replacement therapy, and greater alcohol consumption.

It has been proposed that stress contributes to the progression of some cancers through its effect on the immune system (Reiche et al., 2004). This suggestion is mainly supported by animal research where increased tumour growth and metastases can be observed in animals that have been implanted with tumour cells and then put in stressful situations. Research in humans is much less consistent: the current consensus is that stress has less of an effect on cancer onset than on cancer progression (e.g. Levav et al., 2000).

Support is important for psychological health and adapting to chronic illness (see Chapter 6). Thus, it is not surprising that support can influence the onset and progression of cancer. For example, one longitudinal study found that social isolation was related to an increased likelihood of dying from cancer (Kaplan and Reynolds, 1988). Another study showed that people with late-stage cancer who were married survived longer than those who were unmarried, separated, or divorced (Lai et al., 1999). Studies of this type point to a strong relationship between support and the progression of cancer.

However, this is not necessarily the case for all cancers. Most studies of support have focused on breast cancer where there is clear evidence that poor support affects the progression of cancer. In such studies, the *extent* of support available (i.e. how much support/how many people in support networks) appears to be more important than the *function* of the support (e.g. emotional support/information support) (Nausheen et al., 2009). A review of support in other cancers was less convincing, with ten studies showing a positive relationship and six finding no association (Nausheen et al., 2009). In couple relationships, people with cancer will feel more supported and have greater marital satisfaction when their spouse actively engages in discussions about cancer and helps them find constructive ways of coping with it, rather than being overprotective and hiding their concerns (Hagedoorn et al., 2000).

11.4.2 PSYCHOLOGICAL RESPONSES TO CANCER

Cancer poses a severe threat to health that requires extensive adjustment on the part of individuals and their families. A diagnosis of cancer therefore has to be given carefully and sensitively (see Section 18.4). Between 1 per cent and 58 per cent of people with cancer report clinically significant levels of anxiety, depression, or PTSD (Kangas et al., 2002). The wide variation in the number of people who develop psychological disorders is partly due to medical factors, such as cancer type, severity, and prognosis, and partly due to individual factors, such as a history of psychological problems, life stress, and poor support

(Kangas et al., 2002). The vulnerability-stress model is a useful framework for thinking about how individual vulnerability interacts with medical factors to determine a person's distress (see Figure 3.3).

Psychosocial factors will influence whether a person is more likely to have high levels of distress in response to cancer. As in the general population, women with cancer are more likely than men to report anxiety, depression, or PTSD. Other vulnerability factors include current or previous psychological problems, poor support, and a lower quality of life (Arden-Close et al., 2008).

Although anxiety is often more common than depression in response to cancer diagnosis (Arden-Close et al., 2008), the relationship between cancer and depression has been more widely studied. Depression is associated with cancer onset and mortality, but it is difficult to tease out whether depression causes cancer or is a response to cancer. A meta-analysis of prospective studies in community samples found that people with a history of depression have a slightly increased risk of getting many cancers (Oerlemans et al., 2007). However, depression probably plays a more important role in the *progression* of cancer. A prospective study of over 15,000 men and women showed that people with a history of cancer were almost two times more likely to die during the ten year observation period if they had high levels of psychological distress at baseline (Hamer et al., 2009). This study did not control for severity of cancer at baseline, but the effect of psychological distress remained when people who died in the first year of the study were excluded (as a proxy for cancer severity).

The relationship between depression and cancer is bidirectional and involves physiological and behavioural mechanisms. First, neuroendocrine and immune changes that accompany depression may contribute to the progression of cancer. Second, depression may interact with lifestyle to contribute to the onset and progression of cancer. For example, one 12 year study of over 2,000 people found that smokers were 1.6 times more likely than non-smokers to develop any cancer. However, smokers who were depressed were 2.5 times more likely to develop cancer and 18.5 times more likely to develop smoking-related cancers (Linkins and Comstock, 1990). Third, having cancer may contribute to or exacerbate a depressed mood.

The coping strategies people use are influenced by their appraisal of cancer. As noted in Chapter 3, our appraisal of events determines the extent to which we find them stressful and how we attempt to cope with them. This is also the case in response to cancer (see Case Study 11.2). People who appraise the cancer as a threat or challenge are more likely to use problem-focused coping strategies such as information gathering, problem solving, accepting responsibility, and seeking support. People who appraise the cancer as involving harm or loss are more likely to use avoidant strategies such as denial, distancing, wishful-thinking, and substance use (Franks and Roesch, 2006).

Coping strategies can be either adaptive or maladaptive, depending on the individual and the context. For example, a review of the use of denial by cancer patients found it was more likely to be used by elderly people or those in the terminal phase of cancer. The effect of denial on physical and psychological function was inconsistent, although passive-escape strategies were associated with increased distress (Vos and de Haes, 2007). However, as with depression, it is difficult to determine the direction of causality of this relationship.

CASE STUDY 11.2 Managing the stress of cancer

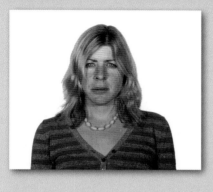

Helen is a 32 year old woman being treated for breast cancer that was diagnosed six months ago. She had a double mastectomy two months ago. There were indications the cancer might have spread so Helen has now started chemotherapy.

She is frightened of cancer, tearful, and does not feel she is coping. She thinks she is going to die, has stopped going out, and does not want to talk about it to anyone. Helen is convinced that no man will want to be in a relationship with her now because of her mastectomy. Chemotherapy makes her feel worse and she can't bear the thought of losing her hair. She has missed two of her chemotherapy appointments recently.

Stress management

Stress management involves education about stress and coping, exploring the person's ways of coping, and facilitating more adaptive coping. Stress management has many forms: in this example we use the transactional model [see Chapter 3] to examine the role of perceived demands, resources, appraisal, and coping:

Demands

Explore the demands of cancer on Helen so they are explicit:

- *What are the triggers to this situation?* e.g. Breast cancer and chemotherapy
- *What demands does it place on her?* Cancer and chemotherapy threaten her health, life, identity, attractiveness (hair), and future.
- *How real are these demands?* Are they based on fact or fears?

Appraisal

Examine her appraisals and how they affect her feelings and coping:

- *When she is feeling overwhelmed and unable to cope, what is she thinking?* This emphasises the role of appraisal in how she feels e.g. 'I am going to die'; 'no man will want me because I have had a mastectomy'.
- *How could she think differently to help her feel and cope better?* This shows how different appraisals and coping strategies might be more adaptive e.g. 'many women go through breast cancer and chemotherapy and are fine'; 'breasts are not the only quality that make women attractive'.

(Cont'd)

Resources to cope

Explore with Helen the resources she has to cope including any she does not recognise because she is feeling overwhelmed. For example:

- *What support does she have available to her?* This includes family, friends, colleagues, and healthcare professionals.
- *How has she coped with previous stressful situations?* This could raise her awareness of her coping strategies and skills.
- *What worked and what didn't work?* This could help her identify the strategies to try again.
- *How can she use these strategies to cope now?* This can help her to realise she has resources to cope.
- *What new ways of coping might help her now?* This encourages her to identify other new coping strategies.

Managing stress

Drawing on the previous stages, you can explore practical steps and strategies that would help Helen manage her cancer and chemotherapy both now and in the future. This is very individual. For example, if talking to people in the same situation helped her in the past, she might join a support group. Or she might realise that in the past she was able to think differently and "talk" herself out of her fears.

Although the way people will cope influences their emotional response to cancer, the role of coping in cancer progression is more controversial. Some research finds a relationship between coping styles and cancer progression and mortality. For example, one study found that women who responded to a diagnosis of breast cancer with acceptance or helplessness were more likely to die over a 5-year period than those who responded with a fighting spirit or denial (Greer et al., 1979). However, subsequent meta-analyses have shown there is little consistent evidence that coping styles play an important part in cancer survival or cancer recurrence (Petticrew et al., 2002).

This does not mean we should dismiss coping as completely unimportant. Coping is important in promoting psychological wellbeing and self-help behaviour. For example, one qualitative study of people with incurable cancer who had outlived their diagnosis by 2-12 years found they had common coping styles of:

- Authenticity – a clear understanding of what was important in their lives.
- Autonomy – a perceived freedom to shape their lives around what they valued.
- Acceptance – more peaceful, joyful experiences and greater emotional closeness to others.

These people were also more involved in their own self help soon after diagnosis than those who did not survive (Cunningham and Watson, 2004).

Responses to cancer are not always negative. There is increasing evidence that many people experience positive personal changes in response to cancer. One review found six important components of psycho-spiritual wellbeing (Lin and Bauer-Wu, 2003):

- Self-awareness.
- Coping and adjusting effectively with stress.
- Connectedness with others.
- A sense of faith.
- A sense of empowerment and confidence.
- Living with meaning and hope.

A meta-analysis of research with people with cancer and HIV showed that personal growth is associated with lower levels of distress, better mental health, and better self-ratings of physical health (Sawyer et al., 2010). Furthermore, the positive aspects of personal growth increased over time: patients who believed their cancer had led to positive changes in their life continued to do well in terms of their mental health and perceived physical health.

11.4.3 INTERVENTIONS FOR CANCER

Research evidence generally confirms that psychological interventions for people with cancer increase adaptation and psychological wellbeing and may lead to improved neuroendocrine and immune function, thereby influencing the progression of cancer (McGregor and Antoni, 2009). A variety of psychosocial interventions for cancer can be used, including counselling, cognitive behaviour therapy, mindfulness interventions, and support groups (see Chapter 19).

Cognitive behavioural therapy (CBT) for cancer usually focuses on reducing stress and depression, helping patients manage pain, fatigue, appetite control, and the side-effects of treatment. This can be done through individual or group programmes and usually involves education, an examination of stress and coping styles, and the use of cognitive and behavioural techniques to improve coping with the difficult and stressful aspects of cancer and its treatment. Research shows that CBT interventions can lead to enduring improved quality of life, reduced distress, reduced fatigue, and an increased perception of benefits (Gielissen et al., 2007).

There has been increasing interest in the use of **mindfulness** interventions, which encourage people to experience life fully by paying attention to moment-to-moment experiences. People are encouraged to be aware of the world, other people, their own thoughts and emotions, and to accept these emotions and thoughts without judgement. Because mindfulness focuses on the present, it is a good way to prevent people ruminating about the past or future. Mindfulness interventions include education and training about mindfulness and meditation. Early evaluations of mindfulness training in people with cancer have shown promising results, suggesting it may lead to improved psychological wellbeing, reduced stress, and better coping (Ott et al., 2009).

Support interventions include individual support, telephone support, support groups, and internet support. The supportive person is usually a peer but can also be a healthcare professional. Early research into support interventions suggested they could prolong survival (Spiegel et al., 1989). However, later research has been mixed. Reviews of the evidence conclude that although support interventions are positively evaluated and lead to high levels of satisfaction, the evidence for psychological and physical benefits is mixed (Gottlieb and Wachala, 2007; Hoey et al., 2008). Mixed findings are probably due to wide variation in support interventions and individuals. Support groups do not appeal to everyone: 20-40 per cent of people with cancer will refuse to attend or drop out. Patients with early or less severe cancer may be more distressed by attending support groups with people who are at the end-stages of the disease. Support interventions are therefore only likely to be beneficial for a subgroup of people, such as those with high levels of distress, poor personal resources, and low available support. People who *do* choose to attend support groups usually report improved psychological wellbeing and quality of life (Gottlieb and Wachala, 2007).

Other interventions have also been used with positive results but it is beyond the scope of this chapter to cover them all. These include physical exercise programmes, which can lead to improved quality of life, physical functioning, and emotional wellbeing (Courneya and Friedenreich, 1999), and massage therapy, which is associated with reduced pain, nausea, distress, and fatigue (Ernst, 2009).

CLINICAL NOTES 11.2

Coping with cancer

- Psychosocial factors influence the onset and progression of many cancers.
- Encourage patients to change risk factors, such as lifestyle, stress, emotions, and psychological problems.
- It is important to treat psychological disorders in patients with cancer.
- Encourage partners and relatives of patients to engage actively in discussions about cancer to find constructive ways of coping with it.
- Generally it is not helpful if the partners of people with cancer hide their concerns.
- Support groups are helpful for some people with cancer, but be aware that many people do not find them to be beneficial.

Summary

- Psychosocial risk factors for cancer include demographic factors, lifestyle, stress, and support.
- Tobacco use, diet, and infections are responsible for up to half of all cancers.

- Poor social support and depression are associated with the onset and progression of some cancers, but it is unclear whether depression causes cancer or is a response to cancer.
- Many people with cancer report clinically significant levels of anxiety, depression, or PTSD.
- Psychosocial interventions for cancer include cognitive behavioural therapy, mindfulness-based interventions, and support groups.
- These interventions usually improve quality of life and psychological wellbeing but there is little consistent evidence that they affect physical outcomes.

📖 FURTHER READING

Ayers, S. et al. (eds) (2007) *Cambridge Handbook of Psychology, Health and Medicine* (2nd edition). Cambridge: Cambridge University Press. Includes short chapters on psychoneuroimmunology, immunisation, and many specific skin disorders or cancers.

Glaser, R. & Kiecolt-Glaser, J.K. (2005) 'Stress-induced immune dysfunction: implications for health'. *Nature Reviews: Immunology, 5*: 243–251. An excellent, authoritative overview of research into the impact of stress on the immune system.

Holland, J.C. (ed.) (1998) *Psycho-Oncology.* New York: Oxford University Press. A slightly dated but comprehensive book covering all aspects of psycho-oncology, including lifestyle factors and risk, screening, responses to treatment, psychiatric comorbidity, psychosocial intervention, cancer in special groups such as children, and those with other special needs.

Walker, C. & Papadopoulos, L. (eds) (2005) *Psychodermatology: The Psychological Impact of Skin Disorders.* Cambridge: Cambridge University Press. Covers the psychological aspects of skin disorders in depth, including chapters on psychoneuroimmunology, psychiatric comorbidity, stigma, and therapy.

❓ REVISION QUESTIONS

1. How do the immune effects of acute stress differ from those of chronic stress?

2. Describe the links between negative emotions and immune function.

3. Describe the links between positive emotions and experiences on immune function.

4. How does stress affect responsiveness to vaccinations?

5. Compare the prevalence of depression in people with immune disorders to the prevalence in the general population. How can we explain the observed differences?

6   What do the results of wound healing studies tell us about the impact of negative psychological states on immune function?

7   Why are psychological interventions useful for treating skin disorders?

8   Outline the important psychosocial risk factors for cancer onset.

9   How do psychosocial factors like coping and social support affect cancer progression?

10   'Every person with cancer should join a support group'. Give arguments for and against this statement.

12 CARDIOVASCULAR AND RESPIRATORY

Research boxes

12.1 Responses to stress and ischaemia in cardiac patients
12.2 Effect of depression on heart rate variability in patients with CHD
12.3 Positive changes following MI

LEARNING OBJECTIVES

This chapter is designed to enable you to:

- Appreciate the role of psychosocial factors in the development of cardiovascular disease.
- Outline the various pathways through which psychosocial factors impact on cardiovascular disease.
- Describe the role of psychosocial factors in the development of respiratory infections and asthma.
- Consider the efficacy of psychological interventions for cardiovascular and respiratory diseases.

Cardiovascular health is affected by a range of psychosocial risk factors, including lifestyle, stress, emotions, and social circumstances. These factors can affect the development of heart disease, as well as the prognosis in people who already have heart disease. Coronary heart disease (CHD) is life-threatening and so requires extensive adjustment and changes in lifestyle. Unsurprisingly, CHD may result in high levels of fear, distress, anxiety, and depression, which in turn may affect both health and prognosis. Cardiac rehabilitation supports people after the onset of heart disease and may help patients reduce their risk of future illness.

The first part of this chapter examines how psychosocial factors can affect the development and progression of heart disease. The second part of this chapter examines psychological factors and respiratory health. Breathing and emotions are in fact highly interlinked. Furthermore, psychosocial factors can influence the onset and progression of respiratory disorders. Given the range and variety of respiratory disorders, it is not possible to cover them all. Here we focus on common examples of respiratory infections and asthma to illustrate the role of psychological factors in acute and chronic respiratory disorders.

12.1 CARDIOVASCULAR HEALTH

Psychosocial factors can affect heart disease through four possible pathways:

☙ Lifestyle factors such as smoking, diet, and exercise can affect the risk of atherosclerosis and CHD.

☙ Psychosocial factors can trigger acute cardiac events in patients with existing coronary pathology.

☙ Socio-demographic factors are associated with risk and the accessibility of services.

☙ Beliefs influence the use of medical care by people with cardiovascular disease.

This section examines the key psychosocial risk factors that influence CHD by looking at lifestyle, stress, depression, hostility or anger, and social isolation.

12.1.1 PSYCHOSOCIAL RISK FACTORS FOR HEART DISEASE

Hundreds of research studies have identified chronic and acute risk factors for CHD (Allan et al., 2007). Chronic risk factors exert their influence over longer periods and include things like smoking, hypertension, and high cholesterol. Acute risk factors are transient physical changes that occur following exposure to physical or psychological triggers, such as exercise or stress, which cause clinical events such as ischaemia, infarction, or sudden death. Chronic and acute risk factors combine to increase the overall risk of a cardiac event. In other words, people with high chronic risk (e.g. a smoker with a family history of CHD) have the greatest risk of a problem occurring when acute risk

---

BOX 12.1   Chronic and acute risk factors for coronary heart disease

	Chronic risk	Acute risk
Physical	Family history	Cardiovascular reactivity
	Cholesterol	
	Hypertension	
	Diabetes	
Demographic	Age (older)	
	Sex (male)	
	Socioeconomic status	
Lifestyle	Smoking	Intense exercise
	Obesity	
	Sedentary lifestyle	
Psychosocial	Stress	Intense stress
	Hostility/anger	Intense anger
	Depression	
	Social isolation	

factors arise (e.g. intense exercise or stress). Box 12.1 shows the main chronic and acute risk factors for CHD.

Many physical and psychosocial risk factors overlap so separating out the impact of physical, lifestyle, and psychological risk factors can be a challenge. For example, a study which followed 2,272 men over ten years found that those with the lowest incomes were three times more likely to die of any cause and more than twice as likely to die of CHD (Lynch et al., 1996). However, the effect of socioeconomic status on CHD was due to 23 different risk factors. These included:

- Physical factors (e.g. fibrinogen, cholesterol, triglycerides, blood pressure, body mass index).
- Lifestyle factors (e.g. smoking, alcohol use, physical activity).
- Psychosocial factors (e.g. depression, hopelessness, and social support).

It is therefore important to consider all areas of risk in prevention and treatment of CHD.

Lifestyle and health behaviours

Lifestyle has a powerful impact on cardiovascular health. A study of more than 20,000 men and women over ten years identified four behaviours that made a dramatic difference to mortality, particularly deaths from cardiovascular causes. People who did not smoke, were physically active, had a moderate alcohol intake, and ate five or more servings of fruit or vegetables a day were four times less likely to die than people who did none of these behaviours (Khaw et al., 2008). This difference remained even after taking into account age, sex, body mass index, and socioeconomic status. In fact, the impact of doing these four health behaviours was the physical equivalent of being 14 years younger.

Changes in lifestyle factors can therefore account for a large proportion of the reduction in CHD over the last twenty years (Ünal et al., 2005). Figure 12.1 shows the contribution of medical treatments and lifestyle to CHD mortality in the UK over recent decades: decreases in smoking, hypertension and high cholesterol made a large contribution to reducing CHD. Reductions in smoking alone have had a greater impact than all the advances in medical treatments during this time (Ünal et al., 2005). Smoking is therefore the single most important lifestyle risk factor to address. Smokers are twice as likely to die from CHD and 2–4 times more likely to have a sudden cardiac arrest. If CHD patients stop smoking their risk of death drops by 36 per cent and risk of another MI drops by 32 per cent when compared to those who continue to smoke (Critchley and Capewell, 2004).

Diet and exercise are important – especially so given the trend for increasing obesity and physical inactivity, which is adversely affecting rates of CHD as shown in Figure 12.1. The British Heart Foundation recommends a diet of at least five portions

Number of life years gained through treatment of CHD and reducing risk factors

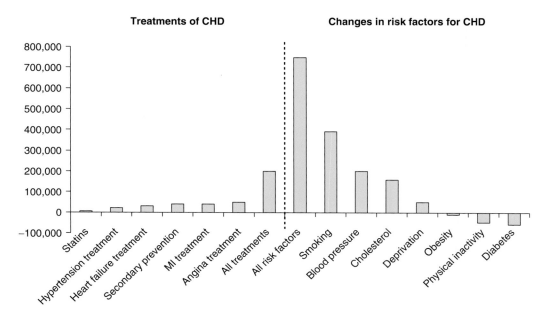

FIGURE 12.1   Role of treatment and risk factors in the decline in CHD (England & Wales 1981–2000). Adapted from Ünal et al. (2005).

of fruit and vegetables a day, reduced fats (including no saturated fats), two portions of fish a week (at least one being an oily fish like salmon or mackerel), reduced salt, and moderate alcohol consumption. Note that either complete abstinence from alcohol or excessive alcohol increases the risk of CHD, whereas moderate consumption appears to reduce the risk (Bagnardi et al., 2008).s Regular moderate exercise helps reduce weight, body fat, blood pressure and cholesterol; improves physical and psychological health; and reduces the risk of CHD and stroke (Vogel et al., 2009).

Being aware of a person's risk factors and helping them to stop smoking, exercise more, and eat healthily are important parts of cardiac disease prevention and rehabilitation. However, one study found that fewer than 20 per cent of cardiology notes covered all the major risk factors (Gravely-Witte et al., 2008). Critical risk factors of smoking and cholesterol were reported in 80 per cent of the notes, but other risks such as obesity and family history were reported in less than 50 per cent of notes.

Careful screening of risk behaviour is an important first step towards reducing CHD and improving the prognosis in CHD patients. Various evidence-based techniques for health behaviour change can contribute to effective intervention and rehabilitation (see Chapter 5).

Stress

The physical and lifestyle risk factors referred to above account for about half the variance in new cases of heart disease (Roig et al., 1987). This is substantial, but it leaves much of the risk unaccounted for. Researchers have therefore focused on other potential risk factors, such as stress, differences in cardiovascular responses to stress, emotions, and social isolation.

ACTIVITY 12.1

- When you are stressed, does this affect your lifestyle e.g. health behaviours like smoking, drinking, diet, sleep, and exercise?
- How do you think we can separate the effect of stress from the effects of lifestyle?

There is substantial evidence from epidemiological, experimental, and animal studies that stress affects CHD. Epidemiological studies show that stressors such as natural disasters, war, terrorism, and even sporting events can be associated with increased cardiac morbidity and mortality. For example, a national survey in the USA showed that diagnosed CHD increased by 53 per cent after the 9/11 terrorist attacks, even after taking into account existing risk factors (Holman et al., 2008). Football matches can have similar effects. Research in Germany and the UK has shown that hospital admissions for cardiac emergencies are more common on World Cup match days, especially in the hours during and after matches (Carroll et al., 2002; Wilbert-Lampen et al., 2008).

Experimental studies have shown that stressful tasks like giving a public speech increase both heart rate and blood pressure and can trigger ischaemia (restricted blood flow to the heart) in patients with CHD (Krantz and McCeney, 2002). Animal studies show that social stress such as subordination or conflict increases athero-sclerosis, accentuates heart rate responses to stress, and lowers the threshold for arrhythmias.

Mental stress and emotion are potent triggers of ischaemia in CHD patients. Ischaemia is easily provoked, reversible and clinically important, so it is a good way to study the effects of stress on the heart. Studies of naturally occurring ischaemia show it is more likely to occur during intense physical activity, stressful mental activity, or when people feel angry. In one study, patients were two times more likely to experience ischaemia when they were tense, sad, or frustrated (Gullette et al., 1997). Research indicates that CHD patients who have strong ischaemia responses to mental stress are more at risk of subsequent cardiac events (see Research Box 12.1) and more likely to die in the three years after an MI (Sheps et al., 2002).

RESEARCH BOX 12.1   Responses to stress and ischaemia in cardiac patients

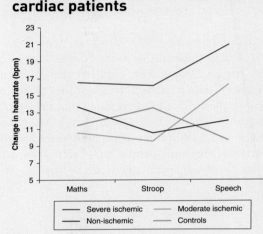

Background

The association between stress and cardiovascular disease is well established and animal research suggests physiological pathways through which this might occur. This was one of the early studies looking at ischemic responses to stress in cardiac patients.

Method and findings

39 cardiac patients were divided into those with severe ischaemia, moderate ischaemia, and non-ischaemia, and compared with 12 non-patient controls. Cardiac function was measured during various stressful tasks and during exercise. Stressful tasks included doing mental arithmetic whilst being mildly harassed and giving a speech about their own personal faults or undesirable habits.

Over half (59 per cent) of patients showed ischaemia during mental stress. This was worst during the personally relevant public speaking task, which resulted in more frequent and more severe ischaemia. Changes in other measures of cardiac function, such as heart rate and blood pressure, were worst in those with moderate and severe ischaemia as can be seen in the figure.

Significance

This study was one of many to confirm results from animal studies and showed that stress could directly affect cardiovascular function in people. This study also demonstrated how people with existing cardiac problems such as ischaemia could be particularly vulnerable to stress.

Krantz, D.S. et al. (1991) Cardiovascular reactivity and mental stress-induced myocardial ischaemia in patients with coronary artery disease, *Psychosomatic Medicine, 53:* 1–12.

Hostility and anger

The study of hostility and anger originated from research into the association between CHD and Type A behaviour pattern. Type A personalities are characterised by excessive competitiveness, impatience, time-consciousness, and hostility or aggression. Research in the 1950s found that Type A men were more at risk of CHD. However, later research revealed that hostility and anger were the most important components of Type A in the development and prognosis of CHD. Meta-analyses show that anger and hostility could be associated with an increased risk of CHD in healthy people, particularly men, and with a poor prognosis in patients with CHD, even after taking into account the severity of the disease (Chida and Steptoe, 2009).

Anger and hostility are therefore chronic risk factors for CHD. However, anger is also a potent trigger of acute cardiac events. In two large studies of MI in the USA and Sweden, anger was found to be a particularly strong trigger. People were between two and four times more likely to have an MI after an angry episode compared to when they were not angry (Steptoe and Brydon, 2009). Interview studies of MI patients show that between 2 and 17 per cent of them reported being angry in the two hours before their MI symptoms. Newton (2009) places the role of anger and hostility in a social context – namely through social dominance and submissiveness. Dominant people have been shown to react more strongly to stress and recover more slowly, particularly if the stressor is a social challenge.

Depression

As with stress, there is substantial evidence that depression is associated with CHD onset and prognosis and that CHD is in turn associated with depression. Between 15 and 30 per cent of patients hospitalised for CHD will be clinically depressed in the year afterwards. This depression can become chronic. For example, a national survey of 30,801 people in the USA found that 9 per cent of people with CHD were depressed compared to 5 per cent of people without any physical illness (Egede, 2007). Depression is more common in CHD patients who are younger, female, socially isolated, or have a history of psychological problems (Bennett, 2007a).

CHD patients with depression have a poorer prognosis. Many studies show a clear dose-response relationship between the severity of depression and cardiac morbidity. This relationship is evident even after physical risk factors are taken into account. For example, one study found that, after controlling for other risk factors, depression was associated with a 2.7 per cent increased risk of death (Surtees et al., 2008). This risk is comparable to other major risk factors for mortality, such as smoking and congestive heart failure. Depression after an acute cardiac event makes people at least twice as likely to have another cardiac event within the following few years (Lichtman et al., 2008).

The link between depression and CHD may be due to both physical and behavioural pathways (see Box 12.2). Depressed patients with CHD show physiological changes that increase their vulnerability to future cardiac problems. For example, Research Box 12.2 shows that depressed patients have a reduced heart rate variability which indicates poor parasympathetic control of the heart. Other studies have shown depression can be associated with HPA axis dysfunction, increased platelet activation and inflammatory responses, and impaired vascular function (Lichtman et al., 2008). An interesting review of twin studies found that nearly 20 per cent of the variability in symptoms of depression and CHD was due to common genetic factors (McCaffery et al., 2006). Thus there may be common genetic determinants of CHD and depression, possibly via inflammatory pathways and serotonin responses.

BOX 12.2   Mechanisms through which depression affects the prognosis of CHD

	Chronic risk
Biological	Hypothalamic-pituitary-adrenal axis dysfunction
	Reduced heart rate variability
	Increased inflammatory response
	Impaired vascular function
	Increased platelet activation
Behavioural	Poor adherence to medication and treatment regimes
	Lack of participation in cardiac rehabilitation
Lifestyle	Smoking
	Diet
	Sedentary lifestyle
Psychosocial	Social isolation
	Chronic stress
	Comorbid anxiety disorders

Given the link between depression and CHD, it is important to identify and treat depression in CHD patients. Yet the evidence suggests the majority of cardiologists do not routinely ask patients about depression, and only half treat depression when it is identified (Feinstein et al., 2006). The American Heart Association recommends that all CHD patients are screened for depression. Patients with mild symptoms should be followed up during subsequent routine visits. Patients with moderate or severe symptoms should be referred for comprehensive evaluation and treatment by a mental health professional (Lichtman et al., 2008). Box 12.3 shows a brief screening questionnaire that can be used with cardiac patients to identify depression and other forms of psychological distress.

RESEARCH BOX 12.2   Effect of depression on heart rate variability in patients with CHD

Background

The association between depression and heart disease is well established but it is not clear what the physiological mechanisms for this is.

Method and findings

A cross-sectional study of whether depression was associated with heart rate variability abnormalities in 56 adults aged 60 or over who had a recent MI (within 72 hours) or unstable angina. Heart rate variability was measured primarily through recording the length of each consecutive R wave in milliseconds and then plotting relative variability in R waves.

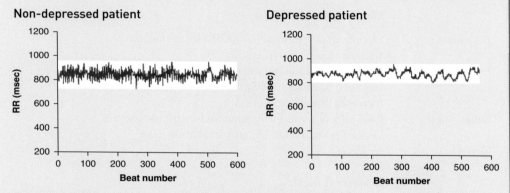

Patients with depression had decreased heart rate variability as shown in the graphs. Increased symptoms of depression were clearly related to decreased heart rate variability in a dose-response fashion.

Significance

Reduced heart rate variability suggests that the parasympathetic control of the heart is impaired in depressed patients. This study clearly illustrates the association between depression and physical vulnerability factors for further cardiac morbidity.

Guinjoan et al. (2004) Cardiac parasympathetic dysfunction related to depression in older adults with acute coronary symptoms, *Journal of Psychosomatic Research, 56:* 83–88.

Social isolation and support

The effect of social support or isolation on cardiovascular disease has been well-established. Early epidemiological research in the 1970s and 1980s found that married men were much less likely to die from heart disease. However, what happens within relationships is also

---

BOX 12.3   Screening Tool for Psychosocial Distress (STOP-D)

Over the last 2 weeks, how much have you been bothered by:

		A little					Moderately				
Feeling sad, down, or uninterested in life?	Not at all	0	1	2	3	4*	5	6	7	8	Extremely
Feeling anxious or nervous?	Not at all	0	1	2	3	4*	5	6	7	8	Extremely
Feeling stressed?	Not at all	0	1	2	3	4	5*	6	7	8	Extremely
Feeling angry?	Not at all	0	1	2	3	4	5*	6	7	8	Extremely
Not having the social support you feel you need?	Not at all	0	1	2	3	4	5*	6	7	8	Extremely

* Recommended cut-off indicating patients who need referral to psychological services for further assessment and treatment for psychological distress.

Reproduced courtesy of Quincy Young from Young et al. (2007) 'Brief screen to identify 5 of the most common forms of psychosocial distress in cardiac patients: validation of the screening tool for psychological distress (STOP-D)', *Journal of Cardiovascular Nursing*, 22: 525–534.

---

important. For example, a study of more than 3,500 adults showed that single men were two times more likely to die from CHD than married men (Eaker et al., 2007). Marital happiness, satisfaction, or the number of disagreements between couples were not associated with CHD morbidity or mortality. However, women who silenced themselves during arguments with their husband were four times more likely to die than women who did not. This influence of marriage and social support on CHD is partly due to single people being more likely to have unhealthy lifestyles and increased distress. For example, a study of over 13,000 Scottish adults showed that 59 per cent of the risk of dying of cardiovascular causes was explained by health behaviours, metabolic dysregulation, and distress (Molloy et al., 2009).

Social isolation is highly pathogenic: it is associated with morbidity and mortality in healthy people and patients with CHD. For example, a study of 430 CHD patients found that people who had less than four close friends or family were more than twice as likely to die from CHD or other causes – even after controlling for disease severity, age, hostility, smoking, and psychological distress (Brummett et al., 2001). The increased risk associated with social isolation is similar to, or greater than, the risk of other major factors such as smoking. However, it seems this is only the case for extreme isolation: there are no differences in risk between people with medium or large support networks.

In sum, psychosocial factors such as stress, depression, anger, and social isolation are influential risk factors for cardiac morbidity or mortality. Depression and social isolation in particular are equivalent to other major risk factors such as smoking. The physical processes through which stress, emotions, and social isolation can affect CHD are likely to include stress-induced autonomic dysfunction, haemodynamic responses, neuroendocrine activation, inflammatory responses, and prothrombotic responses (notably platelet activation). These factors contribute to coronary plaque disruption, ischaemia, cardiac dysrhythmias, and thrombus formation (Steptoe and Brydon, 2009). The role of cardiovascular reactivity and other haemodynamic responses is therefore examined in the next section.

12.1.2 CARDIOVASCULAR REACTIVITY

Efforts to understand the links between psychosocial factors and CHD have focused increasingly on cardiovascular responses to stress and how these are moderated by other risk factors. There is now a wealth of evidence that people vary in the magnitude of their cardiovascular responses to stress. Such research typically involves monitoring changes in blood pressure, heart rate, ischaemia, or endothelial function while people complete stressful tasks like those described in Research Box 12.1. Cardiovascular reactivity appears to be an enduring individual trait because people's responses are fairly consistent over time and with different stressors. The key question is whether hyper-reactivity causes future heart disease or whether it serves as a marker of future risk (without necessarily being causal). A review of prospective studies found that people with hyper-reactive responses to stress were more likely to develop hypertension in subsequent years. Hyper-reactivity may also be associated with atherosclerosis and left ventricular mass, which may be precursors to CHD (Treiber et al., 2003). However, hyper-reactivity was not associated with the development of CHD in healthy populations. This was different in CHD patients, where hyper-reactivity was associated with subsequent cardiac morbidity.

Cardiovascular reactivity therefore differs between people and is associated with long-term risk factors for CHD and a higher clinical risk in patients with CHD. However, reactivity is influenced by a number of other factors, including physical fitness, family history, and support. Being physically fit reduces cardiovascular reactivity to stress and promotes faster heart rate recovery after stress (Forcier et al., 2006). Research also shows that having a friend or ally present when performing stressful tasks can reduce cardiovascular reactivity, particularly if the friend is female (Christenfeld and Gerin, 2000). There is also evidence that people with a family history of hypertension have increased cardiovascular reactivity (Pierce et al., 2005).

Another area of interest is vascular endothelial reactivity. Endothelial function contributes to vessel tone, dilation, platelet aggregation, and inflammation. Stressful situations will typically result in a reduction in endothelial-dependent vasodilation, whereas positive emotion, such as laughing, leads to increases. In one study, people who watched a comedy film had a 22 per cent increase in vasodilation whereas those who watched a harrowing war film had a 35 per cent decrease (Miller et al., 2006). Thus, it has been proposed that vascular reactivity may be the critical link that explains the impact of emotion (both positive and negative) on cardiovascular health.

12.1.3 IMPACT OF HEART DISEASE

MI is a sudden, unexpected, and potentially life-threatening event that can have a severe impact on a person's wellbeing and lifestyle. As noted earlier, up to 30 per cent of patients report depression in the first year after an MI. In addition, up to 40 per cent of patients will report anxiety in the year after MI, and up to 16 per cent will develop post-traumatic stress disorder (PTSD) (Ayers et al., 2009). As with most illnesses, there is little association between the severity of CHD and psychological distress, with the exception of end-stage heart failure when patients are likely to be highly distressed. For example, one study found that the following factors were strong predictors of the development of PTSD:

- A history of psychological problems.
- A belief on the part of the person concerned that the MI had negative consequences (e.g. problems in relationships or dealing with medication and self-care).
- Dysfunctional coping techniques (e.g. trying to numb emotions, distract themselves from upsetting thoughts).

These factors were more strongly associated with PTSD than the perceived severity of the MI (Ayers et al., 2009).

The effect of psychological problems is compounded by the fact that they often occur together. For example, people with PTSD after MI are also more likely to have symptoms of anxiety, depression, and social dysfunction (Ayers et al., 2009). Symptoms of anxiety, such as a racing heart or palpitations, may be a particular issue because they mimic the symptoms of cardiac problems. In keeping with this, patients with depression and anxiety are more likely to contact doctors, have outpatient appointments, attend emergency services, and be re-admitted to hospital (Frasure-Smith et al., 2000). Much of this is due to worry and health concerns rather than cardiac problems.

Psychological problems therefore affect patient wellbeing, quality of life, and their use of health services. They may also affect whether patients change unhealthy behaviours. Some studies have shown that depressed patients are less likely to stop smoking or take exercise and that depression and PTSD are associated with medication nonadherence (Bennett, 2007a), but the evidence is not consistent. However, the effect of heart disease on psychological wellbeing is not always negative. In the last decade, research has increasingly looked at positive changes after illnesses such as MI. An example of this is given in Research Box 12.3, which shows that in the months after MI some patients reported a greater appreciation of life, improved close relationships, and healthy lifestyle changes.

12.1.4 TREATMENT AND REHABILITATION

The prognosis following MI will be much better if treatment is obtained quickly. However, many patients can take several hours to go to hospital for treatment. Surprisingly, people who have had a previous MI will take just as long to get to hospital as those who have not had a previous MI (Yarzebski et al., 1994). Furthermore, the amount of pain a person feels does not affect how quickly they obtain treatment (Walsh et al., 2004). Women are slower to attend hospital, whereas people who believe a heart attack has serious consequences and are active or problem-focused copers are quicker to attend hospital (Walsh et al., 2004).

RESEARCH BOX 12.3　Positive changes following MI

Background

For many years, research looking at the impact of traumatic events focused on the negative impact. This study looked at whether positive changes were reported after MI or cancer.

Method and findings

143 MI patients and 52 breast cancer patients were assessed in hospital and three months later and asked if any positive changes had taken place in their lives following their illness. Responses were then grouped into seven themes.

Three months after MI, 58 per cent of patients reported positive changes in their lives since the illness. The most commonly reported positive changes were lifestyle changes, a greater appreciation of life, improved close relationships, and a change in personal priorities as shown in the figure.

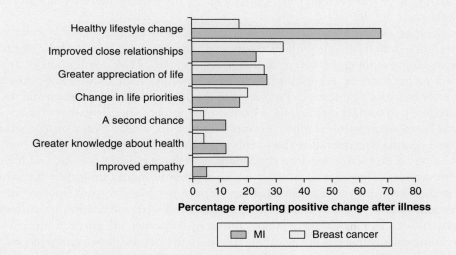

Significance

Until recently, most psychological research focused on the negative repercussions of illness. This study is an example of growing research identifying the positive benefits from adversity. Healthy lifestyle changes are one of the key positive changes reported by MI patients.

Petrie, K.J. et al. (1999) Positive effects of illness reported by myocardial infarction and breast cancer patients, *Journal of Psychosomatic Research, 47:* 537–543.

CLINICAL NOTES 12.1

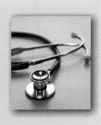

Treating cardiovascular disease

- Careful screening of risk behaviour is an important step towards reducing CHD and improving the prognosis in CHD patients.
- When taking a cardiovascular history it is important to ask about:
  - o Lifestyle factors of smoking, physical activity, alcohol intake and diet.
  - o Current stress, depression, anxiety, anger, and social isolation.
- These factors may be as important as physical risk factors in the progression of illness.
- Depression occurs in 30 per cent of CHD patients and increases the risk of death. Anxiety and PTSD are also prevalent.
- Depression is more likely in younger, female, socially isolated patients or those with a history of psychological problems.
- Guidelines recommend screening for depression using the PHQ-9 and referring moderately or severely depressed people for appropriate treatment.
- Cardiac rehabilitation reduces mortality but attendance is poor. Make sure you refer all patients and strongly encourage them to attend.
- You may want to consider using a home-based psychological rehabilitation programme that can be facilitated by a specialist nurse such as the Heart Manual.

Cardiac rehabilitation

Rehabilitation programmes vary widely between countries and regions. Some are mainly exercise-based whereas others involve psychological components. Given the diversity in rehabilitation programmes it is not surprising that evidence for the efficacy of rehabilitation is mixed. A meta-analysis showed rehabilitation results in a 26 per cent reduction in cardiac mortality in the first five years, as well as reduced smoking, lower cholesterol and triglycerides, and decreased systolic blood pressure (Taylor et al., 2004).

The reality is that rehabilitation programme attendance is poor. For example, although up to 67 per cent of cardiac patients in the UK are referred for rehabilitation, only 13 to 41 per cent will actually attend (Beswick et al., 2004). Lower attendance is seen in people with ischaemic heart disease, older people, women, and

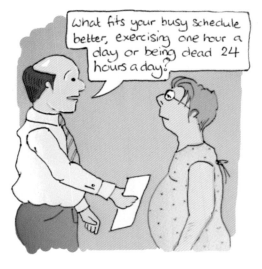

ethnic minority groups. Beliefs about the illness can also influence attendance and other measures of recovery. Patients who believe their illness can be controlled or cured are more likely to attend rehabilitation (see Section 4.4). How severe a person believes the consequences of CHD are will also influence how quickly they return to work, levels of disability, and social impairment – although it is difficult to determine how much of this is due to the actual severity of CHD (Petrie et al., 1996).

Despite the importance of beliefs and emotions in whether patients attend rehabilitation, adhere to treatment and recover, there is mixed evidence about the use of psychological intervention in rehabilitation programmes. A review of 36 trials concluded that although psychological intervention does not influence mortality, it is associated with fewer non-fatal reinfarctions and less depression and anxiety (Rees et al., 2004). Therefore, rehabilitation programmes with psychological components have been proposed, such as the MULTIFIT programme in the USA (Taylor et al., 1997) and the Heart Manual in the UK (Lewin et al., 1992). These are home-based programmes which use CBT or self-efficacy approaches for positive coping, changing maladaptive beliefs, stress management (see Chapter 3), self-management (see Chapter 4) and relaxation (see Chapter 6). Programmes are administered by a facilitator who has undergone brief training. Evaluations of these interventions are broadly positive: patients prefer them to hospital-based programmes and are less likely to drop out (Lewin, 2007), but there is limited evidence of the effect of these programmes on CHD morbidity or mortality. An example of this kind of programme is given in Case Study 12.1.

CASE STUDY 12.1   Cardiac rehabilitation

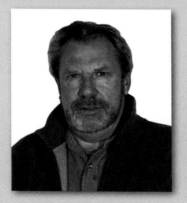 Richard was 42 when he had an MI and surgery to insert a stent into the blocked artery. Since then he has been on aspirin, an ACE inhibitor, and statins to reduce the likelihood it will occur again. He is married with a young daughter and manages a regional finance office. After Richard was discharged from hospital, he participated in a home-based rehabilitation programme using the Heart Manual, with regular check-ups with a nurse to facilitate his progress. The programme was a six-week course based on CBT principles that involve working through manuals and audio recordings to increase understanding and promote lifestyle changes.

First Richard was assessed by a nurse to find out what his needs were with regard to medication adherence and lifestyle changes. Unhealthy behaviours and maladaptive beliefs were explored and Richard was encouraged to challenge these throughout his rehabilitation.

- Part 1 of the Heart Manual provides information and education about heart attacks and heart health. Richard listened to a CD of interviews about heart attacks with doctors, patients, and carers. Part 1 also includes information on common psychological reactions to heart attacks and how to manage distress or seek help if necessary.

- Part 2 of the Heart Manual is a six-week rehabilitation programme, which includes an exercise programme, health education, risk factor reduction, stress management, and sections on low moods, sleep problems, anxiety, and depression. During these six weeks, Richard used a diary to monitor his lifestyle and set his own weekly goals. He was also encouraged to recognise and write down any barriers and benefits to attaining these goals. He also used a CD of relaxation exercises.
- Part 3 of the Heart Manual gives facts and advice to help recovery. Topics include medicines, tests, revascularisation procedures, chest pains, anxiety, stress, and depression.

Richard's wife was involved throughout the rehabilitation programme and encouraged to set joint goals for lifestyle change with Richard. She was given a carers' booklet about the impact of heart attack on relationships, how best to support Richard, and common effects on intimacy and sex. This was particularly useful because Richard admitted taking a lot of his anger and frustration out on his wife. Being able to recognise this and change it helped their relationship.

Richard met the nurse every week for the first few weeks and then continued to complete the heart manual programme on his own. He was followed-up two months later so that any depression or unhealthy behaviour could be picked upon.

Summary

- Psychosocial factors affect heart disease through three pathways: (a) the impact of health-related behaviours, (b) direct or chronic physiological changes that contribute to heart disease, and (c) accessing medical care and treatment.
- The main psychosocial risk factors for heart disease are lifestyle (smoking, exercise, diet), stress, depression, hostility/anger, and social isolation.
- People will differ in their cardiovascular reactivity to stress. Reactivity may be a critical link between stress/emotion and cardiovascular health.
- Heart disease is associated with psychological disorders: many patients will develop depression or anxiety, or experience PTSD.
- Psychological problems are associated with a reduced quality of life, a reduced uptake of rehabilitation programmes, poor adherence to treatment, and the increased use of health services.
- Cardiac rehabilitation programmes significantly reduce cardiac mortality, but are not attended by the majority of patients.
- Psychological interventions for heart disease will reduce non-fatal reinfarctions, depression and anxiety, but will not influence mortality.

12.2 RESPIRATORY HEALTH

In the rest of this chapter we shall consider how psychological factors can contribute to different respiratory disorders and intervention. It is not possible to cover *all* respiratory disorders. Here we will focus on two common examples – acute respiratory infections and chronic asthma – which differ widely in terms of their management and prognosis. These disorders illustrate the different applications of psychological knowledge to respiratory disorders.

12.2.1 BREATHING AND EMOTIONS

Breathing is closely linked to our psychological state: it is the only vital bodily function that can be controlled voluntarily or by reflexes. Controlled slow breathing is the basis for many relaxation exercises and meditation techniques and can reduce physiological arousal, tension, and distress. Fast breathing and hyperventilation are common when we are stressed, anxious, or panicked. Our emotions, thoughts, and behaviour therefore both influence breathing and are influenced *by* breathing. For example, if people are asked to breathe quickly – to hyperventilate voluntarily – they will report a significant increase in anxiety, showing that how we breathe affects our emotions and *vice versa*.

ACTIVITY 12.2

- Take short, shallow breaths – at least 30 per minute – for five minutes.
- What symptoms did you notice? How did you feel physically and emotionally?

Hyperventilation may play a role in panic disorder. Symptoms of hyperventilation (e.g. shortness of breath) are common during panic. Exaggerated respiratory responses are associated with spontaneous panic attacks and people with panic disorder will often have low arterial carbon dioxide (CO_2) caused by chronic hyperventilation. Experimental studies where people are given CO_2 show that people with panic disorder or a family history of panic disorder will respond with greater anxiety (Zvolensky and Eifert, 2001). This effect remains even when they are compared with people with a generalised anxiety disorder or other mood disorders. Thus it may be that people with panic disorder are more sensitive to CO_2. Physical vulnerability to panic is compounded by psychological factors, particularly thoughts and the interpretation of physical symptoms. Panic disorder is strongly associated with anxiety sensitivity – a relatively stable characteristic where people are frightened, worried, or embarrassed by physical symptoms of anxiety.

The reciprocal relationship between breathing and emotion means that controlled breathing can be useful when treating stress-related disorders and panic. It is also useful in promoting emotional wellbeing in chronic lung diseases such as asthma and emphysema (Timmons and Ley, 1994).

12.2.2 UPPER RESPIRATORY TRACT INFECTIONS

Upper respiratory tract infections (URI) such as colds and influenza account for 50 per cent of all acute illnesses and are a major cause of morbidity and mortality worldwide. The economic impact of the common cold is enormous. It is estimated that every year in the USA there are around 1 billion cases of colds that need medical attention and that these cause around 45 million days off work or school (NIAID, 2006). The advent of severe acute respiratory syndrome (SARS) and swine flu (influenza A, H1N1) has increased the impetus to identify which factors are important in whether people 'catch' URIs or not. Colds are the most common URI and are caused by over 200 viruses (Marsland et al., 2007). However, exposure to a virus does not necessarily mean people will develop the clinical symptoms and illness that go with it. In fact, only one in three people exposed to a cold virus will develop a cold (Cohen, 2005).

The most obvious variables to consider are the degree of (a) exposure to a virus and (b) the strength of someone's immune system and overall health. For example, the fact that colds are most prevalent in children may be due to (a) their increased exposure to viruses through contact with other children at school or nursery and (b) a relative lack of resistance. Contrary to common folklore, catching a cold is not affected by cold weather. Evidence shows that putting people in cold conditions has little or no effect on the development or severity of a cold, unless these are extreme conditions. Nor is susceptibility related to factors such as exercise, diet, or enlarged tonsils or adenoids. The use of vitamin C is controversial: a Cochrane review concluded it did not prevent people catching colds but could have a small effect on speeding up recovery (Douglas et al., 2007).

Psychosocial factors associated with susceptibility to URIs include stress, social relationships, sleep, emotions, and socioeconomic status. The evidence is most convincing for stress. The impact of stress on immune function is well established (see Chapter 3), but it seems to be particularly related to a susceptibility to upper respiratory tract infections. For example, one study assessed medical students at several points during their first year. The results showed that during stressful exam periods students had worse immune function and more health problems, most of which were URIs (Glaser et al., 1987). In another series of well-controlled studies, volunteers were given a cold virus by a nasal spray and then quarantined for a number of days. Measures were taken of subjective ratings of illness (e.g. self-reported symptoms) as well as the objective indicators of illness (e.g. immune function and mucus production). Stress was consistently associated with an increased risk of developing a cold: the longer the duration of stressful events, the greater the risk of becoming infected. This effect remained even when controlling for factors such as age, weight, time of year, allergic status, pre-existing immune function or resistance, smoking, diet, and exercise (Cohen, 2005; Marsland et al., 2007).

There is increasing evidence that social relationships can affect our susceptibility to URIs. Interpersonal stress such as conflict with family, friends, or colleagues increases the susceptibility to colds. Furthermore, people with good social networks (both in terms of size of network, integration, and sociability) seem to be protected from the development of colds. It is notable that more sociable people appear to be less at risk of developing colds. This is surprising because it is in direct contrast to the contact hypothesis, where an increased exposure to people is assumed to equate with an increased risk of contracting a virus.

12.2.3 ASTHMA

Asthma is one of the most common chronic diseases in the world and is the most common chronic disease among children in developed countries. Worldwide, the WHO estimate that 300 million people suffer from asthma. The highest prevalence can be found in the UK, Ireland, New Zealand, and Australia – and these rates are increasing. Asthma attacks incur large economic costs in terms of lost productivity, medical treatment, and social security costs. In the past asthma was thought of as a psychosomatic disease i.e. due to, or influenced by, psychological factors. We now know that several factors can contribute to the condition, including a genetic predisposition, diet and lifestyle factors as summarised in Box 12.4. It can be seen that, in comparison to the CHD risk factors in Box 12.1, there are fewer lifestyle and psychosocial causes of asthma. In fact, the role of psychosocial factors is largely limited to triggering asthma attacks in people who already have the disease.

BOX 12.4   Risk factors for developing asthma or triggering asthma episodes

	Asthma onset	Asthma episodes (triggers/exacerbators)
Physical	Genetic vulnerability (family history)	Allergens e.g. pollen, dust mites Food allergies e.g. nuts, shellfish Chest infections Chemical fumes Cold weather
Demographic	Age (younger) Sex (male) Socioeconomic status Ethnic minority Maternal age (younger)	
Lifestyle	Maternal smoking in pregnancy Maternal anxiety Smoking in the home Violence in the home	Smoke Pollution or vehicle exhaust fumes Intense exercise
Psychosocial		Stress Anxiety

Genetic vulnerability and parental smoking are strong risk factors for the initial onset of asthma. Although there is no specific gene that causes asthma, a combination of genes passed from parents to children will approximately double the likelihood of children having asthma. Lifestyle factors are also important, primarily smoking and exposure to other pollutants. For example, if a woman smokes during pregnancy her child has a 35 per cent increased risk of being wheezy or having breathing difficulties. Children whose parents smoke are 1.5 times more likely to develop asthma. Reducing parental smoking is therefore one of the most important, modifiable, risk factors for the development of asthma. Psychological knowledge can be useful in targeting health promotion to encourage parents to give up smoking (see Chapter 5).

There is substantial evidence that symptoms in people who already have asthma are exacerbated by stress (e.g. Sandberg et al., 2000). Research has also shown that children who are exposed to violence report more symptoms and have an increased risk of complications (Wright et al., 2004). The core pathological process of inflammation of the airways has led to the proposal that stress-induced changes in immune responses may contribute to this exacerbation and triggering of asthma (see Chapter 3). For example, in one study children with and without asthma were asked to make a speech and do mental arithmetic in front of an audience (Buske-Kirschbaum et al., 2003). The children did not differ on heart rate responses to this stress, but those with asthma showed a significantly reduced cortisol response. Cortisol is anti-inflammatory so dysregulation of the cortisol response may be important in chronic asthma. There are similar findings for other chronic inflammatory diseases, such as rheumatoid arthritis (see Chapter 11).

In section 12.2.2, we saw that stress makes people much more vulnerable to respiratory infections. The role of respiratory tract infections in triggering asthma is well established: this is another important pathway between stress and asthma attacks (Cohen and Rodriguez, 2001). Section 12.2.1 highlighted the links between breathing and emotions, particularly anxiety. Although breathing training for asthma is not associated with many improved outcomes (Ritz and Roth, 2003), there is emerging evidence that anxiety disorders can exacerbate asthma symptoms. A study of self-reported asthma attacks after the 9/11 New York terrorist attacks showed that among people with asthma, those who also had PTSD were three times more likely to have symptoms and visit their doctor and six times more likely to visit Accident and Emergency departments. This increased risk was irrespective of pre-9/11 asthma symptoms, demographic characteristics, or the amount of exposure to the attacks (Fagan et al., 2003). It therefore appears that anxiety disorders are important in the triggering and perception of asthma symptoms. A meta-analysis found people with asthma were more likely than the rest of the population to have anxiety disorders (Weiser, 2007).

CLINICAL NOTES 12.2

Treating respiratory disorders

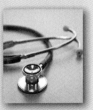

- Smoking and passive smoking are one of the most important, modifiable, risk factors.
- Most people cannot reliably detect changes in their lung function.
  It is important to confirm patients self-report with physical measures such as a spirometer.

(Cont'd)

- Anxiety is strongly implicated in respiratory symptoms. Symptoms can be triggered or exacerbated by stress and anxiety.
- Symptoms are strongly affected by anxiety and beliefs about illness – these factors are more predictive of health outcomes than objective physical health.
- Self-management programmes are very effective at helping people manage their illness better.
- Self-management programmes involve education, the self-monitoring of lung function and triggers, using action plans to cope during episodes, and exploring and changing people's beliefs about illness.
- Guidelines state that self-management programmes should be incorporated into regular medical care.

CASE STUDY 12.2   Illness representations and asthma symptoms

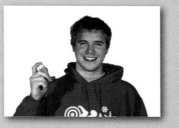 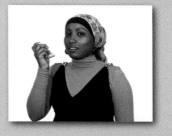

Illness identity	Asthma is a mild condition.	Asthma is a severe condition.
Cause	Caused by infections and a pet allergy.	I inherited it from my dad.
Timeline	It's a remitting condition that some people grow out of.	It'll never go away.
Control	I can control the symptoms and exposure to triggers.	I can't control it.
Consequences	It is unlikely to kill me.	If it gets bad it could kill me.
Management	Relaxed attitude but avoids triggers where possible; will increase medication when he has an infection. Low anxiety so will only visit the doctor when his own attempts to manage his symptoms do not work.	Tense and anxious about asthma symptoms. Has not thought about what might trigger her asthma, so is constantly worried and hypervigilant. Takes regular preventive medication and visits her doctor at the first sign of breathlessness.

Although psychological factors are not strongly implicated in the onset of asthma, they are very important when it comes to managing it. People with asthma are expected to monitor their symptoms and use inhaler medication when they need it. However, up to 60 per cent are unable to reliably detect changes in their lung function (Kendrick et al., 1993). The perception of symptoms and medical outcomes is associated with a variety of psychological factors, including anxiety, pessimism, and perceived stigma. Compared to objective measures of asthma symptoms, these factors are better predictors of outcomes such as the number of times a person is hospitalised for asthma, how long they stay, and their medication prescription. Thus there is a strong role for psychological factors in the management of asthma symptoms and their consequences (Kinsman et al., 1982). This is illustrated in Case Study 12.2 which shows how patients' illness representations will affect how they manage their symptoms (see Section 4.4).

Psychological interventions to help people manage asthma include: education; self-monitoring of lung function and triggers; developing an action plan to help the patient know what to do during an asthma episode; and exploring and modifying illness beliefs. There is plenty of evidence that self-management interventions are highly effective and result in reduced hospitalisation, fewer visits to the doctor, and fewer days off school or work (Wolf et al., 2003). Other positive outcomes include increased self-efficacy in children and reduced nocturnal asthma episodes in adults. Guidelines for asthma therefore explicitly state that self-management should be incorporated into regular medical management and that doctors should encourage patients to use self-management techniques (GINA, 2001).

Summary

- The reciprocal relationship between breathing and emotion means that controlled breathing can be useful when treating stress-related disorders and panic.
- Susceptibility to URIs is affected by stress, social relationships, sleep, emotions, and socioeconomic status. The effect of stress and social relationships on susceptibility to URIs is probably mediated by changes in immune function.
- Traditionally, asthma has been viewed as a psychosomatic illness but the evidence shows the initial onset is mainly determined by biological factors (genetic vulnerability, age, sex) and parental factors (for example having a young mother, being exposed to smoking in the home or to violence).
- Anxiety is strongly implicated in respiratory symptoms. In those who have asthma, symptoms can be triggered or exacerbated by stress and anxiety.
- Although psychological factors are not hugely implicated in the onset of asthma, they are very important when it comes to managing it. Self-management interventions are highly effective and can result in less hospitalisation and fewer visits to the doctor and days off.

CONCLUSION

This chapter has examined the role of psychosocial risk factors in cardiovascular and respiratory disease. There are similarities and differences in the role of psychosocial factors in disorders of these two body systems. Psychosocial factors are extensively associated with heart disease: lifestyle, stress, and negative emotions are critical in the development of disease and the subsequent prognosis. Emotions of depression and anger/hostility are particularly implicated in heart disease. Respiratory disorders are also affected by lifestyle, stress, and emotions, but in this case it is anxiety that research has particularly implicated. In the respiratory disorders addressed here, psychosocial factors are less implicated in the development of pathology than a susceptibility to developing symptoms. Of course, we have only looked at URIs and asthma and it is true to say that lifestyle factors – particularly smoking – are critical in the development of other respiratory diseases such as COPD and lung cancer.

Psychological intervention in cardiac or pulmonary rehabilitation also has various effects. In cardiac rehabilitation, psychological intervention improves psychological well-being but does not influence mortality. In chronic respiratory disorders there is strong evidence that interventions that include psychological components can improve symptom management and healthcare use in disorders that involve significant self-management.

📖 FURTHER READING

Ayers, S. et al. (eds) (2007) *Cambridge Handbook of Psychology, Health and Medicine.* Cambridge: Cambridge University Press. Includes many short chapters on coronary heart disease (impact, surgery, psychological risk factors, rehabilitation, hypertension) and respiratory disorders (asthma, lung cancer, COPD, colds, hyperventilation).

Kaptein, A.A. & Creer, T.L. (eds) (2002) *Respiratory Disorders and Behavioural Medicine.* London: Martin Dunitz. Gives detailed information on psychological risks and the impact and treatment of respiratory disorders. It includes details on asthma, COPD, and cystic fibrosis. It also considers clinical issues such as smoking cessation, adherence, and self-management.

Molinari, E., Compare, A. & Parati, G. (eds) (2006) *Clinical Psychology and Heart Disease.* New York: Springer. Covers psychosocial risk for heart disease and psychological treatment in detail. Includes chapters on depression, anxiety, and various psychological treatments for cardiac rehabilitation.

❓ REVISION QUESTIONS

1 Describe three pathways by which psychosocial factors will influence the onset and progression of heart disease.

2 Outline the major psychosocial risk factors for cardiovascular disease and the size of their effect on the risk of CHD.

3 How do individual differences in a cardiac reactivity to stress affect the risk of cardiovascular disease?

4 Describe the common psychological responses to cardiovascular disease. Outline the impact of psychological interventions on physical and psychological wellbeing.

5 Outline the factors associated with delays to seeking treatment for CHD and non-adherence to treatment regimens.

6 How is the relationship between breathing and emotions reciprocal? What is the clinical relevance of this observation?

7 Describe how psychosocial factors influence the susceptibility to upper respiratory tract infections.

8 Compare the relative importance of psychological and biological factors in asthma.

9 Outline why self-management interventions are effective in treating asthma.

10 Compare and contrast the role of psychosocial factors in cardiovascular and respiratory disease.

13 GASTROINTESTINAL

CHAPTER CONTENTS

LEARNING OBJECTIVES

This chapter is designed to enable you to:

- Outline the physiological basis for the relationship between psychological factors and GI health.
- Appreciate the role of stress in GI function and illness.
- Consider the impact of diet and alcohol use on GI health and illness.
- Outline the role of psychosocial factors in specific GI disorders.

There are clear links between psychology and the gastrointestinal (GI) system. The close relationship is illustrated in common language. Common expressions of psychological states include (to follow the sequence of the GI tract) *choking* on information, not *digesting* difficult news, having butterflies in the *stomach*, someone making us *sick*, having a *gut* feeling, or being scared *shitless*. Direct bi-directional physiological links exist between the brain, autonomic nervous system, and enteric nervous system. This is called the brain-gut axis. The four main areas linking psychological states to the GI system are:

1   The brain-gut axis.
2   The effect of stress on GI function.
3   The effect of lifestyle e.g. diet, alcohol use, smoking.
4   The psychological impact of GI disorders.

The relative importance of these areas varies. Functional GI disorders, such as irritable bowel syndrome and dyspepsia, are more likely to be affected by factors such as stress and symptom perception. Organic disorders, such as cirrhosis or cancer, have stronger associations with lifestyle factors such as diet, drug, and alcohol use. GI medicine is therefore an area that certainly requires a biopsychosocial approach to prevention and treatment (Wilhelmsen, 2000).

We shall start this chapter by examining how psychological factors interact with GI functioning through the brain-gut axis and the role of stress. We shall then examine the role of lifestyle factors on GI health, concentrating on diet and alcohol use. Finally, disorders of the GI system are examined to illustrate the complex interplay between psychology and the gut and the profound impact of GI disorders.

13.1 PSYCHOLOGICAL FACTORS AND THE GI SYSTEM

Physiological responses to stress in our environment involve the central and autonomic nervous systems, immune and neuroendocrine responses (see Chapter 3). All of these are implicated to varying degrees in GI function or disorders (van Oudenhove and Aziz, 2009).

13.1.1 THE BRAIN-GUT AXIS

The **brain-gut axis** comprises the CNS, ANS, and enteric nervous system (see Figure 13.1). The sympathetic and parasympathetic branches of the ANS innervate GI organs such as the stomach, liver, spleen, pancreas, and bowel. Under stress, the sympathetic nervous system and subsequent release of adrenaline will reduce blood flow and peristalsis and inhibit the contraction of the rectum. Sympathetic activation is also associated with reduced food intake and weight loss (Bray, 2000). Under normal conditions, the parasympathetic nervous system restores blood flow and peristalsis to the usual functioning when the stressor is removed.

The **enteric nervous system** is embedded in the lining of the GI system and has been referred to as the *'brain of the gut'* or *'second brain'* because it is large and complex (approximately 100 million neurons) and uses the same neurotransmitters as the CNS. Although it is connected with the CNS, it is able to operate independently. It controls all the functions of the GI tract, including absorption, secretions, motility, microcirculation, and the regulation of immune and inflammatory processes (Benarroch, 2007). Sensory information is sent from the enteric system to the CNS via the vagal nerve, which is thought to comprise 80 per cent afferent fibres (Goyal and Hirano, 1996).

The brain-gut axis means psychological and gastric phenomena influence each other quickly and easily. For example, placebo pills and suggestion may increase or decrease GI activity (see Research Box 13.1) and the symptoms of nausea and vomiting can be classically conditioned, such as when people having chemotherapy develop anticipatory nausea (see Chapter 10). People with functional GI disorders are more likely to have psychological disorders or to have had past traumatic experiences. Furthermore, a high prevalence of

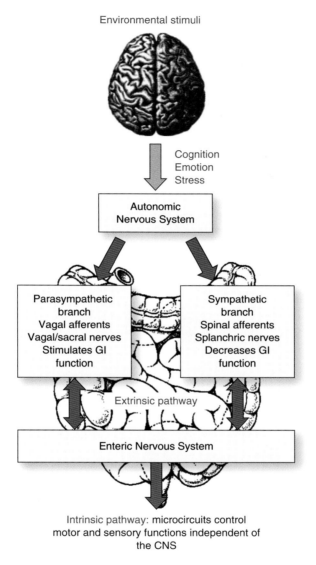

Environmental stimuli

Cognition
Emotion
Stress

Autonomic
Nervous System

| Parasympathetic branch
Vagal afferents
Vagal/sacral nerves
Stimulates GI function | Sympathetic branch
Spinal afferents
Splanchric nerves
Decreases GI function |

Extrinsic pathway

Enteric Nervous System

Intrinsic pathway: microcircuits control
motor and sensory functions independent of
the CNS

FIGURE 13.1   The brain-gut axis

functional GI disorders is found in people with mental health problems, especially depression and anxiety disorders (Garakani et al., 2003).

This reciprocal relationship between emotions and GI function is found not only in people with GI disorders. For all of us, emotions such as anxiety and disgust are linked with GI symptoms. Disgust tends to be accompanied by physiological movements that will mimic retching or vomiting (see Figure 2.1). Products of the GI system (e.g. vomit, faeces)

RESEARCH BOX 13.1   Placebo and GI function

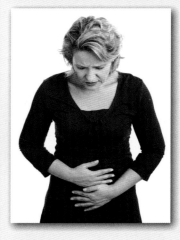

Background

The brain-gut axis suggests a close interplay between psychological factors and GI function. This study used an experimental approach to see whether placebo and suggestion affected GI and autonomic nervous system function.

Methods

18 adults were given placebo pills on three occasions and told either that these would stimulate GI function, relax GI function, or not affect it.

Results

Electrogastrograms were used to measure GI activity and the results showed that GI activity was increased or decreased according to the instructions given with the placebo pill as shown in the figure.

   There were no significant differences in autonomic nervous system activity such as heart rate or skin conductance.

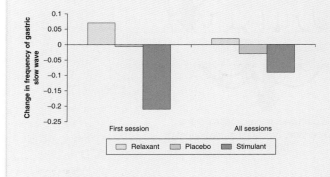

Significance

This study suggests that suggestion and placebo can increase or decrease GI activity – demonstrating a causal influence of psychological factors in GI function, independent of general autonomic nervous system function.

Photograph © Robert Kneschke/ Fotolia

Meissner, K. (2009) Effects of placebo interventions on gastric motility and general autonomic activity, *Journal of Psychosomatic Research*, 66: 391–398.

are universal triggers of disgust in different cultures (Rozin et al., 2000). Anxiety is associated with changes in GI function. In one study, healthy volunteers were asked to recall experiences that had made them feel neutral or anxious. These were recorded and then played back to them while they underwent various tests of gastric function. When listening to the recording of their anxious experience, volunteers had reduced gastric function and more reports of bloating and fullness (Geeraerts et al., 2005).

In functional GI disorders the brain-gut axis may become dysregulated. This is analogous to ANS and HPA-axis dysregulation in stress disorders (see Chapter 3), or dysregulation of immune responses in autoimmune disorders (see Chapter 11). Dysregulation of the brain-gut axis leads to altered sensation, symptoms, motility, and other aspects of GI function. Other alterations include an increased sensitivity to GI symptoms and altered pain pathways. Permanent changes may occur to the distribution of neurons in the enteric nervous system in chronic disease such as Crohn's disease or ulcerative colitis (Villanacci et al., 2008).

13.1.2 STRESS AND THE GI SYSTEM

As the brain-gut axis is intricately connected with stress responses it is not surprising that stress affects GI function in healthy people and exacerbates existing GI disorders, particularly functional disorders such as IBS or ulcers (Leza and Menchen, 2008). Around 70 per cent of the general population report changes in bowel function in response to stress (Drossman et al., 2002). Stress leads to a number of changes in the gut, including increased motility, altered ion secretion, increased intestinal permeability, low-grade inflammation, epithelial abnormalities, and enteric neuron dysfunction. In people with GI disorders, stress can contribute to gastric erosions and ulcers and increase the severity of colitis (Leza and Menchen, 2008). Stress may interact with pathogens such as *Helicobacter pylori* or non-steroidal anti-inflammatory drugs (**NSAIDs**) to increase the likelihood of GI disorders (Caso et al., 2008).

The relationship between stress and GI function is complex because stress is also associated with psychological factors, such as an increased sensitivity to GI sensations and symptoms, a decreased pain tolerance, and changes in lifestyle that will affect GI function (Leza and Menchen, 2008). People with functional GI disorders report more stress and are more likely to perceive major life events as negative or stressful (Hui et al., 1999). Emotional distress, increased sensitivity, and an increased perception of symptoms may play a role in this. For example, in addition to reporting more anxiety, depression, and reduced **quality of life** (**QoL**), people with constipation are also more likely to monitor symptoms, are more sensitive to rectal distension and urge sensations, and are less tolerant of bowel volume (Chan et al., 2005).

Although the relationship between stress and GI symptoms is well established, the exact causal mechanisms through which this occurs are complex and likely to involve many factors, including physiological changes, emotional wellbeing, sensitivity and symptom perception (see Figure 13.2). Stress may interact with other factors such as an exposure to pathogens, lifestyle, and individual differences in coping style. This means that treating GI

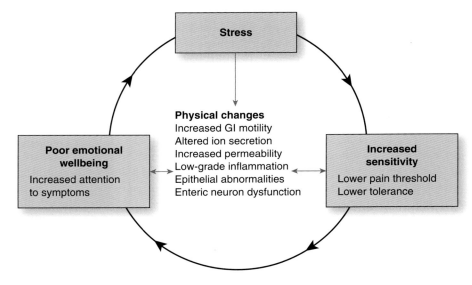

FIGURE 13.2 Stress and GI function

disorders can be particularly challenging: doctors must assess which physical and psycho-social factors are contributing to the disorder and then treat these appropriately.

13.1.3 A BIOPSYCHOSOCIAL APPROACH TO GI DISORDERS: THE CASE OF PEPTIC ULCERS

One clear example of the need to take a biopsychosocial approach is the history of our understanding of peptic ulcers. In the early 1980s Robin Warren and Barry Marshall conducted Nobel Prize-winning research which identified the role of the bacterium *Helicobacter pylori* in stomach ulcers. Marshall used himself as a guinea-pig and infected himself with H. pylori, after which he developed gastritis. This discovery changed our understanding of what causes peptic ulcers. Since then, research has shown that H. pylori can be associated with a range of GI problems, including dyspepsia (heartburn, bloating, and nausea), gastritis, ulcers, and stomach cancer. Treatment of H. pylori with antibiotics has resulted in a steady decline in the incidence of peptic ulcers.

However, not all people with H. pylori develop disease, and 5–20 per cent of people with ulcers do not have H. pylori. It is now thought, therefore, that H. pylori alone does not cause ulcers, but interacts with other factors to create the conditions in which disease may develop. Some researchers focus on how H. pylori prevents healing and encourages chronic disease in exposed or weakened areas of the upper GI tract (Gustafson and Welling, 2009). Other contributing factors include a genetic vulnerability, excess stomach acid, and the use of NSAIDs. Moreover, it has been estimated that psychosocial factors such as stress and lifestyle will contribute to 30–65 per cent of ulcers, regardless of whether these are caused by H. pylori or NSAIDs (Levenstein, 2000). Thus, research into H. pylori and peptic ulcers illustrates how we have moved from a purely biological explanation to a biopsychosocial explanation of peptic ulcer disease.

Summary

- The brain-gut axis comprises the CNS, ANS, and enteric nervous system, which means psychological and GI states influence each other quickly and easily.
- The enteric nervous system is connected with the CNS but able to operate independently.
- In functional GI disorders the brain-gut axis may become dysregulated.
- The relationship between stress and GI function and symptoms is well established, but the relationship is complex and likely to involve many physiological and psychological factors.
- Stress leads to changes in GI motility and physiology. Stress is also associated with decreased pain tolerance, an increased sensitivity to GI sensations, a greater perception of symptoms, and changes in lifestyle that may further impact on GI function.
- A biopsychosocial approach is vital in GI medicine, as illustrated by the interaction between H. pylori and psychosocial factors in peptic ulcers.

13.2 LIFESTYLE AND GI HEALTH

Lifestyle factors such as diet, smoking, alcohol use, and exercise will affect GI health. Smoking is associated with an increased risk of Crohn's disease, peptic ulcers, and cancers of the upper GI tract, but a reduced risk of ulcerative colitis. What we eat influences our risk of developing many disorders including cancer, diabetes, and the intermediate outcomes of obesity: it is estimated that approximately 30 per cent of cancers in developed countries are caused by unhealthy diets (see Figure 11.1). Increased alcohol use is directly related to increased rates of liver disorders and cancers of the GI tract. In this section we shall therefore examine diet and alcohol use in more detail.

13.2.1 HEALTHY AND DISORDERED EATING

Diet and GI health

Diet is important to GI health. However, the links are complex because our diet consists of different nutrients that can affect our health directly or in combination with each other. Various aspects of diet are important to health (see Box 13.1). Although there are some areas where evidence is incomplete or inconsistent, the following aspects of diet are known to be important for GI health:

- **High fibre** reduces bowel cancer risk by up to 40 per cent. This may be due to the effect of fibre on bowel function – i.e. stools spend less time in the bowel, so there is less time for food-related chemicals and antigens to damage the bowel lining. Alternatively, it may be due to the creation of short-chain fatty acids when fibre is broken down which may make it harder for tumours to develop.
- **Fruit and vegetables** reduce the risk of cancers, particularly of the upper GI tract. This may be because they are a good source of fibre (as above) or because they provide vitamins A, B, and C which appear to protect us against cancer.
- **Oily fish** such as salmon and mackerel decrease the risk of cancer and heart disease.
- **Salt** is associated with an increased risk of stomach cancer, which is more prevalent in countries that have a very salty diet, such as Japan (see Figure 11.1).
- **Red meat** increases the risk of stomach and bowel cancer, particularly if the meat is processed e.g. bacon, salami. This increased risk is thought to be due to chemicals contained in red meat, such as haem, that will damage the bowel when broken down. Carcinogens are also created when meat is cooked at high temperatures.

BOX 13.1 Guidelines for a healthy diet

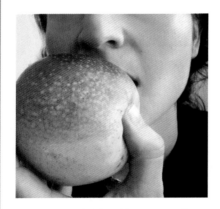

- Diet should be high in fibre: it should include such food-stuffs as fruit, vegetables, pulses, rice, wholegrain foods.
- Eat 5+ portions of fruit and vegetables per day.
- Eat 2+ portions of oily fish a week.
- Decrease the intake of red or processed meat.
- Decrease the salt intake.
- Avoid refined sugar.
- Avoid saturated fats.

Photograph © Pink Shot, www.photoxpress.com

ACTIVITY 13.1

- How does your diet compare to the recommendations given in Box 13.1?
- What kind of factors influence the type of food you eat and when?

Why do we eat what we eat?

Given the evidence outlined above, it is a public health concern that many people do not have a healthy diet. However, a study of more than 40,000 people in Europe showed that there was huge variation to be found between countries: people in Northern European countries have the least healthy diets (Beer-Borst et al., 2000). Whatever the norm for a particular country, women will usually eat more fruit, vegetables, fibre, and less saturated fat than men. This appears to be because women have more concerns about weight and more healthy attitudes and beliefs about food (Wardle et al., 2000).

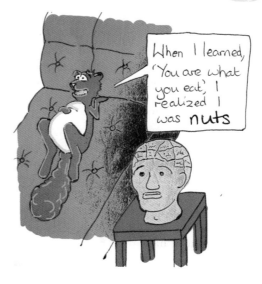

With obesity increasing, it is important to understand how poor dietary habits can develop. Research suggests we are not born with a tendency to over eat or have a poor diet. Studies of infants and young children suggest that if they are offered a variety of healthy food and allowed to eat what they want, they will naturally choose a balanced diet (e.g. Davis, 1939). Poor dietary habits therefore appear to be learnt. This occurs through processes of exposure, reinforcement, modelling, and imitation during childhood (see Chapter 10). Dietary habits are also influenced by attitudes, beliefs, and weight concerns in adolescence and adulthood. Children will eat the food they are exposed to and will prefer those foods they are exposed to regularly. Therefore the more that unhealthy food is available and accessible in the environment (e.g. the sweets aisle in the supermarket), the more likely it is that children will eat and prefer this. Eating habits are also shaped through imitating friends and family. Modelling good eating behaviour can be used to promote healthy eating. One study used videos of 'food dudes' – older children who were filmed enthusiastically eating healthy food – to successfully change children's preferences for foods and increase their fruit and vegetable intake (Lowe et al., 1998).

The meaning of food in interactions between children and parents can shape children's eating behaviour. Food used as a reward or treat will be liked more and preferred over food that is seen as a non-reward. This means that strategies such as telling children they can only have pudding if they eat their vegetables may result in children learning to prefer pudding and dislike vegetables even more! Parental control over what children eat will have different effects depending on how the control is exercised. Hidden control, such as making sure unhealthy food is not available in the child's environment, is associated with less unhealthy eating habits, such as snacking on sweets. Overt control, such as telling the child what they can and cannot eat, is associated with an increased intake of healthy foods like fruit (Ogden et al., 2006). However, parental restrictions may lead to a child eating more 'bad' foods when not in the home environment or under parental control.

In adolescence and adulthood, diet will be increasingly affected by body dissatisfaction and weight concerns. Approximately half of men and three quarters of women will diet at some point during their lifetime, and one in four women will be dieting at any one time (Jeffery et al., 1991). Women at university are particularly likely to be dieting. A study of more than 16,000 students in Europe found that 44 per cent of women were trying to lose weight, even though only 8 per cent were actually overweight (Bellisle et al., 1995).

Dieting, or restrained eating, has its advantages and disadvantages. On the one hand, it is associated with weight loss or reduced weight gain (Tucker and Bates, 2009). On the other hand, restrained eating is associated with a range of negative psychological states, including body dissatisfaction, food cravings, preoccupations with food, guilt about food/eating, over estimating body size, low self-esteem, anxiety and depression (Hawks et al., 2008). Dietary restraint may also contribute to eating disorders such as anorexia and bulimia. Conversely, disinhibited or uncontrolled eating – where people find it hard to control their eating in response to environmental cues – may play a role in overeating and obesity. Some research has examined whether restrained eaters are more or less likely to become disinhibited eaters after they eat a high calorie snack. The results are inconsistent, but for some individuals the combination of restrained eating with difficulty in controlling their eating behaviour may lead to overeating and fluctuations in weight.

Disordered eating: anorexia, bulimia, and binge eating

Paradoxically, as food has become more widely available, disordered eating has increased. Eating disorders include anorexia nervosa, bulimia nervosa, and binge eating disorder. Diagnostic criteria for these disorders are shown in Box 13.2. Estimates of lifetime prevalence range from approximately 0.1 to 3 per cent, but many more people may have symptoms of eating disorders without meeting the full criteria for diagnosis. Eating disorders are associated with an increased risk of other psychiatric problems, such as phobias, anxiety disorders, and substance misuse. For example, in the USA comorbid anxiety disorders occur in 48 per cent of people with anorexia, 81 per cent of people with bulimia, and 65 per cent of people with binge eating disorder (Hudson et al., 2007). Eating disorders can lead to a variety of physical problems, especially GI tract disorders such as gastric reflux, peptic ulcers, and constipation. Severe cases can lead to other problems such as cardiac arrhythmias or arrest.

Anorexia nervosa is a refusal to maintain a healthy body weight – usually defined as less than 85 per cent of expected body weight. Anorexia has a lifetime prevalence of approximately 1 per cent of women and 0.3 per cent of men and cases are increasing. It is most likely to occur in women during their teenage years or early adulthood: it is very rare for new cases to occur after age 25 (see Case Study 13.1). White women from wealthy families are most at risk. Anorexia is also more prevalent in certain occupational

---

BOX 13.2   Eating Disorders (*DSM-IV*)

Anorexia Nervosa	Bulimia Nervosa	Binge Eating Disorder
<ul><li>Refusal to maintain normal body weight</li><li>Intense fear of gaining weight or being fat</li><li>Distorted view of their body shape or denying seriousness of current low body weight</li><li>Amenorrhea for at least three months</li></ul>	<ul><li>Recurrent binge eating</li><li>Recurrent inappropriate methods to compensate e.g. vomiting, use of laxatives, excessive exercise</li><li>Triggers may include stress, trauma, or body dissatisfaction</li><li>Symptoms can occur daily or every few months</li></ul>	<ul><li>Recurrent binge eating associated with feelings of loss of control during eating</li><li>Binge eating associatedwith three or more of the following:<ul><li>Eating until uncomfortably full</li><li>Eating when not hungry</li><li>Eating very fast</li><li>Eating alone because of embarrassment</li><li>Feeling disgusted, depressed or guilty after binge eating</li></ul></li><li>Marked distress over binge eating</li><li>Binge eating at least two days a week for six months</li><li>Not using inappropriate methods to compensate (see bulimia)</li></ul>

---

groups, such as models and dancers, where there is a social pressure to be thin. There are two types of anorexia: the **restricting type**, where weight loss is achieved through dieting or exercise, and the **binge-eating type**, where binge eating and purging are also used to achieve weight loss. Anorexia has the highest mortality rate of any psychiatric disorder, with 3–18 per cent of anorexics dying from related causes or suicide (Herzog et al., 2000).

Many theories have been developed to explain why anorexia occurs, including a genetic vulnerability, biological abnormalities in noradrenaline or serotonin systems, mood disturbances, a need for control, low self-esteem, perfectionism, the internalisation of thin body ideals, dysfunctional family dynamics, and childhood sexual abuse. Although these factors have all been *associated* with anorexia, there is little prospective research that allows us to determine whether such factors are the causes or consequences of anorexia

CASE STUDY 13.1   Anorexia nervosa

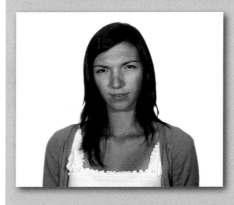

Sally developed anorexia nervosa at the age of 15 and suffered from it for four years before finally putting weight back on. Although she was always slim, Sally said she felt 'deeply uncomfortable about my body and under-confident about who I was'. Comparing herself to girls at school and models in magazines she felt overweight and became determined to get thin. She started to restrict her food intake and exercise excessively. Eventually her weight fell to less than 4.5 stone (28.6 kilos). Her BMI was 10.8.

The anorexia led to heart palpitations. Tests showed extreme malnutrition so Sally was admitted to hospital. After inpatient treatment Sally's weight increased to six stone and she was allowed home. She said being ill and in hospital 'was a turning point as it made me realise the damage I was doing to myself. I had to help myself'. Sally had several months of psychotherapy to help her develop a better relationship with food, a healthier and more realistic view of her body, and a more critical view of media representations of women.

(Stice and Shaw, 2007). Twin studies indicate that genetic and environmental factors are both important (Mazzeo et al., 2009).

Bulimia nervosa affects around 1.5 per cent of women and 0.5 per cent of men (Hudson et al., 2007). Bulimia is characterised by binge eating followed by compensatory behaviours. These usually take the form of **purging** (e.g. self-induced vomiting or the use of laxatives) or **non-purging** (e.g. excessive exercising or fasting). Most people with bulimia are of average weight so this can often go undetected.

Most evidence supports a social-cognitive explanation of bulimia where the promotion of thin body-ideals in the media leads to increased body dissatisfaction, negative feelings, and low self-esteem. These negative feelings can trigger dieting and bulimic behaviours. Bingeing and purging are thought to be used by bulimics to deal with or distract from their negative feelings and thoughts. This then becomes self-reinforcing because it temporarily removes negative feelings. Evidence supports this explanation. For example, exposure to thin models in the media is associated with increased body dissatisfaction, a negative self-concept, and low self-esteem (Striegel-Moore and Franko, 2008). Research also confirms that binge eating is usually preceded by negative emotions, such as anxiety, depression, or loneliness (see Research Box 13.2).

RESEARCH BOX 13.2   Regulating distress by eating

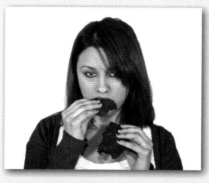

Background

Theories of bingeing and purging argue that it is used by people with eating disorders to deal with and regulate negative emotions.

Methods

This study examined factors that may be used to predict bingeing behaviour in 130 people with bulimia nervosa. The study used interviews and questionnaires to measure a wide range of factors, including impulsivity and people's tendency to act quickly and rashly to avoid negative emotions without thought of the consequences (negative urgency).

Results

Negative urgency was the only variable that predicted binge eating when other factors were controlled for, including anxiety, depression, mood, age, sex, ethnicity, education, premeditation, and functioning.

Significance

This study demonstrated a strong association between the need to act rashly to regulate negative emotions and binge eating in people with bulimia, even after taking into account negative moods such as anxiety and depression.

Anestis et al. (2009) Dysregulated eating and distress: examining the specific role of negative urgency in a clinical sample, *Cognitive Therapy Research, 33*: 390–397.

Binge eating disorder (BED) or **uncontrolled eating** is increasing. The prevalence of BED is around 3.5 per cent of women and 2 per cent of men (Hudson et al., 2007). In contrast to anorexia, new cases of BED will occur throughout adulthood – even up to age 60 (Hudson et al., 2007). People with BED report poor social adjustment, impaired functioning, worse physical health, and more psychological disorders than people without BED (Wilfley et al., 2003).

BED differs from other eating disorders in a number of ways. First, it tends to last longer than anorexia and bulimia (Pope et al., 2006). Second, a vulnerability to BED differs from that of anorexia or bulimia. For example, men are almost as likely to develop this as women and there are no differences between ethnic groups. BED also differs in terms of its course and outcome (Striegel-Moore and Franko, 2008). People with BED are not necessarily obese, although BED is slightly more common in obese people than in the general population.

The concept of BED is relatively new and the diagnosis in DSM-IV is listed under non-specified eating disorders (Striegel-Moore and Franko, 2008). Its aetiology is unclear, but it is thought to be due to factors similar to those associated with bulimia. Prospective studies suggest initial increases in weight can lead to body dissatisfaction, dietary restraint, negative emotions, and emotional eating which will increase risk of BED (Stice and Shaw, 2007). Experimental studies support the role of emotional eating. In one study, women with BED ate faster following a stressful public speaking task, whereas women without BED showed no changes in their eating behaviour (Laessle and Schulz, 2009).

ACTIVITY 13.2

- When are you most likely to overeat and consume a large number of highly calorific foods?
- What factors do you think are important in triggering overeating?

Preventing and treating eating disorders

To be effective, the prevention of eating disorders should be based on our understanding of what causes these disorders. Simple educational approaches are not effective. Prevention programmes are most effective if they are interactive, involve more than one session, promote body acceptance, and are delivered by a healthcare professional. Such programmes will result in reduced risk factors for eating disorders, such as body dissatisfaction, and reduced current or future disordered eating behaviour (Stice et al., 2008).

Treatment of eating disorders varies according to the disorder and usually involves psychotherapy or medication. Relatively little is known about the efficacy of treatments for anorexia. A review of 32 randomised controlled trials found inconclusive evidence for the efficacy of medication or behavioural treatments. Family therapy is an effective treatment for adolescents with anorexia and cognitive behavioural therapy (CBT) appears to reduce the chance of relapse in adults with anorexia once their weight has been restored to normal levels (Bulik et al., 2007).

In contrast, more is known about treatments for bulimia and BED, both of which can be effectively treated with CBT. This counters dysfunctional thoughts about weight and body shape, reduces binge-purge cycles, and enhances self-esteem. Antidepressants can also reduce the symptoms of binge eating and purging in the short term, although this may be a placebo effect. CBT has longer lasting effects. For example, a randomised controlled trial found that CBT alone was more effective (61 per cent cured) than CBT plus antidepressants (50 per cent), antidepressants alone (22 per cent) or a placebo (26 per cent)

(Grilo et al., 2005). CBT for bulimia and BED results in reduced bingeing, dietary restraint, and depression, but not weight loss (Striegle-Moore and Franko, 2008).

Summary

- What we eat affects our risk of many disorders including cancer, diabetes, and the intermediate outcomes of obesity. A healthy diet includes high fibre, fruit, vegetables, and oily fish, and reduced salt, red meat, sugars, and saturated fat.
- Poor dietary habits are learned during childhood though modelling, exposure, reinforcement, and family interactions.
- In adolescence and adulthood dieting and body dissatisfaction is common, even in those who are not overweight.
- Restrained eating is associated with body dissatisfaction, food cravings, preoccupations with food, guilt, over estimating body size, low self-esteem, anxiety and depression.
- Eating disorders occur in approximately 3 per cent of the population and include anorexia nervosa, bulimia nervosa, and binge eating disorder.
- Bulimia and binge eating disorder are influenced by a social pressure to attain the thin-ideal, increased body dissatisfaction, negative emotions, and low self-esteem. Less is known about the causes of anorexia.
- CBT is currently the most effective treatment for bulimia and binge eating disorder.

13.2.2 OBESITY

Obesity has been labelled an epidemic by health organisations. It is defined using the body mass index (BMI; see Box 13.3) and is associated with an increased risk of chronic diseases, including Type 2 diabetes, cardiovascular disease, and cancer. In the UK, obesity has more than doubled in the last twenty-five years (see Figure 13.3). Currently, 25 per cent of adults and 14 per cent of children are obese. Similar prevalences of obesity can be found in other developed countries (CDC, 2008; Thorburn, 2005). It has been predicted that if no action is taken over half of all adults and a quarter of all children in the UK will be obese by 2050, and that obesity-related disorders will cost £50 billion per year (Government Office for Science, 2007).

A simple explanation of weight gain is that it occurs because the intake of energy is greater than the energy expended. This balance is influenced by a complex system of physiological, psychological, and social factors (Government Office for Science, 2007). Such factors include:

- **Genetic vulnerability:** a number of genes have been identified that are associated with obesity. It is thought these genes predispose people to weight gain and interact with other physiological feedback systems, such as the hormone leptin which is released by adipose tissue and has a role in appetite regulation. It is estimated that genes account for 25–40 per cent of obesity (Thomas and Brownell, 2007).

BOX 13.3   Levels of obesity

Classification	BMI (kg/m²)	Treatment
Overweight	BMI ≥ 25	Self-directed diet and exercise: brief weight-management intervention.
Pre-obese	BMI 25 – 29.9	Behavioural weight-loss programmes.
Obese (I)	BMI 30 – 34.9	Behavioural weight-loss programmes.
Obese (II)	BMI 35 – 39.9	Pharmacotherapy; very low calorie diet.
Obese (III)	BMI ≥ 40	Bariatric surgery.

- **Physiological appetite control:** processes of homeostasis should regulate food intake according to need – as seen in the eating behaviour of infants and young children. However, it is clear that many people eat more than they need. This is probably due to food cues in the environment overriding physiological cues.
- **Early development and parental obesity:** parental obesity is strongly associated with children's obesity. This is likely to be due to a combination of genetic and environmental factors. Birth weight and development in early infancy are important in later chronic diseases such as diabetes and heart disease. Rapid weight gain in early childhood is associated with adult obesity.
- **Eating behaviour:** eating behaviour is determined by motivation (see Chapter 2) and the availability of food. Animal research shows that internal drives (i.e. satiety) are overridden when a variety of palatable food is available. In our society, the wide availability of various palatable foods (in large portions) creates an environment where people are more likely to overeat.
- **Diet:** the risk of obesity increases if a person's diet includes foods with high energy density, high fat, sugary drinks, or low fibre.
- **Lack of physical activity:** changes in transport, technology, and work patterns mean there has been a steady reduction in the energy we expend in our daily lives. The majority of the population do not meet current government guidelines for physical activity (Popham and Mitchell, 2006).
- **Work patterns:** increased working hours are associated with obesity; and increased income is associated with spending more on take-away food or dining out.
- **Attitudes and beliefs:** patterns of eating and exercising are influenced by attitudes and beliefs (see Chapter 5). Therefore models of health behaviour can be used to promote more healthy attitudes, beliefs, and eating behaviour (Boudreau and Godin, 2007).
- **Economic factors:** the cost of food as a proportion of our total expenditure has steadily decreased over the last fifty years. In addition, unhealthy foods that are high in sugar or fat tend to be cheaper than healthy foods such as fruit or vegetables.
- **Obesogenic environment:** a range of social, cultural, and infrastructural factors create an environment where obesity is more likely. These include the availability of high energy foods, the design of buildings and workspaces to minimise physical exertion, effort-saving devices, and increases in sedentary entertainment.

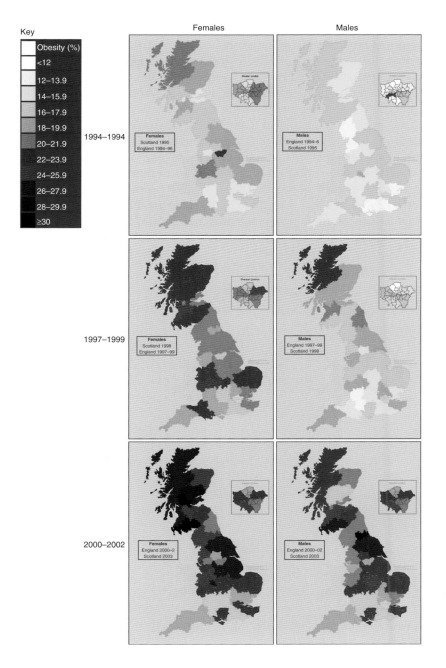

FIGURE 13.3 Trends in obesity in men and women in the UK (1994 to 2002)
Reproduced courtersy of the Government office for Science. Foresight Report (2007). *Tackling Obesities: Future Choices. Project Report* (2nd edition). London: Government Office for Science.

Case Study 13.2 illustrates how some of these different individual, social, and environmental factors might interact to promote obesity. The relative contribution of different causes of obesity may differ between individuals so any treatment should be tailored appropriately. A stepped-care approach should be taken to obesity (see Box 13.3). Group behavioural treatments are more effective than pharmacotherapy at providing sustained weight loss (Thomas and Brownell, 2007). A course of 20 weekly group sessions based on CBT principles results in around a 9 per cent reduction in body weight. Pharmacotherapy results in a 7–10 per cent reduction in body weight, which is superior to placebos. Continued physical activity is one of the best predictors of maintaining weight loss (Thomas and Brownell, 2007). Surgery is only used in severe cases and leads to dramatic and sustained weight loss. However, treating obesity by focusing on individuals ignores the wide range of environmental and social factors that contribute to the epidemic. Prevention is a priority and must tackle social influences, food production and consumption, psychological factors, individual activity, and environmental barriers to activity (Government Office for Science, 2007).

CASE STUDY 13.2   Psychosocial factors and obesity

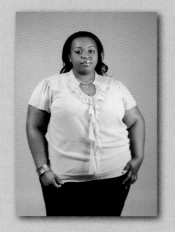

Karen is a 32 year old woman who is morbidly obese at 24 stone (152 kilos). She is unable to work and is largely confined to the home. She finds it hard to be physically active. She has chronic pelvic pain, Type 2 diabetes, and hypertension. She is also being seen by psychiatric services for recurrent depression.

Karen was sexually abused as a child and started putting on weight during this time. She no longer has any contact with her family but her weight gain continued as an adult. She has not had many relationships but recently got married to a man she met through her church.

Karen receives state disability benefits and her husband is her full-time carer. Their diet is very poor – with lots of high fat and sugar-rich foods. They enjoy take-away food in front of the TV and do this at least three times a week.

Karen knows she needs to lose weight. Her husband says he is supportive of this but seems to undermine any attempts at weight loss or changing their diet. Karen does not seem highly motivated to lose weight. The doctor suspects that there are complex reasons why Karen and her husband find it hard to engage in weight reduction programmes.

Photograph © Monteleone/Fotolia

CLINICAL NOTES 13.1

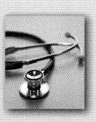

Obesity

- Treating overweight and obese people is challenging because weight regain is common.
- Pharmocological treatment results in weight loss but this is usually regained when drugs are stopped.
- Lifestyle changes of diet and exercise are more likely to lead to a sustained weight loss of approximately 5 per cent.
- Combined lifestyle and pharmacological approaches may be more effective.
- People should be encouraged to build exercise into their daily lives e.g. to walk instead of driving; to take the stairs instead of the escalator.
- Programmes for obese and overweight children can be effective and are increasingly available (e.g. http://www.mendprogramme.org)
- Where possible, families should be involved in weight reduction programmes to address familial influences on eating behaviour.

Summary

- Obesity is defined as a BMI ≥ 30 and is associated with an increased risk of chronic diseases. Its prevalence has increased in recent decades.
- Obesity is caused by a combination of factors, including a genetic vulnerability, physiological appetite control, early development, family context, eating behaviour, attitudes and beliefs, a lack of physical activity, and environmental factors.
- Current interventions include behavioural weight loss programmes, pharmacotherapy, and surgery – all of which vary in effectiveness and cost.

13.2.3 ALCOHOL USE

Alcohol-related problems are common in developed countries and account for 9 per cent of the disease burden (WHO, 2005; see also Chapter 2). Alcohol misuse is associated with a wide range of health problems and pathologies, including liver damage, hypertension, stroke, breast and GI cancer, accidents, sexually transmitted diseases, memory loss, anxiety disorders, personality disorders, depression, and drug use. In the UK, alcohol misuse is increasing and alcohol-related deaths have approximately doubled in the last twenty years.

Alcohol affects the liver in a number of ways. Alcohol is a toxin so even small amounts put a strain on the liver. Acute alcohol poisoning is caused by binge drinking and can be fatal. Chronic alcoholic liver disease starts with inflammation (hepatitis), then a fatty liver, both of which are potentially reversible if alcohol use is stopped. The final stage of alcohol liver disease is cirrhosis, where the scarring of the liver is largely permanent. Symptoms will often only arise when liver disease is advanced. They include abdominal pain, tenderness, thirst, fatigue, jaundice, a loss of appetite, fever, mental confusion, weight gain, and nausea. Alcoholic liver disease is the main reason for liver transplants in many developed countries.

Screening for alcohol use in primary care is important and simple screening tools such as the AUDIT (see Box 13.4) are available for this. Alcohol *dependence* has physical, psychological, and social components. It usually involves an increased physical tolerance, withdrawal symptoms when intake is stopped, the increasingly dominant role of alcohol in a person's life, difficulty in controlling alcohol intake (e.g. consuming more than intended, unsuccessful attempts to reduce intake), and continued drinking despite the knowledge that this is a problem (Sayette, 2007). Alcohol *abuse* is where people have at least one of the following behaviours:

* Continued drinking that interferes with a major role or obligation such as work.
* Continued drinking despite legal, social, or interpersonal problems related to alcohol use.
* Recurrent drinking in situations where intoxication is dangerous.

ACTIVITY 13.3

* How much do you think someone has to drink to become dependent on alcohol?
* Do you think this varies between individuals?

Alcoholism is determined by an interaction of genetic, psychological, and cultural factors. Twin and family studies confirm that the children of alcoholics are at greater risk of developing alcohol problems. This may be partly due to a greater sensitivity to the positive effects of alcohol or a decreased sensitivity to its negative effects (Sayette, 2007). Explanations of alcoholism draw on learning theory (see Chapter 10): alcohol use is reinforced by increasing positive emotions (positive reinforcement) or decreasing negative emotions (negative reinforcement). Alcohol use may become associated with a particular social context or cues, which can make it hard for individuals to abstain when exposed to these cues.

BOX 13.4 SCREENING FOR ALCOHOL PROBLEMS (AUDIT)

Read questions as written. Record answers carefully. Begin AUDIT by saying 'Now I am going to ask you some questions about your use of alcoholic beverages during this past year'. Explain what is meant by 'alcoholic beverages' by using local examples of beer, wine, vodka etc. Code answers in terms of standard drinks. Place the correct number in the box at the right.

1. How often do you have a drink containing alcohol?
(0) Never [Skip to Qs 9–10]
(1) Monthly or less
(2) 2 to 4 times a month
(3) 2 to 3 times a week
(4) 4 or more times a week

4. How often during the last year have you found that you were not able to stop drinking once you had started?
(0) Never
(1) Less than monthly
(2) Monthly
(3) Weekly
(4) Daily or almost daily

2. How many drinks containing alcohol do you have on a typical day when you are drinking?
(0) 1 or 2
(1) 3 or 4
(2) 5 or 6
(3) 7, 8, or 9
(4) 10 or more

5. How often during the last year have you failed to do what was normally expected from you because of drinking?
(0) Never
(1) Less than monthly
(2) Monthly
(3) Weekly
(4) Daily or almost daily

3. How often do you have six or more drinks on one occasion?
(0) Never
(1) Less than monthly
(2) Monthly
(3) Weekly
(4) Daily or almost daily
*Skip to Questions 9
and 10 if Total score
for Questions 2
and 3 = 0*

6. How often during the last year have you needed a first drink in the morning to get yourself going after a heavy drinking session?
(0) Never
(1) Less than monthly
(2) Monthly
(3) Weekly
(4) Daily or almost daily

7. How often during the last year have you had a feeling of guilt or remorse after drinking?
(0) Never
(1) Less than monthly
(2) Monthly
(3) Weekly
(4) Daily or almost daily

9. Have you or someone else been injured as a result of your drinking?
(0) No
(2) Yes, but not in the last year
(4) Yes, during the last year

8. How often during the last year have you been unable to remember what happened the night before because you had been drinking?
(0) Never
(1) Less than monthly
(2) Monthly
(3) Weekly
(4) Daily or almost daily

10. Has a relative or friend or a doctor or another health worker been concerned about your drinking or suggested you cut down?
(0) No
(2) Yes, but not in the last year
(4) Yes, during the last year

Record total of specific items here

Totals ≥ 8 indicate harmful or hazardous drinking. Totals ≥ 20 indicate possible alcohol dependence. Consult user manual in all of these cases.

Babor, T.F., Higgins-Biddle, J.C., Saunders, J.B. & Monteiro, M.G. (2007) *AUDIT: The Alcohol Use Disorders Identification Test: Guidelines for use in primary care* (2nd edition). Geneva: World Health Organisation (available at: http://whqlibdoc.who.int/hq/2001/WHO_MSD_MSB_01.6a.pdf)

Treatments for alcohol disorders should therefore address the physical, psychological, and social aspects of the disorder. Pharmacotherapy can be used to reduce the positive effects of alcohol, increase negative effects, or reduce craving. Effective psychological interventions include motivational interviewing (see Case Study 2.2), skills training, CBT, self-help groups, and couples therapy. The importance of addressing social factors is illustrated by the finding that, for married or cohabiting people, couples therapy is more effective than individual therapy in reducing short- and long-term alcohol intake and increasing satisfaction with the relationship (Powers et al., 2008). Reviews show the outcome of treatment is also better if the initial alcohol dependence is less severe and if the individual has no comorbid psychopathology, greater self-efficacy, a greater motivation to quit, and a treatment goal (Adamson et al., 2009).

CLINICAL NOTES 13.2

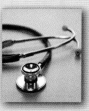

Helping people with alcohol problems

- The AUDIT tool can be used to screen people for alcohol problems (Box 13.4):
  - (a) AUDIT scores of 8–15: give advice on alcohol use, the health risks, and importance of staying within recommended limits.
  - (b) AUDIT scores of 16–19: refer for counselling and monitoring of alcohol use.
  - (c) AUDIT scores of 20+: refer to specialist alcohol services for evaluation and treatment.
- Remember that people will often under-report their alcohol use.
- People with a history of alcohol dependence should be treated at lower levels of use.
- Use your clinical judgement if what the patient reports is not consistent with other evidence.

Summary

- Alcohol misuse is associated with a wide range of health problems, including liver damage, hypertension, strokes, cancer, accidents, sexually transmitted diseases, and psychological disorders.
- Acute alcoholic hepatitis is caused by binge drinking and can be fatal. Chronic alcoholic liver disease includes inflammation (hepatitis), a fatty liver and, cirrhosis.
- Alcohol *dependence* involves an increased physical tolerance, withdrawal symptoms, a dominant role for alcohol in a person's life, difficulty in controlling alcohol intake, and continued drinking despite the knowledge that it is a problem.
- Alcohol *abuse* occurs when drinking interferes with a person's major roles or obligations; causes legal, social or interpersonal problems; or continues in situations where intoxication is dangerous.
- Alcoholism is determined by the interaction between genetic, psychological, and cultural factors.
- Couples therapy is an effective treatment for alcoholism but the outcome of treatment is partly determined by the severity of alcohol dependence, a comorbid psychopathology, alcohol-related self-efficacy, and a motivation to quit.

13.3 GI DISORDERS

13.3.1 IRRITABLE BOWEL SYNDROME

Irritable Bowel Syndrome (IBS) is a functional bowel disorder that is diagnosed when no organic disorder is identified. It is one of the most common GI disorders, affecting 3 to 18 per cent of the population. Physiological risk factors include genetic vulnerability, gastroenteritis, and sex, with women twice as likely to have IBS (Rey and Talley, 2009). Symptoms are shown in Box 13.5.

BOX 13.5   Rome criteria for Irritable Bowel Syndrome

Three months of continuous or recurrent abdominal pain or discomfort that is:
  Relieved by defecation
  Accompanied by a change in frequency of defecation or consistency of stools
AND at least two of the following symptoms for at least three days a week:
  Changes in stool frequency
  Changes in stool form
  Passage of mucous
  Feelings of bloating or abdominal distension

IBS is associated with increased stress, psychological disorders, and childhood or sexual abuse (Van Oudenhove and Aziz, 2009). People with IBS have an increased prevalence of depression, generalised anxiety disorder, panic, phobias, and somatisation disorders. They are also hypersensitive to GI symptoms such as rectal distension (Naliboff et al., 1997). This appears to be due to a greater vigilance for these symptoms and a greater likelihood of labelling such symptoms as negative or painful (Van Oudenhove and Aziz, 2009). Functional MRI studies show that people with IBS do not have the same pattern of cortical response to painful stimuli. Most notably, they have increased activation in areas of the brain associated with emotional processes such as anxiety and hypervigilance (Silverman et al., 1997). This and other research findings have led some to conclude that IBS is best conceptualised as a hyper-reactivity of the brain-gut axis that can be triggered by psychological or biological factors (Pae et al., 2007).

The role of psychological factors in IBS is illustrated by the fact that it is responsive to placebo and suggestion. One study used a placebo 'analgesia' gel during rectal distention and found it led to less pain and less cortical activity in the neural pain matrix. This reduced activity was the same as if the rectal distention was smaller (Price et al., 2007).

Antidepressants have been used to treat the physical symptoms of IBS and reviews of the evidence suggest these can have a small effect, mostly on abdominal pain or discomfort (Ford et al., 2009). This effect appears to be independent of associated changes in depression and anxiety (Hashash et al., 2008). However, the treatment of psychological distress is important in itself. People with IBS are more likely than people with inflammatory bowel disease or healthy people to consider or attempt suicide: the risk of suicide is positively correlated with more severe or chronic IBS (Spiegel et al., 2007).

Psychological intervention may be a useful adjunct to medical treatment of IBS (Lackner et al., 2004). Hypnotherapy, meditation, stress management, and CBT have all been found to produce improvements in IBS symptoms. For example, one study of individuals who did not respond to initial medication found that the addition of six sessions of CBT to their medication regimen led to a greater improvement in IBS symptoms up to six months later (Kennedy et al., 2006).

13.3.2 INFLAMMATORY BOWEL DISORDERS

Inflammatory Bowel Disorders (IBD) include Crohn's disease and ulcerative colitis, which are chronic diseases characterised by periods of remission and relapse. Main symptoms include abdominal pain, vomiting, blood in stools, weight loss, and diarrhoea. IBD is thought to be caused by an interaction between the environment and a genetic susceptibility that leads to immune dysfunction in the GI tract.

Up to 74 per cent of people with IBD think lifestyle and psychological factors such as diet and stress are important for the course of their IBD (Moser et al., 1993). Although the evidence as to whether stress plays a causal role in the onset of IBD is mixed (e.g. Singh et al., 2009), there is stronger evidence that major or chronic stress predicts relapse (e.g. Garrett et al., 1991). The influence of stress on IBD may be due to any of the physical effects of stress on the GI system (see Figure 13.2), but a key pathway appears to be through triggering increased mucosal inflammation in people with IBD (Santos et al., 2008).

Aspects of someone's lifestyle are important, though the role these play is unclear. Smoking is associated with an increased risk of Crohn's disease but with a decreased risk of ulcerative colitis. Use of oral contraceptives increases the risk of IBD. Diet is generally thought to be important because food-related antigens in the gut may trigger inflammatory responses. However, it is not clear whether diet is a causal factor or just exacerbates the disease once it has developed. Reviews of dietary treatments for IBD have found no consistent evidence that changing the amount of fat, sugar, fruit, vegetables, or fibre in the diet improves IBD symptoms (Yamamoto et al., 2009).

IBD has a profound impact on QoL. The majority of patients find that symptoms affect their work (66 per cent) and leisure activities (75 per cent) (Ghosh and Mitchell, 2007). Psychological and social problems predict both QoL and whether symptoms will worsen over time (Hart and Kamm, 2002). The relationship between IBD and psychological distress is not as strong as in functional disorders, such as Irritable Bowel Syndrome. However, anxiety increases as IBD gets worse (Porcelli et al., 1996). The progressive nature of IBD means many people will require surgery – up to 40 per cent of people with ulcerative colitis will have a colectomy (Hancock et al., 2006). Although surgery reduces the severity of symptoms it can lead to other difficulties such as faecal incontinence, pouch failure, and female infertility (Hanauer, 2008).

Adjusting to IBD is a significant challenge. However, comparatively little attention has been paid to this in the psychological literature. One study found that if patients blamed themselves for IBD they were more likely to use avoidant coping (i.e. to avoid thinking or talking about it which in turn was related to poor adjustment (Voth and Sirois, 2009). In contrast, taking responsibility for IBD resulted in less avoidance and better adjustment. People with most severe IBD were more likely to use avoidance and have poor adjustment. It is difficult to know whether the disease severity leads to avoidance or *vice versa*. However, this study suggests that encouraging patients to take responsibility and not blame themselves or use avoidant coping might be helpful.

Psychological interventions for IBD include CBT, stress management, and support groups. There is inconsistent evidence that these interventions can affect the physical symptoms of IBD. However, they do help people manage their symptoms better. Psychological interventions can lead to a reduction in symptom-related stress, disease-related worries, depression, anxiety, pain, and the use of anti-inflammatory drugs (Bennett, 2007b). Interventions that combine psychological and physical care may be even more effective but there is insufficient evidence at present. A pilot study of an intervention for ulcerative colitis that included stress management, diet, exercise, and self-care strategies found it led to better mental health and decreased bowel symptoms. However, it did not lead to changes in physiological factors such as circulating lymphocytes (Elsenbruch et al., 2005).

13.3.3 CANCER OF THE GI TRACT

Gastro-intestinal cancers are common and deadly. Cancer of the lower GI tract (colon and rectum) is the second most common cancer in developed countries, surpassed only by lung cancer (see Figure 11.1). Cancer of the upper GI tract (oesophagus, stomach, pancreas) is less common but has high mortality rates because it tends to be asymptomatic in the early stages. Survival rates therefore tend to be low. Symptoms and challenges of cancer in the upper and lower GI tract differ. Cancer of the upper GI tract may lead to problems eating, swallowing, dysphagia, nausea, and vomiting; whereas cancer of the lower GI tract leads to symptoms associated with bowel function and treatment may involve ostomies.

Cancer of the upper GI tract

Cancer of the upper GI tract is associated with gender, age, H. Pylori infection, dietary factors, and smoking. In addition, genetic vulnerability may play a role in some stomach and pancreatic cancers. Cancer of the upper GI tract is more common in older adults and men. Epidemiological research shows that diets high in salt and processed meat will increase the risk of stomach cancer, whereas a high fruit intake decreases risk (Bae et al., 2008; Larsson and Wolk, 2006). High alcohol consumption increases the risk of oesophageal cancer.

The prognosis is poor because there are very few symptoms in the early stages of upper GI tract cancer. It is common for the cancer to have metastasised before diagnosis. Six month survival rates for stomach and oesophageal cancer therefore range from

15 to 65 per cent depending on the stage of the cancer. Treatment nearly always involves surgery such as a partial or total removal of the oesophagus or stomach. These surgical procedures are difficult and can have a range of side effects. Symptoms and side effects include pain, difficulty in swallowing, weight loss, malnourishment, acid reflux, and abdominal discomfort. Unfortunately, curative surgery is often not an option for patients with gastric cancer. These patients are offered palliative care to manage the pain and surgical intervention to manage perforation or obstruction.

Given the poor prognosis, it is understandable that many patients will have high levels of anxiety and depression. The relationship between depression and cancer is particularly strong in pancreatic cancer, where survival rates are approximately 5 per cent over five years. Between 50 and 76 per cent of patients with pancreatic cancer have severe depression (Manne, 2007). Depression is so common in these patients that it is often listed as a presenting symptom of pancreatic cancer and prospective studies suggest that depression often precedes cancer of the pancreas (Manne, 2007).

Studies of QoL show that physical functioning, work, and home life are strongly affected by upper GI tract cancers. Quality of life generally decreases immediately after surgery but may improve in the long term, especially if treatment is curative. QoL is better in patients who have less invasive or toxic treatments and who feel involved in decision making about their treatment (Kim et al., 2008; Manne, 2007). For those receiving palliative care, QoL steadily deteriorates towards death (Manne, 2007). However, one aspect of QoL that is not consistently affected is emotional functioning (Conroy et al., 2006). This may reflect individual differences in emotional responses to stress (see Chapter 3). Psychological wellbeing and coping are important in adjusting to disease and can affect disease outcomes (e.g. Tian et al., 2009; see also Chapter 6).

Cancer of the lower GI tract

Cancer of the lower GI tract is associated with genetic vulnerability, older age, diet, smoking, being sedentary and overweight. It is estimated that lifestyle changes such as increasing physical activity, establishing good dietary habits, and maintaining a healthy body weight could decrease the risk of GI cancers by as much as 80 per cent (CRUK, 2010; Cummings and Bingham, 1998).

Exercise and body weight can have a dose-response effect on bowel cancer. For example, a 5-point increase in BMI increases the risk of colon cancer by up to 30 per cent (Larsson and Wolk, 2007). Many studies have shown that physical activity decreases the risk of developing bowel cancer and improves the prognosis in people who have bowel cancer. The underlying mechanisms are unclear, but may involve increased insulin-like growth factor-binding protein and reduced prostaglandins. Exercise in people with bowel cancer is associated with increased QoL and reduced mortality from cancer and other causes (Trojian et al., 2007).

Much of the literature on QoL in colorectal cancer focuses on the impact of ostomy surgery. This shows that ostomies can have a significant impact on emotional wellbeing, QoL, sexuality, and body image (Brown and Randle, 2005). Most people will experience a sharp decline in their body image after surgery, but this then gradually improves over time. People with ostomies are more likely to be depressed than people with the same illness but without ostomies, particularly if they are younger, female, less educated, or have poor support. For many aspects of QoL, the effect of ostomies is bimodal: people are either not very affected or severely affected (Brown and Randle, 2005). This highlights the importance of individual differences in coping and levels of support in helping people adapt to ostomies and accept changes in their body image (Manne, 2007).

CLINICAL NOTES 13.3

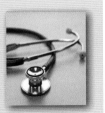

Working with GI disorders

- Patients with GI disorders such as IBS or GI cancers are at a high risk of psychological problems.
- Be alert for patients who have psychological and/or social problems because this is associated with poor QoL and may influence the course of the disease.
- Although IBS is strongly associated with psychological factors it is not helpful to portray it as 'all in the mind'.
- Explaining the close connection of the brain-gut axis can help patients understand the impact of psychological, lifestyle, and physical factors.
- It may be helpful to encourage patients not to blame themselves or use avoidant coping but to take responsibility for the course of their illness.
- Encouraging lifestyle changes such as increased exercise, a healthy diet, and reduced alcohol use can improve patients' emotional wellbeing and in some cases improve the prognosis.
- Screen for psychological disorders and offer support or psychological intervention where appropriate.

Summary

- Irritable bowel syndrome (IBS) is one of the most common GI disorders, affecting 3–18 per cent of the population. It is associated with stress, psychological disorders, and past psychological trauma.
- Psychological intervention and antidepressants can result in some improvement in IBS symptoms.

- Inflammatory Bowel Disorders (IBD) include Crohn's disease and ulcerative colitis are caused by an interaction between the environment and a genetic susceptibility that result in immune dysfunction in the GI tract.
- Stress is associated with a relapse in IBD. Psychological and social problems predict quality of life and whether symptoms will worsen over time.
- Psychological interventions for IBD result in less symptom-related stress, disease-related worries, depression, anxiety, pain, and the use of anti-inflammatory drugs.
- Gastro-intestinal cancers are strongly associated with lifestyle factors, including H Pylori infection, diet, smoking, and being sedentary and overweight.
- Anxiety and depression are common in people with GI cancer. This is particularly the case for pancreatic cancer, where depression is a possible presenting symptom.
- Ostomies can have a significant impact on emotional wellbeing, quality of life, sexuality, and body image, but there are large individual differences in how people cope and adjust.

FURTHER READING

Ayers, S. et al. (eds) (2007) *Cambridge Handbook of Psychology, Health and Medicine* (2nd edition). Cambridge: Cambridge University Press. Includes short chapters on many relevant topics including cancers of the digestive tract, obesity, eating disorders, vomiting and nausea, irritable bowel syndrome, inflammatory bowel disease, gastric and duodenal ulcers, etc.

Toner et al. (2000) *Cognitive-Behavioral Treatment of Irritable Bowel Syndrome: The Brain-Gut Connection*. New York: Guilford. A guide to individual and group CBT for IBS.

REVISION QUESTIONS

1 Describe the brain-gut axis.

2 What is the relationship between stress and GI function?

3 Why is a biopsychosocial approach important in GI illness? Illustrate your answer with reference to one specific GI illness.

4 How does diet affect health?

5 What constitutes a healthy diet?

6 Outline three eating disorders and discuss what causes them.

7 How do we define obesity? Outline five different types of causes of obesity.

8 How does alcohol abuse affect health?

9 What is the difference between alcohol dependence and alcohol abuse?

10 Discuss the role of psychosocial factors in one GI disorder.

14 REPRODUCTION AND ENDOCRINOLOGY

LEARNING OBJECTIVES

This chapter is designed to enable you to:

- Outline the psychological and mood changes associated with (a) the menstrual cycle and (b) menopause.
- Discuss the psychological impact of pregnancy and birth.
- Recognise the impact of miscarriage and stillbirth.
- Describe the main postnatal psychological problems that can occur.
- Outline the major links between endocrine disorders and psychosocial wellbeing.
- Consider the ethical issues associated with the use of hormonal treatment.

In this chapter we shall consider reproduction and endocrinology together, primarily through focusing on reproductive events and disorders. We shall also consider (in Section 14.2) non-reproductive endocrine disorders, such as Cushing's syndrome. The emphasis of the chapter is on the psychological, behavioural, and social factors that can influence, and are influenced by, the reproductive and endocrine systems.

14.1 REPRODUCTION

Reproductive events include the onset of menstruation (menarche), conception, pregnancy, miscarriage, childbirth, and menopause. Although these events mostly focus on physical changes in women, they also involve issues that affect both men and women, such as sexual dysfunction and infertility. Procedures and treatments associated with reproduction that are particularly common include contraception, cervical smear tests, hysterectomy, and hormone replacement therapy (HRT). Reproductive issues raise unique ethical dilemmas such as: at what point terminating a pregnancy is morally defensible; the rights of donor parents and the children of donors; the use of IVF for pregnancy in older women; and whether a subsequent pregnancy should be used by parents to provide a child with the right genetic make-up to be an organ or tissue donor for a sick older sibling.

These events can be viewed using different perspectives: biomedical, psychological, social, and cultural. The perspective we choose to take has implications for our understanding of the disorder and the treatment we use (see Chapter 1). For example, from a biomedical perspective, treatment for pre-menstrual syndrome (PMS) would involve pharmacological methods to counteract hormonal fluctuations. From a psychological perspective, treatment might involve identifying maladaptive behaviour and thoughts and finding more helpful ways of coping. A social perspective of PMS might examine social stress and available support for women, as well as considering cultural expectations and narratives about PMS. It should be apparent that no single perspective would offer an adequate explanation for, or treatment of, PMS. Therefore it is important to take a biopsychosocial approach where we consider all the different perspectives outlined above. This in turn will lead to a more informed and holistic approach to consultation and treatment.

In this chapter it is not possible to examine the wide range of reproductive and endocrine events and disorders. We shall therefore concentrate on menstruation, menopause, pregnancy, and childbirth. We then look at a selection of endocrine disorders. You will also find relevant information in other chapters covering such subjects as puberty (Chapter 8), Cushing's syndrome (Chapter 3), and diabetes (Chapter 11).

14.1.1 MENSTRUATION AND MENOPAUSE

The age at which girls start menstruating – **menarche** – has fallen markedly throughout the twentieth century. This change is thought to be due to better health and basic nutrition, but also to increased weight and obesity in young girls (see Chapter 8, Chapter 13). Figure 14.1 shows biological events and changes during the menstrual cycle.

The effect of the **menstrual cycle** has been examined in relation to a range of behaviours such as sexual behaviour, sleep, and diet. The follicular phase prior to and during ovulation has been associated with an increased libido (Gangestad and Cousins, 2001). From an evolutionary perspective, increased sexual behaviour at this time increases a woman's chances of conception. The menstrual cycle can also influence our choices of mate: women in the fertile phase of the menstrual cycle have a greater preference for men with more typically masculine characteristics (e.g. taller, with more masculine faces and bodies, and more social presence and sexual competitiveness: Little et al., 2007). However, this is only the case when women are asked to rate or choose men for short-term relationships, and not when they are instructed to choose men for long-term relationships.

The menstrual cycle does not affect sleep and diet as much as is commonly believed. One study in which women kept detailed daily sleep records found that although women rated their quality of sleep as worse in the days before and during menstruation, there was no actual difference in the amount of sleep or waking during the night (Baker and Driver, 2004). Similarly, research suggests that changes in food preferences are more strongly influenced by cultural norms than biological changes. For example, chocolate cravings during the menstrual cycle differ strongly between cultures (Zellner et al., 2004), suggesting that any effect of the menstrual cycle on food preferences is culturally defined.

Premenstrual Syndrome (PMS)

Physical and psychological symptoms often occur in the luteal stage, just before menstruation. These symptoms are commonly referred to as **pre-menstrual tension (PMT)** or **pre-menstrual syndrome (PMS)**. PMS includes a range of symptoms such as irritability, sleep problems, depression, labile mood, and abdominal bloating. PMS is reported by up to 30 per cent of women and is most common among those aged 25–35. Around 1-2 per cent of

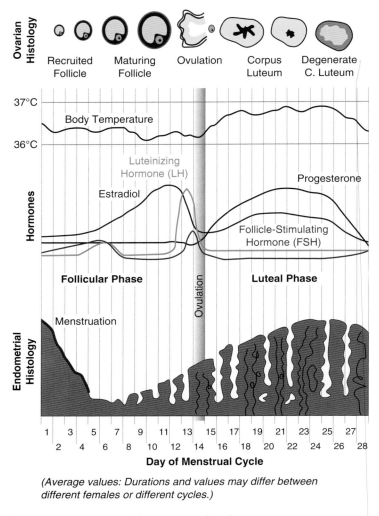

FIGURE 14.1 Physiological events of the menstrual cycle

women experience a severe form of PMS referred to as premenstrual dysphoric disorder (PMDD: see Gehlert et al., 2008). PMDD is diagnosed when there are marked disturbances in home life, social life, and work due to significant changes in sleep, appetite, energy, concentration, mood, and anxiety which appear during most of the last week of the luteal phase and abate in the week after menses (American Psychiatric Association, 2004). PMDD is not simply the exacerbation of an existing mood disorder during the premenstrual period: it is supposed to be 'switched on' during certain days within the menstrual cycle, and 'switched off' for the remainder of the cycle. However, women with a past history of depression are more likely to suffer from PMDD and PMDD is also associated with poor overall health. There is evidence of higher rates of suicide attempts in the luteal phase (Saunders and Hawton, 2001).

The relative contribution of physical and psychological factors to PMS and PMDD is unclear and the diagnosis remains controversial. Timing of symptoms suggests fluctuations in hormone levels play some causal role in psychological symptoms (Rapkin, 2003). The increased vulnerability of women with a history of depression suggests that predisposing factors can be exacerbated by the menstrual cycle. However, cultural differences in PMS suggest that the interpretation of symptoms is influenced by cultural norms. Interventions should therefore take into account biological, psychological, and cultural factors.

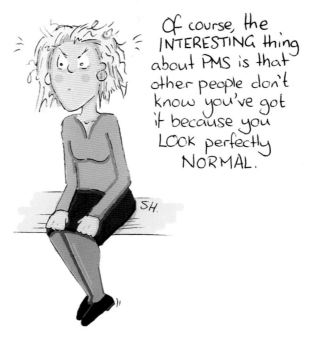

Of course, the INTERESTING thing about PMS is that other people don't know you've got it because you LOOK perfectly NORMAL.

Proper diagnosis of PMS entails monitoring a woman's symptoms over the course of at least one menstrual cycle. Various aids have been developed to help with this, such as the PMT-Cator (Magos and Studd, 1988) – a simple wheel on which women record their experiences of five common symptoms every day for six weeks.

The recommended treatment of PMS in the UK and USA is anti-depressants. Meta-analyses have shown that progesterone or progestogen treatment is not clinically effective (Wyatt et al., 2001). Despite this, practices still vary between countries. A study of patterns of PMS and PMDD in different countries found that very few doctors had actually diagnosed these syndromes (Weisz and Knaapen, 2009). When women were diagnosed, they were most commonly treated with medication. In this study, doctors in the USA, UK, and Canada favoured anti-depressants, French doctors favoured hormone and analgesic treatment, and German doctors favoured complementary medicine (Weisz and Knaapen, 2009).

Psychological intervention for PMS is effective. Meta-analyses of intervention trials show that education and monitoring are of limited use, but cognitive behaviour therapy (CBT) and CBT-based interventions can result in reduced depression and anxiety, less interference of symptoms on daily functioning, and more positive behaviour changes (Busse et al., 2008). Standard intervention packages are now available. Case Study 14.1 gives an example of an 8-session intervention. One trial found this intervention to be as effective as antidepressants over six months and more effective over the first year (Hunter et al., 2002).

CASE STUDY 14.1 Narrative therapy for premenstrual syndrome

Margo's symptoms are intolerance, impatience, and angry outbursts. Anything and everything annoys her during PMS. Anger alternates with feelings of vulnerability, insecurity, depression, and the guilt of knowing she has hurt others.

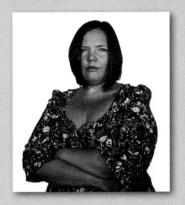

She does not 'own' her PMS self, whom she strongly dislikes. It makes her feel like a Jekyll and Hyde character where she is normally gentle and loving yet PMS makes her angry, aggressive, and horrible. She is very open about having PMS and uses it to explain her behaviour. She thinks PMS is due to hormones and diet, but she recognises that the symptoms can be worse if she is stressed or feeling down.

Margo had eight sessions of psychotherapy as follows:

Session 1: Explored Margo's history of PMS and the effect on her life. The therapist and Margo put together a working model of her PMS that included physical factors (hormones, diet), psychological factors (mood, stress, relationship issues), and narrative factors (blaming PMS, seeing her PMS self as someone else).

Session 2: Explored the influence of stress and talked through angry outbursts so Margo could see that stress played an important role in triggering her impatience and anger. Margo was taught relaxation exercises to help her deal with stress and began keeping a diary of triggers and thoughts before and during angry episodes.

Session 3: Considered relationships and PMS – how they are affected or contribute by towards certain patterns of behaviour. Margo learnt how to deal with issues assertively rather than aggressively, and how to say no. Expectations of other people were also examined (are they realistic/helpful).

Session 4: Considered self-care through expressing needs and doing things Margo enjoyed. Barriers to self-care were challenged. Margo learnt about the importance of diet and exercise and developed an activity schedule which had something positive every day and included regular exercise. Margo was given information about positive thinking.

Session 5: Examined how Margo could help herself by thinking positively and by re-'writing' her PMS experience so she would be more in control. First the therapist showed Margo how her previous symptoms were made worse by a vicious cycle of negative thoughts, feelings, and behaviour. Then Margo thought of ways to challenge or change her thoughts to be more positive. In between sessions Margo tried this out and completed a diary to see whether it helped her feel better.

Sessions 6 & 7: Continued to help Margo redefine her PMS, practise positive thinking, and use more adaptive coping strategies.

(adapted from Ussher et al., 2002)

Session 8: Reviewed the therapy, how Margo had changed, how she might continue to change, and what she had learned that would help in the future.

At the end of the therapy Margo felt more in control; her relationships and self-esteem had improved greatly, and she was more aware of how her behaviour was affecting other people. She realised that stress had played a big role in her symptoms. She also felt more ownership of her PMS: *'I have a lot of relief knowing that it's all under my control really; that it isn't something apart from me'*. After therapy, the symptoms were not as intense and she was usually able to stop herself before exploding.

Menopause

Menopause is defined as the last menstrual period. There is variation in when this occurs but it is usually between 45 and 55 years of age. The physical changes of menopause result in an increased risk of diseases like osteoporosis. Menopause has been associated with a variety of symptoms that vary between cultures. Between 50–70 per cent of women in western cultures experience symptoms such as hot flushes and night sweats. Reporting of hot flushes in cultures such as Japan has increased as cultural awareness of the menopause, or *kônenki*, has also increased (Melby et al., 2005). Thus, as noted for PMS, cultural discourses influence the interpretation of menopause symptoms. Other symptoms include poor memory, a loss of libido, irritability, problems with skin or hair, vaginal dryness, anxiety, and headaches.

In terms of mental health, there is mixed evidence as to whether women are more vulnerable to depression during this time. A review concluded that fluctuations and declines in ovarian hormones may influence the onset and progression of depression (Deecher et al., 2008). Ovarian hormones are known to have specific modulatory effects on the serotonergic and noradrenergic systems, both of which are involved in depression. Furthermore, a meta-analysis revealed that women who use **hormone replacement therapy (HRT)** have lower levels of depression than other post-menopausal women (Zweifel and O'Brien, 1997).

However, there are likely to be multiple physical, psychological, and cultural causes of depressed mood during menopause. For example, one study found that depressed mood in menopausal women was strongly influenced by a history of depression, a history of premenstrual complaints, negative attitudes toward ageing or menopause, and poor current health (Dennerstein et al., 2004). In cultures where menopause is viewed positively and increases the prestige of the women concerned, much lower levels of symptoms are reported (Freeman and Sherif, 2007). In Western cultures, however, it has been found that concurrent stressful events are important predictors of women's wellbeing during menopause. Menopause also often coincides with significant role changes, such as children leaving home. A combined biopsychosocial approach is necessary to provide a better understanding of wellbeing during menopause.

The use of HRT to treat the symptoms of menopause has been controversial and is a good illustration of the importance of research methods when examining treatment effects. Early studies of HRT were methodologically weak (for example, they did not control for the baseline health status or have a placebo group as a comparison). However, in recent large-scale placebo-controlled clinical trials, use of HRT was stopped early when it became apparent that it was associated with an increased risk of breast cancer and thromboembolism and did not protect against heart disease as originally thought (WHI, 2009).

Summary

- The menstrual cycle is associated with changes in behaviours and mood, but these vary between cultures.
- PMS and PMDD are psychological symptoms associated with the luteal phase of the menstrual cycle. PMS affects up to 30 per cent of women and PMDD up to 2 per cent.
- The relative contribution of physical, psychological, and cultural factors to PMS/PMDD is unclear but it is likely all of these factors are involved.
- A psychological intervention for PMS/PMDD can be as effective as anti-depressants.
- Menopause is often associated with hot flushes and a range of other physical and psychological symptoms.
- There is some evidence that menopause can be associated with depressed mood, which is probably also due to physical, psychological, and cultural factors.

14.1.2 PREGNANCY AND CHILDBIRTH

Over recent decades fertility rates in developed countries have declined. Today, around 20 per cent of women will have no biological children, compared to 10 per cent of women born in the mid-1940s. The average age for women to have their first baby has steadily risen. In the UK the average age for a woman to have her first baby has risen from 24 to 29 in the last forty years. These changes are strongly influenced by more women continuing in higher education and wanting to develop a career and have financial security (Brewster and Rindfuss, 2000), but may also be influenced by fertility problems that delay conception.

Infertility is usually defined as a failure to conceive after three years in normal couples where there are no known problems with the man or woman's fertility. Approximately one in eight couples will seek help for infertility and it is known to be a stressful and difficult time. Women with fertility problems consistently report more negative emotions: 25 per cent have clinically relevant depression (Oddens et al., 1999). Sexuality and relationships may also be affected, but this is variable and influenced by the quality of the relationship (Mahajan et al., 2009).

Pregnancy

Pregnancy is a time of huge physical and psychosocial transition. It is undoubtedly a positive time for many women, but is also associated with impaired physical functioning, health, and wellbeing (Haas et al., 2004). In early pregnancy most women experience nausea and vomiting. Although this is commonly referred to as 'morning sickness' only 2 per cent of women have such symptoms restricted to the morning – 80 per cent experience nausea and vomiting all day. These symptoms resolve by week 14 of pregnancy for 50 per cent of women and by week 22 for most remaining women. Although postnatal depression is most well known, mental health problems are almost as frequent in pregnancy as they are after birth. Severe depression occurs in approximately 10 per cent of women during pregnancy and 12–15 per cent of women after birth (O'Hara and Swain, 1996). Anxiety disorders are prevalent in 15 per cent of women during pregnancy and approximately 10 per cent of women after birth (Ross and McLean, 2006).

Stress and distress in pregnancy influence birth outcomes, foetal development, and infant characteristics. There is substantial evidence that stress in pregnancy is associated with a premature birth and a low birth weight. For example, women who are the victims of domestic abuse are 1.4 times more likely to have a low birth weight baby (Murphy et al., 2001). Job stress can also result in adverse outcomes. Women who work in physically demanding jobs, do shift work, or report work fatigue are more likely to have a premature birth, hypertension, and birth complications (Mozurkewich et al., 2000). Emotional distress in pregnancy has a similar effect. Depression and anxiety are associated with obstetric complications, pregnancy symptoms, a preterm labour, more requests for delivery by caesarean section, and an increased use of pain relief during labour (Alder et al., 2007; Wiklund et al., 2007).

Antenatal stress can affect foetal and infant development. Ultrasound studies have shown various effects of maternal anxiety on foetal behaviour, such as reduced foetal movement (Van den Bergh et al., 2005). Longitudinal research has shown that stress and anxiety in pregnancy are associated with poor cognitive, behavioural, and emotional development in children and that these effects remain even after controlling for prenatal, obstetric, and other psychosocial factors (O'Connor et al., 2002; Talge et al., 2007). Further evidence comes from animal research. The offspring of pregnant rats or monkeys exposed to stressors are significantly more likely to be stillborn or have low birth weight and are more likely to have impaired neuromotor functioning, impaired learning, greater behavioural disturbance, and HPA axis dysfunction in response to stress (Chapillon et al., 2002; Schneider et al., 2001).

The effect of stress and distress on infant characteristics could be due to a range of factors. First, it may be that the mother and child have genes that will increase the likelihood of anxiety and emotional problems. Second, women exposed to stress during pregnancy may live in adverse circumstances. If adversity continues after the birth it will also influence the emotional development of the infant. Related to this, adversity may be associated with lifestyle factors that affect the developing foetus (e.g. poor nutrition). A third explanation is that there are critical periods during pregnancy during which foetal stress responses are programmed or 'hard wired'. This *foetal programming hypothesis* proposes that the foetus is particularly sensitive to maternal stress during mid-pregnancy (19–26 weeks) and at the end of pregnancy (30+ weeks). The effect of stress on foetal development is thought to occur through (a) a reduced blood supply to the uterus; (b) reduced nutrients; (c) an increased transmission of stress hormones to the foetus. However, it is important to note that research shows that if infants have a nurturing early environment or positive attachment then the impact of antenatal stress is reversible (Rice et al., 2007).

In terms of medical care there are two main implications. The first is that if we reduce stress and anxiety in pregnancy it may have the potential to reduce caesarean sections and improve maternal and infant outcomes. For example, providing counselling to antenatal women with a severe fear of childbirth can reduce requests for elective caesarean deliveries (Halvorsen et al., 2008). Yet the importance of anxiety in pregnancy is not widely recognised so it is rarely screened for or treated.

The second issue is the impact of stress on female doctors who are pregnant. As we have seen, stressful and physically demanding jobs are related to adverse outcomes. Research on women doctors has shown they are at increased risk of pregnancy complications, especially in late pregnancy. During pregnancy, female doctors working in hospitals report that the physical demands of the job (e.g. night shifts, standing for long periods) are stressful and there is poor support from colleagues. Institutional support for doctors during pregnancy is lacking and needs to be properly examined (Finch, 2003).

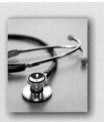

CLINICAL NOTES 14.1

Antenatal care

- It is important to identify pregnant women with high levels of distress or anxiety and offer appropriate intervention.
- Reducing stress and anxiety in pregnant women benefits the well-being of women and their unborn babies.
- It may also lead to fewer requests for elective caesarean deliveries.
- Referral to perinatal psychology services may be appropriate. They can provide psychological support for women and their families in pregnancy and after birth.
- Such services are increasing as health services realise the long-term impact maternal mental health can have on both the mother, and the health and development of children.

Birth

In birth, the greatest change in recent years has been the type of delivery. In the UK, caesarean delivery rates have risen from under 5 per cent in the 1950s to almost 30 per cent today.

The reasons for this increase are not clear. One suggestion is that more women are requesting a caesarean section in preference to a vaginal birth. However, an Australian study found that only 6 per cent of pregnant women wanted a caesarean delivery – and most of these women had obstetric complications or a previous complicated delivery (Gamble and Creedy, 2001). In the UK most caesareans are performed as emergency deliveries after labour has started, suggesting that the rise in caesarean sections is due to increased complications during labour and/or an increased tendency for doctors to carry out caesareans rather than continue with non-operative births.

Around 10 per cent of women would prefer a home delivery and most of these women want a home birth because they think they will have more control (Davies et al., 1996). Research has shown that choice and control during birth are related to postnatal psychological outcomes such as satisfaction with the birth. There are also indications that a lack of control during birth might be a risk factor for postnatal depression and post-traumatic stress disorder (PTSD) (Czarnocka and Slade, 2000). However, research in the Netherlands, where approximately 30 per cent of women give birth at home, suggests the place of birth makes no difference to the proportion of women who find giving birth traumatic (Stramrood et al., 2009).

Because birth is a common 'normal' event, it may be difficult to understand how it can be traumatic. However, 20-30 per cent of women find giving birth traumatic and around 2 per cent develop **postnatal PTSD** (Ayers and Ford, 2010). Women who have assisted deliveries or caesarean sections are more likely to develop PTSD but it is not a straightforward relationship: individual risk factors interact with what happens during birth to determine whether women find it traumatic. Risk factors include previous psychological problems or sexual trauma, the type of delivery, and a lack of support during labour and after birth (Ayers et al., 2008). The symptoms of women who develop PTSD include flashbacks to the birth, intrusive thoughts about what happened, an avoidance of reminders of the birth, and hyperarousal including increased anger and irritability (American Psychiatric Association, 2004). Women who have a stillbirth are particularly at risk: approximately 20 per cent report PTSD in the initial months after a stillbirth (Turton et al., 2001). Most women with PTSD also develop depression. An example of CBT treatment for a woman with postnatal PTSD and depression is given in Case Study 19.1.

Support during labour has a critical influence on birth outcomes and psychological wellbeing. Women are more likely to be traumatised by giving birth if they feel poorly informed, not listened to, inadequately cared for, and have little support from staff or their partner (Ayers and Ford, 2010). The provision of support for women during labour is not standard in many poorly resourced countries. This means experimental studies have been possible, where women are randomly allocated a person to support them or not. An example of one of these studies is given in Research Box 14.1. A meta-analysis of these studies shows that simply providing a lay person (a 'Doula') to support a woman during labour results in better physical outcomes for both mother and baby, including shorter labours, less analgesia, fewer assisted or operative deliveries, and higher maternal satisfaction with the birth experience (Hodnett et al., 2007).

RESEARCH BOX 14.1   Support in labour

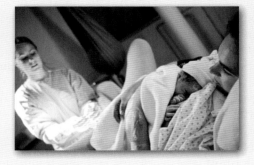

Background

Experimental studies in countries where women do not usually have a companion with them during labour clearly show that providing a lay person to support women results in better outcomes for both mother and baby. However, it is not ethically possible to replicate these kinds of studies in countries where women usually have a partner or other supportive person with them during labour.

Methods and findings

This study included 16,610 women giving birth in the same year, excluding women who had planned caesarean sections. A range of health and psychosocial variables were measured during pregnancy, birth, and the postnatal period.

Women who did not have anyone accompanying them during labour were more likely to have a preterm birth, an emergency caesarean section, pain relief, a short labour, and low satisfaction with life nine months after the birth.

Their babies had a lower birth weight, were more likely to be in intensive care, and had delayed motor development.

Women were less likely to have a supportive companion during labour if they were single, from ethnic minority groups, from poor households, and with low levels of education.

Significance

Support during labour is as critical for women in Western countries as in non-Western countries where experimental research has been done. This study identified groups of women who are at a greater risk of being alone and unsupported while giving birth. Such women may benefit from more support from healthcare professionals during labour and after birth.

Photograph © Raphaël Goetter, www.flickr.com

Essex, H. & Pickett, K. (2008) Mothers without companionship during childbirth: Analysis within Millennium cohort study, *Birth, 35*: 266–276.

14.1.3 POSTNATAL PSYCHOLOGICAL PROBLEMS

The transition to parenthood involves a huge adjustment with many new demands and stressors, including sleep deprivation. Having a baby is associated with an initial decline in the quality of a couple's relationship and an increased risk of psychological problems. In addition to PTSD, other disorders that occur after birth include baby blues, puerperal psychosis, anxiety and bonding disorders.

Up to 70 per cent of women have the 'baby blues' in the first week after a birth, which may be linked to large fluctuations in hormones during this time. Between 10-15 per cent of women develop depression in the first postnatal year, usually within two months of the birth (O'Hara and Swain, 1996). **Postnatal depression** is associated with prenatal and postnatal factors, in particular a history of psychological problems, anxiety, or depression in pregnancy, difficult sociodemographic circumstances and low support (O'Hara and Swain, 1996). Recent research suggests men may also be more likely to develop depression during this period.

Anxiety disorders appear to be more common than depression but are less well researched. Recent research suggests up to one in five women may be affected by anxiety disorders in pregnancy or after giving birth (Ross and McLean, 2006).

Puerperal psychosis occurs in only 0.1 per cent of women but is a severe disorder in which both mother and baby are at high risk of injury or harm. Women with this disorder will usually require inpatient treatment at a mother and baby psychiatric unit. Women with a personal or family history of psychosis or bipolar disorder are more likely to develop puerperal psychosis. Women who have had one episode of puerperal psychosis are also four times more likely to develop it again after a subsequent pregnancy. This suggests a strong familial and biological cause.

One important issue with postnatal psychological problems is determining whether these are present before the birth. For example, women with anxiety or depression in pregnancy are more likely to have postnatal depression. In addition, research suggests that the prevalence of depression during pregnancy is not significantly different to depression after birth. Thus, some people would question whether the notion of 'postnatal' psychological disorders is appropriate. It may be that pregnancy, birth, and adjusting to parenthood can exacerbate or initiate a wide range of different mental health problems, similar to those observed after other stressful events like bereavement or divorce.

CLINICAL NOTES 14.2

Postnatal care

- Birth can be experienced as traumatic and, following difficult births, some women will develop PTSD.
- Watch out for high levels of anxiety and re-experiencing symptoms such as nightmares, intrusive thoughts, and flashbacks.
- Postnatal PTSD is usually successfully treated if women are referred to psychotherapy in the first few months after birth.
- Be vigilant for signs of postnatal depression, but be aware that many women will have depressive symptoms prior to, or during, pregnancy.

(Cont'd)

- A proportion of women may develop other anxiety disorders such as OCD, panic, or social phobia.
- Peuperal psychosis is very severe and women should be given *immediate* inpatient treatment – preferably in a mother-baby unit so an infant can go as well.
- Make sure you are aware of the availability of psychological interventions for women with postnatal PTSD, postnatal depression, or puerperal psychosis.

Miscarriage and stillbirth

Approximately 20 per cent of pregnancies will end in a miscarriage, which may be caused by foetal or placental abnormalities. While often thought of as a lesser event, miscarriage can be as distressing to some women as a stillbirth (Friedman and Gath, 1989). Between 10-50 per cent of women experience depression after a miscarriage and the symptoms can persist for up to one year afterward (Lok and Neugebauer, 2007). The experience of miscarriage can be traumatic, involving sudden pain, blood loss, and possibly an emergency admission to hospital. Up to 25 per cent of women may have symptoms of post-traumatic stress disorder (PTSD) one month after miscarriage. This drops to around 7 per cent four months after a miscarriage, with half of these cases being chronic (Engelhard et al., 2001).

Around 0.5% of babies are stillborn (after 24 weeks gestation). In about 70 per cent of cases the reason for death is unexplained. Parents develop an attachment to their child throughout pregnancy, so this is usually an intensely painful loss: 20-30 per cent of women experience depression during the first year, and 33 per cent of parents have marital difficulties after the loss. Subsequent pregnancies will also be very stressful and understandably will involve high levels of worry and anxiety over the health of the baby. Current medical practice offers parents the chance to see and hold their dead infants on the premise that it will help the grieving process. However, there is conflicting evidence as to whether this increases or decreases the risk of PTSD (Turton et al., 2001).

Summary

- Fertility rates are generally declining in developed countries and the age at which women have their first baby is increasing.
- Antenatal stress and distress are associated with premature birth, foetal, and infant characteristics.
- There has been a steady increase in the number of caesarean section deliveries.
- Supporting women during labour results in better physical outcomes and maternal psychological wellbeing.

- The transition to parenthood is associated with increases in depression, anxiety, and psychotic disorders. Anxiety disorders may be more prevalent than depression but are remarkably under-recognised.
- Psychological problems following a birth can have an adverse impact on the woman, their relationships, and the infant.
- Miscarriage and stillbirth can be associated with high levels of distress, such as depression and PTSD.

14.2 ENDOCRINE DISORDERS AND PSYCHOSOCIAL WELLBEING

Psychoneuroendocrinology is the study of how psychological states are influenced by changes in hormone secretion. It is playing an increasing role in the diagnosis and treatment of affective disorders and anxiety disorders. One of the most obvious reasons for this change is the observation that patients with primary endocrine disorders are more likely than the general population to experience psychiatric morbidity. Alongside this observation, there is increasing understanding of the synergies between the neural and endocrine systems and the differing roles of hormonal and neuronal control of the function of the pituitary (which is often referred to as the 'master gland') by the hypothalamus. Dysfunction in brain regions such as the hypothalamus can affect the functioning of the endocrine system, which is in turn associated with psychiatric symptoms.

The notion of the 'psychopharmacological bridge' has also guided work in this area. If a drug produces a therapeutic effect (e.g. relieving symptoms) and has specific biochemical actions (e.g. modifying hormone secretion), then this suggests a casual link between the therapeutic effects, the biochemical changes, and the cause of the syndrome. For example, if a drug known to treat cortisol hypersecretion also reduces the psychiatric symptoms of depression, this suggests that cortisol hypersecretion is a casual factor in the onset and progression of the depression.

Hypothalamic-Pituitary-Adrenal axis (HPA)

There is a wealth of research evidence documenting HPA axis hyperactivity in drug-free depressed patients. Changes in HPA axis in depressed people include elevated CRH in cerebrospinal fluid, enlarged pituitary and/or adrenal glands, and increased production of ACTH and/or cortisol during periods of depression. It is not completely clear whether these HPA changes are a cause or symptom of depression. For example, dysregulation of the HPA axis can occur after periods of chronic or severe stress. This is also observed in other stress-related illnesses such as PTSD where conversely there is a reduced cortisol response (see Chapter 3).

Cortisol hypersecretion (Cushing's syndrome)

Common psychiatric aspects of cortisol hypersecretion include depression and irritability. In the initial description of his eponymous syndrome, Cushing (1932) described a relationship between cortisol hypersecretion and depression, irritability, an inability to concentrate, and sleeplessness. People with Cushing's syndrome have a consistent constellation of psychological symptoms, predominantly impaired affect: around three-quarters are depressed, 90 per cent are irritable. Fatigue is universal and may be explained by common insomnia. Many patients also report a decreased libido. Cognitive symptoms include decreased concentration and poor problem solving and memory. These factors combine to influence social withdrawal, which may also be affected by changes in physical appearance such as truncal obesity, a round face and a 'buffalo hump'.

In patients with cortisol hypersecretion there may be problems of **differential diagnosis**: it may be difficult to decide whether a patient with hypercortisolemia has primary depression or early Cushing's syndrome.

Cortisol hyposecretion (Addison's disease)

Addison's disease results from destruction of the adrenal glands. In the past, the most common cause of this was tuberculosis. Today the vast majority of cases are due to the idiopathic autoimmune destruction of the adrenal glands. The major behavioural manifestations of cortisol hyposecretion are lethargy and apathy. Other behavioural manifestations include irritability, crying, and impaired sleep. Patients may also have problems with memory and concentration and report tachycardia. In patients with cortisol hyposecretion there may be problems of differential diagnosis because the patient may show non-specific symptoms that will wax and wane. In addition, periods of stress will exacerbate symptoms – because the adrenal glands are called on to increase secretion (see Chapter 3) – and these symptoms will decrease when the stress abates. These presenting symptoms mean hypocortisolism can be misdiagnosed as a primary psychiatric condition. For example, tachycardia, dizziness, and complaints of lethargy may be seen as signs of anxiety disorders or may be misdiagnosed as chronic fatigue syndrome.

For both of the cortisol-related syndromes just described, there is evidence that changes in cortisol levels produce the original psychiatric symptoms. The effective treatment of cortisol hypersecretion is associated with improvements in mood and cognitive function. The effective treatment of cortisol hyposecretion leads to an alleviation of psychological and behavioural symptoms.

ACTIVITY 14.1   DIFFERENTIAL DIAGNOSIS

- What is meant by differential diagnosis?
- Why may differential diagnosis be difficult in patients with cortisol hyposecretion or hypersecretion?

Hypothalamic-Pituitary-Thyroid axis (HPT)

The link between thyroid function and behaviour was first documented nearly two hundred years ago. Parry (1825) noted that hyperfunction of the thyroid was associated with 'various nervous affectations' and symptoms such as restlessness, hyperactivity, and impaired concentration. A causative role of hypothyroidism in psychopathology was demonstrated by Asher (1949) in a case series suggesting that thyroid hormone deficiency may lead to depression and psychosis and that the administration of desiccated thyroid alleviated these psychological symptoms. Abnormal thyroid function is more common among patients with psychiatric illnesses than in the general population. However, part of this difference is iatrogenic: various psychotropic medications (e.g., lithium, neuroleptics, and antidepressants) will disturb the HPT axis function to varying degrees.

In recent decades, there has been an increase in understanding of links between thyroid function and psychological wellbeing. Most people with thyroid disorders complain of a mental disturbance that remits on correction of the thyroid illness. This indicates the involvement of the HPT system in psychological states.

Hyperthyroidism

The behavioural states observed in hyperthyroidism include intense dysphoria, usually with pronounced anxiety. Other common complaints include nervousness, emotional lability, restlessness, and impaired concentration. Insomnia and fatigue are common and patients may feel too weak and tired to carry out planned activities. Decreased concentration and impaired memory are correlated with thyrotoxicosis.

Hypothyroidism

Hypothyroidism is the most common clinical disorder of thyroid function. The most common psychiatric symptoms can be grouped into cognitive dysfunction (impaired memory, inattentiveness, slower and poorer problem solving) and mood changes (predominantly depressed mood, but also anxiety, insomnia, irritability, and confusion). Psychosis may be present in approximately 5 per cent of hypothyroid patients, but is linked to more severe hypothyroidism.

For both the thyroid-related syndromes just described, there is evidence that psychological symptoms follow the hormonal abnormality. In hyperthyroidism, scores on measures of mood, anxiety, and cognitive function will return to normal after a return to euthyroid status. Similarly, in hypothyroidism, most psychiatric symptoms are reversible following effective treatment of the thyroid disorder.

Growth hormone

Excess secretion of growth hormone results in gigantism in children and acromegaly in adults. The most common cause of growth hormone hypersecretion is pituitary adenoma. Physical symptoms are usually obvious e.g., abnormal growth of the hands and feet, changes in bony and soft tissue including an altered facial appearance. Psychiatric symptoms are rare although depression may occasionally occur. Although clinical psychiatric symptoms are rare, people with acromegaly have lower scores on measures of quality of life, which appear to be related to lower self-esteem due to changes in body image (e.g. Pantanetti et al., 2002; Rowles et al., 2005). These changes can lead to social withdrawal, disruption in interpersonal relations, mood swings, and a loss of initiative and spontaneity.

Growth hormone deficiency causes an absence or delay in the lengthening and widening of the skeletal bones. In some cases the onset of the disorder occurs prenatally and in others the condition occurs months or years later. Clinical psychiatric symptoms of growth hormone deficiency are rare. However it has clear impacts on self-esteem and a distorted body image. Children with growth hormone deficiency have higher rates of anxiety, depression, social phobia, and attentional dysfunction than their peers. In adults, quality of life is lower in those with growth hormone deficiencies (Hull and Harvey, 2003). This may be displayed as social phobia, fear of negative evaluation, decreased interest or pleasure in activities, depression, fatigue, and irritability. In addition, there are lower marriage rates and higher rates of unemployment.

Some impacts of growth hormone deficiency are height-related, especially for men (Jackson and Ervin, 1992). However, the observed differences can not be explained solely on the basis of short stature. Comparisons among adults of a very short stature show that people who are short but do not have a growth hormone deficiency have fewer psychosocial problems than people who have growth hormone deficiencies (Hull and Harvey, 2003). Furthermore, effective treatment of a growth hormone deficiency in adults does not increase height, but does tend to improve quality of life (Hull and Harvey, 2003).

CLINICAL NOTES 14.3

Endocrine disorders

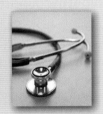

- Given the common occurrence of psychological symptoms in endocrine disorders, it is important to make an accurate diagnosis.
- Don't assume that psychological symptoms are 'just psychological' – they may be the result of endocrine disorders
- A differential diagnosis is important for ensuring that an appropriate treatment is administered.

Sex hormones and psychosocial wellbeing

Testosterone has two effects on the body: androgen effects (the development and maintenance of secondary male sexual characteristics) and anabolic effects (the promotion of muscle growth). **Anabolic androgenic steroids** (AAS) are synthetic compounds structurally related to testosterone. Bodybuilders and many athletes use androgenic anabolic steroids to develop a more muscular physique. This practice is generally banned in competitive sports because of concerns that competition should be fair and based on natural ability.

Long-term AAS use can have serious consequences for physical and psychological well-being (Kanayama et al., 2008). It can lead to irreversible toxicity in the cardiovascular system and organ systems. AAS misuse also appears to be associated with psychosocial problems such as dependence syndromes, mood disorders, psychotic syndromes, and progression to other forms of substance abuse (Kanayama et al., 2008). Most research has focused on young men, but attention has also been given to AAS use among adult women (Gruber and Pope, 2000) and adolescents (Bahrke et al., 1998).

In men, use of AAS has unwanted physical side-effects such as testicular atrophy, reduced sperm production, acne, and the development of abnormally large mammary glands (Thiblin and Petersson, 2004). There is also concern about the psychological side-effects of using androgenic anabolic steroids, particularly the phenomenon colloquially known as 'roid rage' as illustrated in Case Study 14.2. A recent review of published research revealed inconsistent evidence of increased rates of hypomania and increased aggressiveness and violence among steroid users (Thiblin and Petersson, 2004). Research in this area is hampered by the fact that because non-prescribed steroid use is illegal it is difficult to estimate the size of the population at risk, or to recruit large numbers of steroid users into controlled trials. In addition, men who decide to use steroids may differ from other men in important ways, including their propensity for aggression. Furthermore, as noted in the section on aggression, there is no simple explanation for all aggressive or violent behaviour (see Chapter 9).

CASE STUDY 14.2   'Roid rage': the impact of steroids on behaviour

The story of David Bieber is cited as an example of 'roid rage' – aggression and violence linked to use of anabolic steroids. In 2004 *The Times* newspaper carried a report on how Bieber's misuse of steroids resulted in 'a trail of lives shattered by an American dream turned sour'.

Bieber came from a comfortable middle-class background and was remembered by his school friends as happy and even-tempered. In his late teens, Bieber began using steroids, ostensibly to make him a stronger footballer. The drugs changed Bieber's physique, but also altered his temper. A little over ten years after he began using steroids, Bieber was responsible for the contract killing of a business rival, the attempted murder of a former lover, and violent assaults against a string of girlfriends. Some people – including Bieber's father - blamed steroid misuse for his violent behaviour.

14.2.1 ETHICAL ISSUES IN HORMONE THERAPY

The sections above highlight how the treatment of hormonal abnormalities can improve psychological wellbeing. However, it is also true that hormonal treatment can be used to treat problems that do not have a hormonal cause. Research Box 14.2 highlights some of the ethical issues involved in using medical treatments to treat what are essentially social problems. The study elaborated in the research box was part of a series which showed that oestrogen treatment for adolescent girls to reduce their adult height was a negative experience for many of the girls involved (Pyett et al., 2005), that it was associated with fertility problems in adulthood (Venn et al., 2004), and that it did not lead to better psychosocial wellbeing (Bruinsma et al., 2006).

RESEARCH BOX 14.2   Endocrine treatment for tall girls

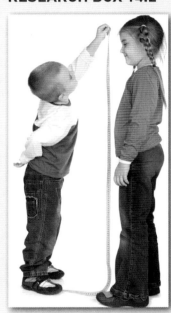

Background

Until quite recently, some doctors and parents who were concerned that girls may grow too tall used hormonal treatment to reduce their adult height. Oestrogen treatment reduces final adult height because it brings forward the earlier fusion of the epiphyseal plates of long bones, thereby stopping any further growth in bone length.

This treatment was given because of concerns about psychosocial problems such as: feeling different and/or being teased; adopting a bad posture (e.g. stooping); withdrawing socially; being less able to find a husband (it was assumed that a man would not want to be shorter than his wife); having difficulty in finding suitable clothing; and being excluded from some 'feminine' careers (e.g. classical ballet, flight attendant).

Oestrogen treatment could reduce someone's height by 5cm (2") or more.

Methods and findings

The growth patterns of 844 Australian girls were assessed between the late 1950s and early 1990s. All were assessed because of concerns that they would be over 178 cm (5'10"). Half of these girls had oestrogen treatment and were compared to those who were not treated.

There were no differences between treated and untreated women in depression, eating disorders, psychological wellbeing, and social support. Depression was more likely if women had had negative experiences of the treatment and/or the assessment process (assessment involved examining markers of pubertal growth such as the development of breasts and pubic hair).

Significance

Most of the girls treated were still taller than average. There were no psychosocial benefits from the treatment. On the contrary, the processes of assessment and treatment
appeared to have impaired psychological wellbeing. These findings are striking given
changes in the social desirability of height in women and a move away from many prior
stereotypes about femininity.

Photo © Sandra Gligorijevic/Fotolia

Bruinsma, F. et al. (2006) Concern about tall stature during adolescence and depression in
later life, *Journal of Affective Disorders, 91*:145–152.

Use of hormonal treatment raises a range of other
ethical issues. For example, in our society tallness is
usually desirable and the treatment of growth hormone deficiencies can be used to increase final adult
height. However, its potential use by people without
growth hormone deficiencies raises important questions about where we draw the line between medical
therapy and psychosocial enhancement.

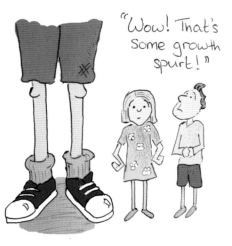

14.2.2 STRESS AND ENDOCRINE FUNCTIONING

As well as considering how changes in endocrine
function can affect psychological wellbeing, it is
important to note that psychological states can affect
endocrine function. A key focus of research in this
domain is the study of responses to stress. All stressors – be they physical threats or
psychological stress – will produce a two-phase pattern of endocrine response (Pinel,
2007). In the first phase, stress prompts adaptive changes in the endocrine system to help
the person (or animal) to deal with physical threats e.g. the mobilisation of energy
resources, the inhibition of inflammatory responses, and increased resistance to infections. However, where stress is prolonged or repeated, it can produce maladaptive changes
in the endocrine system such as enlarged adrenal glands.

Prolonged stress can lead to the dysregulation of endocrine function and increased wear
and tear in systems regulated by the endocrine system, labelled allostatic load (McEwen,
1998). Prolonged stress can also lead to impaired immune function because of interactions between the endocrine and immune systems: cortisol inhibits the production of pro-
inflammatory molecules by macrophages and other immune cells and adrenalin and
noradrenalin can modulate the production of cytokines by immune cells (Griffin and
Ojeda, 2004). The influence of stress on immunity is addressed in detail in Chapter 3.

Summary

- Psychoneuroendocrinology is the study of how psychological states are influenced by changes in hormone secretion.
- Disorders of the HPA axis, thyroid function, and sex hormones all have associated psychological symptoms, suggesting some biological basis for these symptoms.
- Growth hormone disorders are less associated with psychological symptoms.
- Use of hormonal treatment reduces psychological symptoms, suggesting a biological basis.
- Use of hormonal treatment for social problems, such as height, raises a range of ethical issues, especially if it does not improve psychological wellbeing.
- Endocrine function is strongly affected by stress, which can result in dysregulated responses such as those observed in depression and PTSD.

FURTHER READING

Ayers, S. et al. (eds) (2007) *Cambridge Handbook of Psychology, Health and Medicine* (2nd edition). Cambridge: Cambridge University Press. Includes short chapters on many topics including HRT, infertility, antenatal care, breastfeeding, chromosomal abnormalities, contraception, foetal wellbeing, postnatal depression, endocrine disorders, growth retardation, hyperthyroidism, etc.

Martin, C. (ed.) (2010) *Perinatal Mental Health*. Keswick, Cumbria: M&K. A comprehensive up-to-date book that covers a wide range of psychological disorders in pregnancy and after birth.

Wolkowitz, O.M. & Rothschild, J. (eds) (2003) *Psychoneuroendocrinology: The Scientific Basis of Clinical Practice*. New York: American Psychiatric Press. A comprehensive text that covers a wide range of topics including the effects of steroids on mood and cognition, Cushing's syndrome, Addison's disease, contraceptives, HRT, PMS, PMDD, anabolic steroid use, thyroid function, and psychiatric disorders.

REVISION QUESTIONS

1 Describe the psychosocial characteristics of hormonal changes during the menstrual cycle.

2 Outline the similarities and differences between Pre-Menstrual Syndrome (PMS) and Pre-Menstrual Dysphoric Disorder (PMDD).

3   What strategies can be used to help women manage Pre-Menstrual Syndrome (PMS)?

4   Describe the psychosocial impact of menopause.

5   Discuss strategies that could be used to reduce psychological distress during pregnancy and birth.

6   Outline women's psychological responses to miscarriage and stillbirth. Why do these responses occur?

7   Describe the main psychological problems that can occur during the postnatal period.

8   Choose one endocrine disorder. Outline its common psychosocial symptoms.

9   Consider the evidence that 'Anabolic steroid use makes men more violent'.

10 How might prolonged stress lead to endocrine disorders?

15 GENITOURINARY MEDICINE

> **Figure**
>
> 15.1 The ABC of safe sex: a billboard in Botswana
>
> **Research boxes**
>
> 15.1 Does promoting sexual abstinence work?
> 15.2 Improving adherence among dialysis patients

LEARNING OBJECTIVES

This chapter is designed to enable you to:

- Understand sexual health from a biopsychosocial perspective.
- Outline psychological approaches to limiting the spread of sexually transmitted infections.
- Appreciate how concerns about personal reputation, embarrassment, and gender identity can affect the experience of illness and help-seeking behaviour in genitourinary medicine.
- Outline patient experiences and concerns in kidney disease.

Genitourinary medicine is an umbrella term that covers aspects of andrology (men's reproductive health), gynaecology (women's reproductive health), and urology. Genitourinary medicine is primarily related to diagnosing and treating **sexually transmitted infections (STIs)**. Thus much of this chapter will focus on STIs. First, however, we shall consider broader issues related to sexual health. The closing sections of this chapter will deal with problems in the urinary and renal systems.

15.1 SEXUAL HEALTH

People commonly equate **sexual health** with **reproductive health** (see Chapter 14). However, sexual health is much broader. If we were to equate 'sexual health' with 'reproductive health', we would exclude a consideration of the sexual health needs of people who (a) are infertile, (b) choose not to reproduce, (c) are post-reproductive, or (d) are homosexual. The WHO definition of health (see Chapter 1) has therefore been adapted to define sexual health as:

> A state of physical, emotional, mental and social well-being in relation to sexuality; it is not merely the absence of disease, dysfunction or infirmity. Sexual health requires a

positive and respectful approach to sexuality and sexual relationships, as well as the possibility of having pleasurable and safe sexual experiences, free of coercion, discrimination and violence. (World Association for Sexual Health, 2007)

This is a broad, biopsychosocial conceptualisation of sexual health which includes a consideration of sexual freedom, sexual pleasure, and sexual safety. These three domains are outlined below.

15.1.1 SEXUAL FREEDOM

Unfortunately, **sexual coercion** and abuse is widespread. Twenty per cent of women and 5 per cent of men report that they have had unwanted sexual activity because of actual or threatened force (de Visser et al., 2007; Laumann et al., 1994). Experience of sexual coercion is related to a range of subsequent difficulties. People who have been coerced have poorer psychological wellbeing, poorer physical health, greater health anxiety, and use health services more. They are more likely to engage in health-compromising behaviours like smoking, heavy drinking, and illicit drug use. They are also more likely to have been diagnosed with an STI. They are also more likely to experience sexual problems such as a fear of intimacy, a lack of sexual pleasure, and anxiety about sexual performance. Research reveals that any sexual coercion – not just early, repeated or more severe coercion – leads to poorer health and less healthy patterns of behaviour (de Visser et al., 2007). It is clear there is a need for support services for people who experience sexual coercion in order to minimise its impact.

Treating the aftermath of sexual coercion or abuse requires sensitivity and excellent communication skills (see Chapter 18). More broadly, health professionals need to be aware that patients' understandings of sex and related issues may differ (see Box 15.1). Patients may report a diverse array of sexual orientations and sexual behaviours. As long as these behaviours are consensual and legal, any judgemental attitudes or discrimination from health professionals are inappropriate and may be a barrier to promoting sexual health.

BOX 15.1   What is sex?

Although people will usually assume that 'sex' means 'vaginal intercourse', it is important when taking a medical history to be very clear about what patients mean when they talk about sex.

During his presidency, Bill Clinton was questioned several times about whether he had had a sexual relationship with White House intern Monica Lewinsky. Clinton publicly stated 'I did not have sexual relations with that woman', but later revealed that his use of the term 'sexual relations' excluded his receiving oral sex. It is interesting to note that many people agree with Bill Clinton that oral sex does not count as sex (Rissel et al., 2003; Sanders and Reinisch, 1999).

ACTIVITY 15.1   HOW DO WE TALK ABOUT SEX?

- Take a few minutes to write different colloquial or "slang" terms for different sexual behaviours.
- Now write down the terms that you would use if you were talking to a medical professional about your own sexual behaviour.
- It is important to be aware of the terms that patients may use to refer to sexual behaviour. Some may prefer slang terms. Others may prefer euphemisms or will refer indirectly to their sexual behaviour.

15.1.2 SEXUAL PLEASURE AND SEXUAL PROBLEMS

The vast majority of adults believe that an active sex life is important for their overall wellbeing and relationships (e.g. Rissel et al., 2003). However, **sexual problems** or **sexual dysfunctions** are remarkably common and many become more common with age. A large population-representative study in Australia found that over 70 per cent of women and nearly 50 per cent of men had reported at least one sexual problem in the previous year. Some sexual problems have an organic cause, while others are primarily psychological in nature. Whatever their causes, sexual problems can impair quality of life. For example, many people report that they feel anxious about their sexual performance or do not find sex pleasurable.

Many men report that they achieve orgasm too quickly and many experience problems in achieving or maintaining an erection. Rapid ejaculation has a strong psychological component and psychological interventions can therefore be effective treatments. Erectile dysfunction may be caused by psychological factors, but commonly has an organic cause. The likelihood of erectile dysfunction is significantly greater in older men, particularly if they have cardiovascular disease, diabetes, or undiagnosed hyperglycemia (Grover et al., 2006; Richters et al., 2003a). It is notable that since treatments for erectile problems became available in the late 1990s, the number of men reporting erectile dysfunction appears to have increased (Kaye and Jick, 2003). It has been suggested that this has been due to pharmaceutical companies marketing drugs that were designed to treat erectile problems due to organic causes, such as diabetes or prostate surgery, as 'lifestyle' drugs that may be desirable to all men (Lexchin, 2006). Such findings indicate that a biopsychosocial approach (see Chapter 1) is just as important in genitourinary medicine as in other medical domains.

ACTIVITY 15.2   HOW YOUNG IS TOO YOUNG? HOW OLD IS TOO OLD?

- What would you think – and what would you say – if a 15 year old patient asked you for a prescription for oral contraception?
- What would you think – and what would you say – if an 80 year old patient asked you for a prescription for medication to treat erectile dysfunction?

Common sexual problems among women include vaginal dryness and pain during intercourse or an inability to orgasm (Laumann et al., 1999; Mercer et al., 2005; Richters et al., 2003a). Some of these problems are more common among older women, particularly vaginal dryness, which is influenced by hormonal changes associated with menopause (see Chapter 14). However, others, such as painful intercourse are more common in younger women.

When treating sexual problems it is often useful to distinguish between Desire for sex, Arousal once sex is initiated, and obtaining Orgasm (DAO). Dysfunction is often limited to one of these stages and an accurate diagnosis can aid the appropriate targeting of treatment. Sexual difficulties are an important focus of treatment because they are related to less satisfaction with physical and emotional aspects of relationships and a lower level of general happiness (Laumann et al., 1999; Richters et al., 2003b).

Chronic Pelvic Pain

Chronic Pelvic Pain (CPP) is not a diagnosis of a single disease, rather it is a symptom which may be the result of underlying processes in one or more different organ systems. CPP is defined as constant or intermittent pain in the pelvis or lower abdomen not associated with menstruation, pregnancy, or sexual intercourse. It is believed to affect around 24 per cent of women (Zondervan et al., 2001). However, the actual prevalence may be higher than this: many women accept the symptoms as part of being female and when they do seek medical help the lack of a clear cause of CPP means that it may be diagnosed in different ways. Numerous potential causes of CPP in different organs systems have been proposed (Howard, 2003):

- Gynaecological (e.g. endometriosis, chronic pelvic inflammatory disease).
- Gastrointestinal (e.g. Irritable Bowel Syndrome, Inflammatory Bowel Disease).
- Urological (e.g. interstitial cystitis).
- Musculoskeletal (e.g. fibromyalgia, pelvic floor abnormalities).
- Psychoneurological (e.g. nerve entrapment).

Women with CPP are more likely than other women to have a history of sexual abuse. They are also more likely to experience depression, anxiety, and catastrophic thinking. These psychological phenomena could be implicated in CPP as either causes or consequences. Whatever their role is in CPP, it should be noted that such negative states influence the perception of pain (see Chapter 4), and that they should be addressed by suitably qualified professionals.

Research suggests that simply providing time to listen to a woman's experiences of CPP can have a therapeutic benefit (Price et al., 2006). However, it should be noted that patients will usually want a diagnosis or explanation of their symptoms and that meeting these expectations in the case of CPP may not be straightforward. Because of the complex nature of CPP and the large number of different causes with similar or overlapping symptoms, it is important to conduct a thorough patient history which will allow a differential diagnosis and the selection of the appropriate treatment (Howard, 2003). This can be time consuming and demanding, particularly given the need to focus on experiences of sexual abuse as potential aetiological factors.

A systematic review of trials of the efficacy of treatments for CPP revealed that a multi-disciplinary approach addressing physical and psychological symptoms was most effective (Stones et al., 2005). Counselling and writing therapy were found to be beneficial for many patients. However, it is important to note that treatment for CPP is directed more toward managing symptoms than curing the disease.

Although much of the research into CPP has focused on women, men may also experience chronic pelvic pain and this is often a symptom of prostate cancer (see 15.3.1).

15.1.3 SEXUAL SAFETY

Sexual safety is important: it protects against unwanted pregnancy and STIs. Teenage birth rates in many developed countries are high. The highest teenage birth rates are found in the USA and UK, with other English-speaking countries recording higher teenage birth rates than European nations (UNICEF, 2001). Although some teenagers are happy to become parents, most teenage pregnancies are unplanned. Teenage motherhood is associated with fewer educational qualifications and poor employment prospects (UNICEF, 2001). When teenage birth rates are combined with the high rates of termination of pregnancy in teenagers, it is clear that many young people do not take adequate precautions to avoid an unintended pregnancy. A failure to practise **safer sex** consistently also explains why STIs are widespread. We shall examine this in the following section.

Summary

- Sexual health is broader than reproductive health and includes sexual freedom, sexual pleasure, and sexual safety.
- Sexual problems are remarkably common, with the majority of adult women and men reporting at least one sexual problem in the previous year.
- A substantial minority of women and men have experienced sexual coercion or abuse. This is associated with poor psychological and physical wellbeing, increased health anxiety, increased health service use, and more health-compromising behaviours.
- Chronic Pelvic Pain may arise from dysfunction in several different organ systems. Because its underlying causes may be difficult to determine, it may not be possible to give patients the accurate diagnosis or effective treatment they are seeking.
- Sexual risks include unwanted pregnancies and contracting STIs, both of which can be avoided by practising safer sex.

15.2 SEXUALLY TRANSMITTED INFECTIONS

15.2.1 HIV/AIDS

Human Immunodeficiency Virus (HIV) is a retrovirus which causes **Acquired Immune Deficiency Syndrome (AIDS)**. The predominant mode of transmission is unprotected sexual activity. It is estimated that approximately 33 million people worldwide are infected with HIV, with over 2.5 million new infections per year: the vast majority of these are in sub-Saharan Africa (UNAIDS/WHO, 2009). The prevalence of HIV infection varies widely between regions: 5.2 per cent in sub-Saharan Africa; 1.0 per cent in the Caribbean; 0.6 per cent in North America; 0.3 per cent in Western Europe.

In many regions, sex between men and women is the primary route of transmission. Even in those areas where sex between men and injection drug use are the major transmission routes, the importance of heterosexual transmission is increasing (UNAIDS/WHO, 2009). For example, in Europe in 2008 approximately 38 per cent of new infections with a known cause were attributed to heterosexual activity (European CDPC, 2009).

Although the virus was identified in the early 1980s, no vaccine or cure has been developed. Since the mid-1990s antiretroviral medications which can suppress viral replication have been available. For many people, HIV/AIDS is now a chronic illness rather than a death sentence. However, these medications are expensive and so are often unavailable in the poorer countries which have been hardest hit by the global AIDS epidemic. Although antiretroviral medications are effective at prolonging life, the treatment regimens can be quite complicated and burdensome in terms of the timing of doses and changes to food and fluid intake. This means that adherence is often a problem. A meta analysis found that various behavioural interventions can improve adherence and produce lower viral loads, but that more research is needed to determine exactly which components of these interventions produce the desired changes (Simoni et al., 2006). The data suggest that providing information about the importance of adherence and discussing patients' beliefs, motivations, and expectations about treatment are important for improving adherence, but that interventions based on reminders or rewards are not effective (see Chapter 19, Research Box 19.1).

The complexity of antiretroviral medication regimens combined with impaired health and uncertainty about the future combine to impair quality of life in people living with HIV (e.g. Dray-Spira et al., 2003; Ezzy et al., 1999; Ezzy, 2000). The psychological impacts of HIV infection are addressed in the chapter on immunology (see Chapter 11; Section 11.2; Case Study 11.1), and include higher rates of depression than in the general population (Ciesla and Roberts, 2001). Interventions designed to treat depression among people with HIV/AIDS are effective at both reducing depression and improving immune function (Antoni et al., 2006).

In the absence of a vaccine or cure for HIV infection, behaviour change is the only way to contain the further spread of the epidemic. Behavioural means for preventing sexual transmission of HIV are the same as those for other STIs. The epidemiology, psychosocial impacts, and prevention of STIs are addressed in the following section.

15.2.2 SEXUALLY TRANSMITTED INFECTIONS

After notable declines during the late 1980s and early 1990s, the prevalence and incidence of numerous sexually transmitted infections (STIs) have risen and continue to rise in many developed countries (Fenton et al., 2004; Gavin et al., 2009; Miller and Zenilman, 2005). However, these increases have not been observed in all countries. The large cross-national differences can not be explained by differences in rates of sexual behaviour *per se*, but reflect instead different patterns of preventive behaviours, different cultural attitudes toward sex, and different provision of sexual health services.

Between 10-20 per cent of adults report having been diagnosed with an STI (Fenton et al., 2001; Grulich et al., 2003). However, many more people have STIs that are, because of a lack of knowledge or consultation, undiagnosed. Young people are particularly likely to have undiagnosed STIs. For example, the UK National Chlamydia Screening Programme, which consists of the opportunistic screening of under-25s, had found that 13 per cent of men and 10 per cent of women tested positive. Furthermore, human papillomavirus DNA (indicating a current infection) has been found in 10 per cent of all women and 20 per cent of women aged under 25 (de Sanjosé et al., 2007). Many STIs can be prevented by the consistent and correct use of condoms. However, as we shall see in the next section, rates of condom use are not as high as is desired by health professionals.

Although young people are a key focus of STI prevention activities, the rates of increase in STIs observed among people aged 45+ in recent years are as high as those among young people (Bodley-Tickell et al., 2008). Older people are now more likely than in past generations to be single or undergoing relationship change. The availability of drugs to treat erectile dysfunction may also contribute to greater levels of sexual activity and a corresponding increase in the likelihood of STI transmission (Paniagua, 1999). An important influence on the quality of sexual health care for older people is that doctors and older patients often find it embarrassing to talk about sexual issues (Gott, 2006).

The terms STI and **STD** are used interchangeably, but it is important to note that these two acronyms can refer to quite different things. The term STD refers to disease, and physical manifestations of infection. An STD-focused sexual health programme would only target those people who had physical manifestations of disease. In contrast, all people infected or at risk of infection would be the targets of an STI-focused programme. This distinction is important because asymptomatic STIs may still damage the reproductive organs.

Treatment with antibiotics is available for many bacterial STIs (e.g., Chlamydia, gonorrhoea). However, cures for viral STIs are not available, although symptomatic treatment is available (e.g. for blisters or sores due to genital herpes). Untreated STIs can lead to serious complications, including infertility in women. Many STIs can be unsymptomatic for some time. This explains why the proportions of people treated for STIs are often lower than the prevalence rates found in population-based screening. Furthermore, people may delay seeking treatment because of embarrassment about talking to others about their sexual behaviour (Stone and Ingham, 2003).

15.2.3 PROMOTING CONDOM USE

In the absence of vaccines or curative treatments for HIV and many other STIs, it is vital to encourage those behaviours that will limit the spread of STIs between people. These are sometimes split into the **'ABC' of STI prevention:**

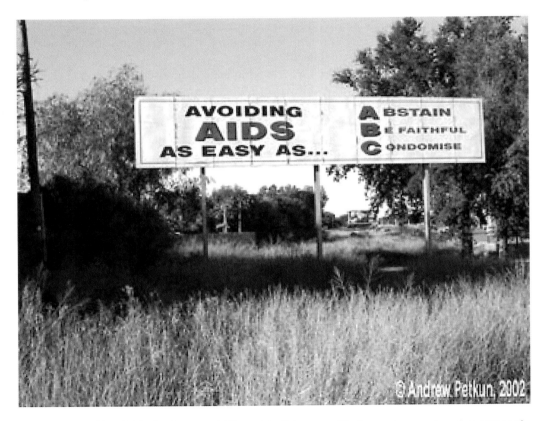

FIGURE 15.1   The ABC of safe sex: a billboard in Botswana. Photograph reproduced courtesy of Andrew Petkun.

BOX 15.2   The ABC of safe sex

A	Abstain from sex	If you don't have sex, you can't get an STI.
B	Be faithful	If you are in a monogamous relationship with a partner who has no STIs, you can't get an STI.
C	Use condoms	If you use condoms, the risk of acquiring an STI is reduced.

Most attention within public health and health promotion has been given to (to use the labels from Box 15.2) Part C, because A and B require more fundamental changes in sexual behaviour. Indeed, research into abstinence-based sexual health programmes indicates that they have no overall impact on the delay of initiating sex, limiting sexual partners, or the increasing use of condoms or other contraception. Indeed, there is concern that abstinence-only programmes may be counter productive in the long run, because such programmes do not teach people how to have safer sex if they cease to abstain from sex (Research Box 15.1).

RESEARCH BOX 15.1   Does promoting sexual abstinence work?

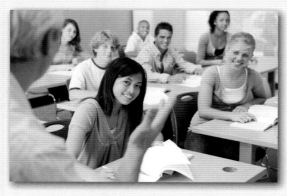

Background

During the Bush administration in the United States, sexuality education programmes were eligible for special funding if they agreed to promote the message that abstinence was the only certain way to avoid pregnancy and STIs and agreed not to promote the use of contraception or provide instructions in using contraception.

Methods and findings

This study aimed to determine whether abstinence-only programmes run using the special funding had the intended positive effects on young people's sexual health. Four different abstinence-only programmes run in four States were evaluated: 1,209 adolescents were randomly allocated to abstinence-only programmes and 848 were assigned to control-group programmes. Follow-up data were gathered 4-6 years after the programmes began.

The results revealed that abstinence-only programmes did not reduce sexual activity among adolescents. Indeed, the average age at first sexual intercourse and the average number of sexual partners were the same regardless of which education programme the teenagers received. There was no evidence that the abstinence-only programmes had better outcomes related to the risks of teenage pregnancy or STIs. Adolescents in all programmes (abstinence-only or control) had poor knowledge about healthy sexual behaviours.

Significance

Abstinence-only programmes provide outcomes that are no better or worse than conventional sexuality education. However, given the high levels of STIs and unplanned pregnancies

(Cont'd)

among teenagers and young adults, comprehensive sexuality education programmes aimed at improving knowledge and skills are likely to provide the best long-term outcomes.

Photo © Monkey Business/Fotolia

Trenholm, C. et al. (2008) Impacts of abstinence education on teen sexual activity, risk of pregnancy, and risk of sexually transmitted diseases, *Journal of Policy Analysis and Management,* 27: 255–276.

Although the vast majority of people do use condoms sometimes, rates of consistent condom use are low. For example, when people are asked about their most recent sexual experiences, fewer than a quarter report that they used a condom (de Visser et al., 2003). Furthermore, among people who do use condoms, around one in seven do not put the condom on before genital contact, thereby exposing themselves to infection with a range of STIs. It is therefore necessary to promote correct and consistent condom use.

Impact of behavioural interventions

Research based on social cognitive models of behaviour (see Chapter 5) shows that people's condom use may be predicted from their attitudes, subjective norms, self-efficacy, and intentions to use condoms (Albarracín et al., 2001; Sheeran et al., 1999). Condom use tends not to be influenced by knowledge about HIV/STIs, a perceived susceptibility to infection, or the perceived severity of infection. Thus, scare campaigns may be ineffective in promoting condom use (Witte and Allen, 2000). It is better to focus on attitudes, beliefs, skills, and confidence. Indeed, because condom use involves more than one person, it is important that people develop the skills to communicate about condom use with their partners. Condom-promotion interventions are more effective when they include a skills component rather than only focusing on changing individuals' knowledge and attitudes (Albarracín et al., 2003; Carey et al., 2000).

A Cochrane review found that significant reductions in HIV risk behaviours among homosexually active men can be achieved via behavioural interventions, be they individual interventions (e.g. promoting personal skills), small group interventions (e.g. group counselling), or community-level interventions (e.g. community-building empowerment activities) (Johnson et al., 2009).

The observed low rates of condom use among heterosexual people are influenced by the availability of hormonal contraception. People tend to be more concerned about unplanned pregnancy than STIs and will often make a trade-off between condoms and other contraception (e.g. Ott et al., 2002). This means that if people are using the contraceptive pill to prevent pregnancy, then they tend not to use condoms. Among young couples, the shift from condoms to the pill is often a marker of the seriousness of the relationship and mutual trust. Condom use is much less common between regular partners than between new partners or in 'one night stands', and the reasons for condom use differ in these different contexts – people tend to be less worried about STIs with regular partners (de Visser and Smith, 2001). However, the decision not to use condoms in regular relationships is not always based on accurate knowledge of partners' STI status.

Rates of condom use may continue to decline in response to the increasing availability and use of the oral contraceptive pill, long-lasting hormonal contraception implants, and post-coital contraception (the 'morning-after pill'). Because hormonal contraception offers no barrier to STI transmission, it could be argued that it is irresponsible to prescribe the pill without also giving condoms to protect against STI transmission. However, it has also been found that few people using the pill also use condoms, so there is a need to find out how to encourage condom use among people who use hormonal contraception.

CLINICAL NOTES 15.1

Sexual behaviour and contraception

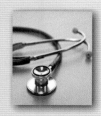

- Many people feel embarrassed talking about sexual behaviour and sexual problems. Let patients know that you are comfortable talking about these issues in a non-judgemental way.
- When prescribing oral contraception, ensure that patients are aware that non-barrier methods offer no protection against STIs. Encourage individuals and their sexual partners to be tested (and treated) for STIs.
- People are more likely to use condoms if you address their attitudes and beliefs. However, it is also important to help people develop the skills needed to negotiate condom use with sexual partners.

Given that unplanned pregnancy and STIs are both attributable to sexual activity without adequate precautions, it makes sense to address both outcomes in settings which traditionally addressed only one of these outcomes e.g. family planning services or STI clinics. However, a review of studies of the integration of STI and HIV within family planning services concluded there was too little research available to determine whether this leads to better outcomes for patients (Church and Mayhew, 2009). However, an important potential pathway for integrated care is adding HIV/STI testing to family planning services. The authors of the review identified several important domains for the integration of services:

- 🐦 The provider level i.e. medical professionals offering both family planning and STI services.
- 🐦 The facility level i.e. internal referral between family planning specialists and STI specialists.
- 🐦 Referral services i.e. external referrals from family planning to STI services and vice versa.

Within primary care, brief interventions can be an efficient way of addressing sexual health issues in patients who may not otherwise attend specialist sexual health services.

CASE STUDY 15.1   A Sexually Transmitted Infection

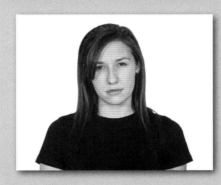

Lucy is a 19 year old retail sales assistant who was recently diagnosed for the first time with an STI. Several months ago she went to a party where she met Tom. There was an obvious spark between them, and they ended up going back to his house and having intercourse. They did not use a condom. Lucy was using oral contraception, and she didn't want to spoil the moment by asking Tom to use a condom. She was worried he would think she was suggesting he wasn't clean.

A few weeks later, Lucy noticed discharge from her vagina and a soreness/ itchiness when urinating. She was embarrassed about this and even more embarrassed about seeing her usual doctor, so she waited for a few days hoping that the symptoms would clear up. When they didn't, she decided to visit a specialist STI clinic.

I was a bit embarrassed going in to get tested ... I was worried that there would be real matron type nurses telling me off for being stupid ... or dirty old men in the waiting room. I didn't want to see anyone I knew, because it wouldn't be good for my reputation. So I didn't make eye contact with anyone in the waiting room. I think most other people there felt the same way.

She said that it was very reassuring to be treated by staff who did not judge her but simply addressed the facts and offered reassurance. Lucy was diagnosed with gonorrhoea and treated with a single dose of antibiotics.

Lucy was relieved that treatment was so quick and effective, but the information she was given by the clinic staff made her more concerned about other STIs and the impact they could have on her reproductive capacity:

It did get me thinking about condoms, but it's hard when you're getting carried away. I know that I need to get better at asking guys to use condoms. One tip a friend gave me was to say that you aren't on the pill even if you are. That way you can get a guy to use a condom without saying anything about diseases.

Summary

- In addition to its physical effects, HIV has detrimental effects on psychological wellbeing and quality of life. Quality of life can also be affected by complex treatment regimens which can suppress viral replication, but do not offer a cure.
- Rates of STIs have increased in recent years in many countries. This increase has not been limited to young people, but has also occurred among older adults.
- Although condoms offer effective protection against HIV, other STIs, and unwanted pregnancy, only a quarter of people will regularly use condoms.
- Among heterosexual people there is often a trade-off between condom use and oral contraceptives.
- Condom use can be increased by targeting people's knowledge and attitudes. However, it is also important to equip people with the necessary skills to negotiate and use condoms.

15.3 PROSTATE AND TESTICULAR CANCER

Cancers of the prostate and testicles are common and may affect, and be affected by, men's views of masculinity or sexuality. Many men endorse and embody traditional definitions of masculinity according to which men are supposed to be 'strong silent types'. These beliefs may help to explain why men are less likely to use medical services (Broom and Tovey, 2009). Men's reluctance to seek screening and treatment may be particularly marked for health conditions which affect sexual potency, because sexual potency is a central aspect of common definitions of strong masculinity.

15.3.1 PROSTATE CANCER

Epidemiology and screening

The prostate gland surrounds part of the urethra of men and produces a fluid component of semen. **Prostate cancer** is one of the most common cancers in men, accounting for about a quarter of all diagnosed cancers among men in developed countries (see Figure 11.1). Although the causal mechanisms involved in prostate cancer are not precisely known, risk factors include age, a family history of prostate cancer or breast cancer (especially breast cancer due to BRCA2 mutations), and physical inactivity. Specific concerns related to prostate cancer include its potential impact on masculinity and sexuality (Kunkel et al., 2000; Lintz et al., 2003).

At the time of diagnosis with prostate cancer, many men are asymptomatic. Symptoms become more prominent when the cancer is advanced. A common symptom is urinary incontinence. Pain in the lower back, hips, or thighs may be experienced if the cancer has metastasised. As with any cancer, a diagnosis of prostate cancer may lead to anxiety or depression and a desire for information about the prognosis and treatment options. However, anxiety and depression often go unnoticed and many men feel they have needs which they believe are not being met by the services available to them (Lintz et al., 2003).

Medical professionals must be aware of the psychological aspects of screening, diagnosis, and treatment for prostate cancer. **Prostate Specific Antigen** (**PSA**) levels are a widely used marker for prostate cancer. However, PSA screening is somewhat controversial because it may not always detect cancer or reduce mortality, but may increase anxiety (Kunkel et al., 2000). Digital rectal examination (DRE) is another form of screening where a physician feels for abnormalities that may indicate prostate cancer. However, many men find rectal examinations difficult because of perceived links between anal penetration and homosexuality: indeed DRE is perceived more negatively than are colonoscopies and many men find the insertion of a finger more difficult than the insertion of a piece of equipment (Winterich et al., 2009).

Treatment

Treatment options vary depending on whether the cancer is restricted to the prostate or has metastasised. Men with low risk localised tumours may be offered active monitoring or 'watchful waiting' rather than treatment. Higher risk localised cancers may be treated by a **radical prostatectomy** – surgery to remove the prostate gland, external radiotherapy, or internal radiotherapy.

Surgery, radiation, and hormone treatment commonly have side effects which reduce quality of life. Radical prostatectomy and radiotherapy often lead to transient or permanent urinary incontinence and impotence. Urinary incontinence is experienced by the majority of men post-surgery and can lead to embarrassment, a loss of a sense of control, depression, and reduced social interactions (Ko and Sawatzky, 2008; see also Section 15.4.1). The impact of impotence due to nerve damage during surgery is influenced by men's pre-surgery levels of sexual activity and their partners' levels of concern about impotence (Kirschner-Hermanns and Jakse, 2002). Modern nerve-sparing surgery can reduce the likelihood and severity of urinary incontinence and impotence.

It is important to include concerns about urinary incontinence and sexual function when decisions are made about surgery, radiation therapy, or watchful waiting. The choice of therapy is not simple, because there is a lack of conclusive evidence that any single approach offers better long-term prospects. This means that it may be particularly important to consider the impact of different treatments on quality of life (Kunkel et al., 2000). For example, men's willingness to undergo a radical prostatectomy may be influenced by the extent to which they are concerned about potential impairments to sexual function due to nerve damage. The adverse psychosocial impacts of diagnosis and treatment for prostate cancer can be reduced via effective psychological intervention (see Research Box 15.2). Counselling and providing erectile aids or medication may be beneficial.

If a tumour has spread beyond the capsule surrounding the prostate, surgery or radiotherapy may be combined with a course of hormone treatment – the growth and function of the prostate is affected by testosterone, so some treatments work by reducing the testosterone levels. A recent systematic review of research revealed that androgen-ablation therapy is associated with significant (but subtle) declines in cognitive capacity (Nelson et al., 2008). Research with animals and studies of older men also indicates that lower levels of testosterone are related to cognitive impairments.

CASE STUDY 15.2 Prostate cancer diagnosis and treatment

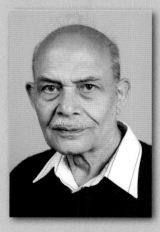

Jim is a 69 year old retired teacher. He was diagnosed with prostate cancer when he was 67. His experiences highlight a number of important psychosocial issues related to the care and treatment of men with prostate cancer.

Jim found some of the screening processes and tests difficult to go through. This was partly due to the uncertainty of some of the test results. It was also because some of the tests were challenging, particularly the digital-rectal examination in which the doctor inserted a gloved finger into Jim's rectum to feel for lumps, hardness, or other abnormalities in the prostate gland:

Some parts of the whole diagnosis process were pretty strange. I mean, having another man put his finger up your back passage is not something that had happened to me before ... and I won't be rushing back to do it again!

(Cont'd)

Jim said the doctor was very reassuring at this time, but the experience of diagnosis was made worse by the insensitivity of some staff. There were times when unknown staff walked in and out of the room without introducing themselves or having any apparent reason to come in when he was (and felt) so exposed.

Once the diagnosis had been made, Jim faced the difficult decision of choice of treatment – surgery, radiotherapy, or 'watchful waiting'. He found it hard to make a decision: the outcomes and side-effects associated with each option were quite varied. Furthermore, he felt he was having to deal with probabilities rather than certainties:

> I found it hard to decide which approach to take. A friend of mine is hyper-logical and he suggested I draw up a table of different pros and cons and give each treatment option a score and decide that way ... but I mean, how can you really weigh up the different options? What's more important – living, having sex, or not wetting myself? I was tempted to take the "wait and see" approach just to avoid having to decide.

Jim found it useful to attend a group support network for men with prostate cancer. Although he was apprehensive about talking to other men about his concerns, he appreciated the benefits after attending a few sessions:

> I went to a group for men in my situation. It was great because all the people there had cancer, and some were worse off than me, but they were all very genuine. They weren't so concerned any more about how much money they earned, or what car they drove, or those kinds of things. Everyone was on a very genuine level. This made it easier to join the group and gave me a lot of support.

After talking to his wife and family Jim opted for radical prostatectomy surgery, and was pleased that he was able to have robot-assisted surgery which reduces the likelihood of nerve damage that can cause impotence and incontinence.

Photo © YellowCrest/Fotolia

15.3.2 TESTICULAR CANCER

Epidemiology and screening

The testicles produce sperm so are vital for men's reproductive capacity. They also produce testosterone, which is the principal male sex hormone. **Testicular cancer** is relatively rare, accounting for around 1-2 per cent of cancers in men. However, it is most common among men in their twenties and thirties, and it is one of the most common cancers among young men. It is more common in Caucasian men than men with Asian and African ethnic backgrounds.

Testicular self-examination (TSE) is an important element of diagnosing and treating testicular cancer because (as for other cancers) early detection and treatment are associated with better outcomes. Because it is unusual to develop cancer in both testicles at the same time, men can compare one testicle to the other to identify any lumps or swellings which should be checked by a medical professional. Although TSE may be an important part of monitoring, very few men practise this behaviour and many are unaware of the importance of TSE (Rudberg et al., 2005; Wardle et al., 1994). We therefore need to increase awareness of the issue and identify strategies to increase rates of TSE.

The Health Belief Model and Theory of Planned Behaviour (see Chapter 5) have been shown to be useful in predicting TSE (McClenahan et al., 2007). One study of young men revealed that rates of TSE could be improved significantly by a brief intervention which encouraged men to develop **implementation intentions** specifying 'when', 'where', and 'how' they would perform TSE (Steadman and Quine, 2004).

Treatment

It is sometimes possible surgically to remove small tumours from a testicle. However, the most common surgical response is removal of the affected testicle (an orchidectomy or orchiectomy). This procedure reduces the risk that pre-cancerous cells may remain in the testis and is possible because men with only one testicle can maintain their fertility and hormone production. Modern treatments can cure most testicular cancer patients and may involve an orchidectomy with or without radiotherapy or chemotherapy (Huddart et al., 2005).

Although most patients treated for testicular cancer are cured, treatment side-effects include impairments to sexual function and fertility. These issues are important to consider given the epidemiology of testicular cancer – diagnosis and treatment often occur before men have become fathers and at an age when sexual activity is important to them. Men may be concerned that the removal of a testicle will make them impotent (i.e. unable to get or maintain an erection) and infertile (i.e. unable to produce children). However, a man with one healthy testicle can still have normal erections and produce healthy sperm. Nevertheless, problems with impotence and fertility do often occur in men post-orchidectomy.

A meta-analysis of outcomes of testicular cancer treatment found that the prevalence of sexual difficulties varied widely (Jonker-Pool et al., 2001). The most common problem was ejaculatory dysfunction (45 per cent of men), and this was clearly related to surgery in the retro perineal region. At least 10 per cent of men reported erectile problems or decreases in sexual desire, sexual activity, orgasm intensity, or sexual satisfaction. Although erectile disorders were the least common of these problems (12 per cent of men), they were significantly related to reductions in satisfaction, sexual activity, desire, and orgasmic intensity. The authors of this meta analysis concluded that physiological outcomes (impaired ejaculation and erection) were clearly related to treatments that affect the neurological systems involved. In contrast, psychological outcomes (desire, activity, orgasm, and satisfaction) did not vary according to treatment modality. Thus, although sexual problems appear to be more common among men treated for testicular cancer, not all of the observed impairments can be attributed to disease or treatment factors. Instead psychosocial factors are important. The symbolic importance men and society in general give to men's genitals mean that removal of a testicle can be a challenge to their perceived masculinity (Gurevich et al., 2004).

CLINICAL NOTES 15.2

Prostate and testicular health

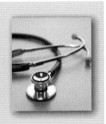

- Encouraging men to say exactly how, when, and where they will perform testicular self-examination is a simple way to increase self-screening behaviour for testicular cancer.
- When diagnosing and treating cancers of the prostate and testicles, be aware of how men's beliefs about their masculinity may be affected by the cancer itself and symptoms and side-effects such as urinary continence and impaired sexual functioning.

Summary

- Prostate cancer is one of the most common cancers in men.
- Treatment options for prostate cancer depend on how advanced the cancer is and men's evaluations of the side effects of treatment.
- Many men experience transient or permanent urinary incontinence and erectile problems following surgery or radiotherapy. The importance of maintaining normal functioning in these domains may influence men's decision to be treated or to undertake 'watchful waiting'.
- Testicular cancer is not as common as prostate cancer. However it is more common among younger men than older men.
- Treatment of testicular cancer often involves removal of the affected testicle. Although this need not affect men's sexual or reproductive capacity, men often experience impairments in these domains after treatment. Psychological factors are important because of beliefs about intact genitalia, sexual potency, and masculinity.
- Psychological interventions can be effective in treating the psychological distress arising from the diagnosis and treatment for cancers of the prostate and testicles. This includes psychological treatment for the common impairments to sexual wellbeing.

15.4 URINARY INCONTINENCE AND RENAL FAILURE

This section will outline two common disorders of the renal and urinary systems. The first (urinary incontinence) is not life-threatening, whereas the second (renal failure) often is. In both cases, psychosocial factors must be considered in treatment and management plans.

15.4.1 URINARY INCONTINENCE

Urinary incontinence (UI) is the involuntary leakage of urine which can have different causes. The population prevalence of any form of UI is 20-30 per cent among young adults, 30-40 per cent among middle-aged people, and 30-50 per cent among elderly people (Nitti, 2001). It is more common among women than men. The severity of urinary incontinence tends to increase with age. UI is the result of bladder dysfunction (urge incontinence) or sphincter dysfunction (stress incontinence). It is not possible to determine accurately whether patients have urge-, stress-, or mixed-incontinence simply by studying the symptoms.

Urge incontinence is the involuntary loss of urine occurring for no apparent reason while suddenly feeling the need or urge to urinate. It occurs when bladder muscles inappropriately contract to expel urine, often regardless of the amount of urine that is in the bladder. It may be called 'reflex incontinence' if it results from overactive nerves controlling the bladder. Patients with urge incontinence may be described as having an 'unstable' or 'overactive' bladder. In addition to surgical and medical treatments, there may be a role for psychological and behavioural therapies. These include exercises to strengthen the pelvic floor muscles and 'bladder training', whereby people are taught to 'hold on' to their urine for increasingly longer times and to empty their bladders at regular, scheduled intervals so that they can increase their capacity to resist the urge to void their bladders (NICE, 2006).

Stress incontinence arises when the pelvic floor muscles have insufficient strength. It involves the loss of small amounts of urine when people cough, laugh, sneeze, exercise, or perform other movements that increase pressure on the bladder. Among women, stress incontinence is more common during pregnancy (because of greater pressure on the bladder), as well as during the pre-menstrual period and during menopause (because lowered oestrogen levels can lead to lower muscular pressure around the urethra). Among men, stress incontinence is a common side effect of prostatectomy. Because stress incontinence arises from muscle weakness, it can be treated via psychological and behavioural means such as pelvic floor muscle training and bladder training (Hay-Smith and Dumoulin, 2006).

UI may cause embarrassment, distress, and discomfort. It has measurable detrimental effects on quality of life (Gil et al., 2009; Monz et al., 2005). Many people with UI report that it limits their ability to engage in activities which either increase the strain on the bladder (e.g. physical exercise) or those where the availability of toilets may be uncertain, intermittent, or restricted (e.g. long-distance travel, vacations, theatre/cinema, etc.). One interesting aid for people in this situation is the Australian Continence Management Strategy's National Toilet Map (http://www.toiletmap.gov.au), which aims to help people with urinary incontinence engage in social activities with less concern about being 'caught short' and unable to find a toilet.

Discussions of problems related to urinary function and sexuality can be difficult and embarrassing for many patients. Many doctors also find these issues difficult (Tomlinson, 2004). Clinical Note 15.3 outlines some important points to bear in mind when carrying out intimate examinations. Legal, cultural, and religious factors may influence what patients believe to be appropriate physician behaviour.

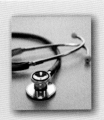

CLINICAL NOTES 15.3

Carrying out intimate examinations

- Embarrassment and anxiety tend to be 'contagious'. The more calm and professional you are, the easier the examination will be for you and the patient.
- Guidelines for intimate examinations include:
  o Explain why the examination is necessary.
  o Explain exactly what it involves and what you will be doing.
  o Get the patient's consent.
  o Offer a chaperone if appropriate.
  o Make sure the room is private and that people will not walk in during the examination.
  o Treat the patient with respect and dignity (e.g. cover exposed parts of the body when you have finished).
  o Keep all discussion *relevant*. Avoid unnecessary personal comments.
  o Be prepared to stop the examination at any time if the patient asks you to.

15.4.2 RENAL FAILURE AND DIALYSIS

Chronic kidney disease (CKD) is the gradual loss of kidney function over time. The early stages of CKD may be asymptomatic, but symptoms do appear as the capacity of the kidneys to remove toxins, wastes, and excess water from the body becomes more impaired. CKD often develops into **end-stage renal disease (ESRD)**, which is when the kidneys no longer function. Patients with ESRD require a kidney transplant or must undergo **dialysis** to remove wastes and excess water from the body.

Kidney disease is becoming more common and is a major public health problem worldwide. A recent review of 26 population-based studies found that the median prevalence of CKD in all adults is around 7 per cent but increases to around 25 per cent in adults aged 64 years or more (Zhang and Rothenbacher, 2008). This increase can be explained in large part by the increasing prevalence of diabetes and hypertension, which are major risk factors for CKD (Coresh et al., 2007). Obesity is also associated with an increased risk of advanced CKD. However, it appears to be the cardiovascular risk factors that accompany obesity – rather than obesity *per se* – which make overweight people more likely to develop CKD (Foster et al., 2008).

Psychosocial aspects of kidney disease and treatment

Patients with CKD and ESRD often have impaired quality of life (QoL), especially emotional wellbeing (Mapes et al., 2004; Perlman et al., 2005). Particular challenges for people with kidney disease are depression arising from their current poor health and the prospect of further declines in health. Depression is more common among CKD and ESRD patients than among the general population. It appears to be more common or severe when illness interferes with important aspects of people's lives such as work or family life. Poorer QoL is important because it is an independent predictor of adverse outcomes and mortality among patients with CKD and ESRD (Mapes et al., 2004; Tsai et al., in press).

ESRD patients with impaired affect may benefit from antidepressant medication, but many antidepressants have side effects that are difficult for ESRD patients to tolerate. In this context psychological interventions are appealing and there is evidence that supportive psychotherapy and cognitive behavioural therapy (CBT) are both effective for reducing the symptoms of depression in people undergoing dialysis (Christensen and Ehlers, 2002). The results of one small-scale intervention indicated that exercise coaching and rehabilitation counselling can improve QoL in people undergoing dialysis, but that rehabilitation programmes are most effective if they are initiated before patients begin dialysis (Fitts et al., 1999).

Treatment of kidney disease also entails restrictions to the diet and fluid intake. ESRD patients undergoing dialysis must regulate their fluid intake in order to avoid fluid overload which can lead to congestive heart failure, hypertension, pulmonary oedema, and a shortened life span. The demands of intensive treatment regimens can impair QoL. Time demands are particularly marked for patients undergoing clinic-based dialysis, which entails 3-4 hour sessions three times per week. For these reasons, home dialysis or peritoneal dialysis (involving the use of a catheter and portable bags of dialysis fluids) may be more appealing to patients. All dialysis patients must also adjust to their dependence on artificial means for survival and a lack of control over their health (Christensen and Ehlers, 2002). For these reasons, kidney transplantation may appear more appealing than ongoing dialysis. **Kidney transplantation** should not be thought of as a cure for ESRD, but a new phase of treatment, because although transplant recipients are free from the dietary restrictions of dialysis, they must adhere to strict regimens of immunosuppressant drugs and be alert to any physical changes that may indicate infection or the rejection of the organ (Christensen and Ehlers, 2002).

Comparisons of people with ESRD indicate that QoL tends to be better among transplant recipients than among patients undergoing dialysis (Ogutmen et al., 2006). However, when looking at different aspects of QoL, it has been found that transplant recipients have more pain and discomfort and a poorer body image. Other studies have failed to find differences in QoL according to treatment modality, but have highlighted the importance of psychological wellbeing and better treatment/illness knowledge for better overall QoL (Sayin et al., 2007).

In addition to being of concern in their own right, impaired affect and QoL are important because they may affect adherence to treatment requirements for dialysis or organ transplantation. Lower adherence may also be affected by certain health beliefs (e.g. low self-efficacy, external locus of control) and less social support (Christensen and Ehlers, 2002). Intervention research indicates that adherence can be improved by behavioural strategies such as self-monitoring, forming behavioural contracts, and positive reinforcement reward systems (Christensen and Ehlers, 2002; Welch and Thomas-Hawkins, 2005) (see Research Box 15.3).

RESEARCH BOX 15.2 Improving adherence among dialysis patients

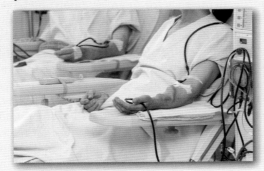

Background

Dialysis patients must regulate their diets and fluid intake to avoid the problems arising from electrolyte imbalances and fluid accumulation. This study was designed to address a lack of experimental evidence about effective interventions to improve adherence to fluid restrictions.

Methods and results

Twenty dialysis patients undertook a behavioural self-regulation intervention. They were compared to 20 control group participants who were matched in terms of age, sex, diabetic status, and average interdialysis weight gain (a marker of adherence to fluid intake guidelines). The intervention was delivered to groups of 4–6 participants. It consisted of seven weekly hour-long sessions with homework between sessions. The contents of the intervention session are listed below:

- Review of the importance of adherence to fluid-intake guidelines (Session 1).
- Description of the self-regulation approach and its application to dialysis (Session 1).
- Overview of behaviour of self-regulatory processes such as self-monitoring, self-evaluation and self-reinforcement (Session 2).
- Instruction in self-monitoring skills. Initiation of homework using a diary to monitor fluid intake, mood, and behaviour (Session 3).
- Personalised goal-setting for fluid intake and weight gain between treatments (Session 4).
- Establishment of self-reinforcement strategies, including rewards (Session 5).
- Teaching stimulus control, self-instruction, and related behavioural coping skills to promote regulation of fluid intake (Session 6).

- Daily monitoring of fluid intake, which was discussed during weekly group meetings (Sessions 3–7).
- Weekly self-evaluation of fluid intake and weight gain relative to goals. Weekly review of self-regulatory coping skills and difficulties in meeting goals (Sessions 3–7).

Immediately following the intervention, there were no differences in adherence between the control and intervention groups. However, whereas adherence in the control group declined over the 8-week follow-up period, adherence improved in the group taught behavioural monitoring skills.

Significance

This study shows that behavioural self-regulation interventions can reverse natural patterns of worsening adherence to fluid intake restrictions over time. This study contributes to a growing body of evidence that multifaceted theory-based, group-administered behavioural interventions can improve adherence in haemodialysis patients.

Photo © Picsfive/Fotolia

Christensen, A.J. et al. (2002) Effect of a behavioral self-regulation intervention on patient adherence in hemodialysis, *Health Psychology*, 21: 393–397.

Summary

- Urinary incontinence (UI) may be caused by muscle weakness or a lack of control over an inappropriate urge to urinate.
- The prevalence and severity of UI increase with age. UI is often a cause of embarrassment and can lead people to restrict their social activities.
- Psychological and behavioural factors are important in treating UI. Treatment may involve muscle-strengthening exercises and bladder training designed to improve patients' control over their urge to urinate.
- Chronic Kidney Disease and End-Stage Renal Disease are becoming increasingly common. Part of this increase can be explained by increases in disease that are risk factors for CKD such as diabetes and hypertension.
- Patients with ESRD will rely on kidney transplants or dialysis. Transplantation is associated with a better quality of life.
- Dialysis places large demands on patients' lifestyles and is associated with depression and impaired quality of life.
- Psychological interventions are effective for alleviating impairments to psychological wellbeing among patients with ESRD. Psychological interventions are also effective for improving patients' adherence to the dietary requirements of their treatment.

📖 FURTHER READING

Ayers, S. et al. (eds)(2007) *Cambridge Handbook of Psychology, Health and Medicine* (2nd edition). Cambridge: Cambridge University Press. Includes short chapters on prostate cancer, contraception, herpes, HIV/AIDS, incontinence, pelvic pain, sexual assault, testicular self-examination, sexual dysfunction, sexually transmitted infections, and urinary tract symptoms.

Tomlinson, J. (ed.) (2004) *ABC of Sexual Health* (2nd edition). London: Wiley. Developed specifically for doctors, this book covers a wide range of topics. It addresses a range of physical and psychological aspects of sexual health and sexual relationships and includes a useful chapter on taking a sexual history.

❓ REVISION QUESTIONS

1   What is sexual health? Describe three components of sexual health.

2   What impact – according to the evidence – does sexual coercion or abuse have on people?

3   What are the possible causes of chronic pelvic pain? What impact does chronic pelvic pain have on women?

4   What psychological interventions are effective at promoting safer sex?

5   How has the prevalence of STIs changed over time? What factors may contribute to this?

6   Discuss the specific psychological challenges that may occur in men with prostate or testicular cancer.

7   Outline the psychological interventions that might be effective in the treatment of urinary incontinence.

8   What is the psychological impact of chronic kidney disease and end-stage renal disease?

9   Which psychological interventions are effective adjunctive treatments for chronic kidney disease and end-stage renal disease? What aspects of patient wellbeing and behaviour do they affect?

16 PSYCHIATRY AND NEUROLOGY

> **Figure**
>
> 16.1   Predisposing, precipitating, and perpetuating factors in psychiatric disorders
>
> **Research box**
>
> 16.1   What does 'consent' mean in practice?

LEARNING OBJECTIVES

This chapter is designed to enable you to:

- Appreciate how predisposing, precipitating, and perpetuating factors influence the development of psychiatric disorders.
- Outline the major features and causes of, and treatment options for, common psychiatric and neurological disorders.
- Identify the methods for assessing psychiatric wellbeing and cognitive function.
- Describe various treatment options for psychiatric illnesses and neurological disorders.

16.1 PSYCHIATRY

Many primary care patients present with complaints that are primarily psychological rather than physical. Furthermore, as noted in previous chapters, many physical illnesses are accompanied by psychological symptoms. One large study across 14 different countries and cultures found a strong association between higher rates of psychiatric morbidity and higher numbers of physical symptoms, especially for physical symptoms that did not have a medical explanation: psychiatric morbidity was present in 4 per cent of people with no unexplained symptoms, but 69 per cent of those with five or more unexplained symptoms (Kisely et al., 1997).

Rather than appearing as obvious illnesses, many psychiatric disorders present combinations of similar symptoms. For example anxiety may appear in and of itself, but is also a component of some forms of depression, schizophrenia, dementia, and personality disorders. For this reason it may be helpful to think of psychiatric disorders as syndromes rather than clear diagnostic entities.

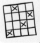

ACTIVITY 16.1   WHAT IS A MENTAL ILLNESS?

- Take a few minutes to write your own definition of what a psychiatric disorder is.
- At what point does abnormal behaviour constitute illness?
- Do psychiatric disorders always have an underlying physiological cause?

16.1.1 MODELS OF PSYCHIATRIC DISORDERS

Until the 1800s in Europe and North America, witchcraft and demonic possession were common explanations for psychopathology. Such beliefs still persist in many traditional cultures. Modern medicine has a more sophisticated understanding of mental illness based on research findings. However, different explanations assign varying importance to bio-medical and psychosocial factors.

Biomedical explanations

According to the biomedical model, psychiatric disorders result from dysfunctions in the biochemistry and physiology of the brain and body or damage to the brain. The implication of biomedical models is that once we identify the biological causes of psychiatric disorders, we can develop effective treatments. Although this model is clearly useful for some disorders, it cannot explain all disorders. A major limitation of this model is its assumption that physical or physiological abnormalities underlie all psychiatric disorders. Some disorders (e.g., phobias) may simply be extreme forms of normal behaviour.

Psychological explanations

In contrast to biomedical models, psychological models argue that people's experiences – and responses to these experiences – may cause mental disorders without there being any physiological abnormality. Three such models are (a) psychoanalysis, (b) learning theory, and (c) cognitive behaviour theory.

Psychoanalytic approaches explain psychiatric disorders as the result of conscious and unconscious responses to experiences rather than abnormalities in brain functioning. Therapy based on this approach would seek to identify the unconscious processes producing the symptoms and try to help the patient to manage these.

Learning theory approaches argue that many psychiatric disorders result from mala-daptive learning. Treatment based on this approach would use approaches such as oper-ant and classical conditioning (see Chapter 10) to 'unlearn' maladaptive responses such as phobias.

Cognitive behavioural approaches are the most commonly used psychological approaches. They are based on the idea that psychopathology arises when people acquire irrational beliefs or dysfunctional ways of thinking about themselves, their behaviour, or other people's responses to them. Cognitive behavioural therapy (CBT) is aimed at chal-lenging and changing maladaptive patterns of thinking.

Psychosocial models

Psychiatric disorders often involve biomedical and psychological factors. As a result, the biopsychosocial model (see Chapter 1) is applicable to psychiatry. This approach recognises that physiological and psychological factors may be involved in the onset and progression of psychiatric disorders. For example, recent research has used fMRI to study psychoanalytic concepts and phenomena like repression, thereby linking medical and psychological models of normal and abnormal mental processes (Mancia, 2006). The biopsychosocial model also emphasises the importance of social responses to psychiatric disorders: do we lock 'mad' people in asylums or provide care for 'ill' people in the community?

The causes of psychiatric disorders vary between conditions and the causes for a particular mental illness vary from person to person. Rather than assuming that all cases of particular psychiatric disorders can be explained by a single cause, it is important to think of how a range of factors can combine over time to affect the onset and course of an illness. We can think of these in terms of three Ps: Predisposing factors, Precipitating factors, and Perpetuating factors (see Figure 16.1).

Predisposing factors are things which make people more susceptible to mental illness. Genetic factors, experiences *in utero*, a traumatic birth, and childhood experiences such as neglect and abuse can increase the risk of some mental disorders.

Precipitating factors are events or experiences which influence whether a predisposition to a mental illness is 'activated'. Not every person with the same predisposing factors will develop a psychiatric disorder – precipitating factors may interact with predisposing factors to bring about psychopathology. A useful analogy is the interaction of genes and behaviour in lung cancer: whether a person smokes cigarettes influences whether a genetic predisposition results in the development of lung cancer. Precipitating factors known to influence the onset of psychiatric disorders include diseases such as brain tumours (Mainio et al., 2005), illicit drug use, and psychosocial factors such as traumatic events, bereavement, and social isolation or difficult relationships (Arseneault et al., 2004; Brewin et al.,

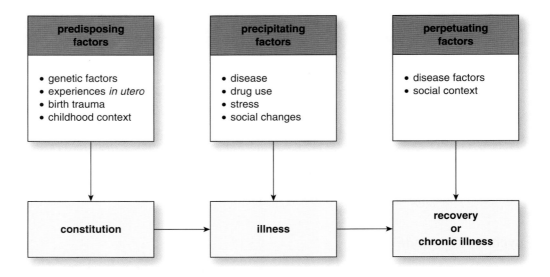

FIGURE 16.1 Predisposing, precipitating, and perpetuating factors in psychiatric disorders (adapted from Gelder et al., 2005)

2000). The interaction between predisposing factors and precipitating factors is often referred to as a **diathesis-stress model**, in which diathesis refers to predisposing factors (see Chapter 3).

Perpetuating factors act after the onset of mental illness to prolong its duration. Sometimes diseases are self-perpetuating. For example, maladaptive coping behaviours in people with anxiety disorders may perpetuate the illness (McManus et al., 2008). As noted elsewhere (see Chapter 17), non-compliance with treatment regimens can prolong illness, particularly if patients do not understand or believe that they are unwell (Osterberg and Blaschke, 2005). Social factors may also prolong illness. For example, family members or friends may not facilitate someone's recovery. In addition, individuals may derive secondary gains such as attention, care, and time off work from inhabiting the sick role (see Chapter 9): a reluctance to give up these gains may prolong a illness.

16.1.2 CLASSIFICATIONS OF PSYCHIATRIC DISORDERS

Definitions of mental illness have changed over time to reflect changes in our understanding of different psychiatric disorders and their causes. Changes in social attitudes can also lead to changes in what is considered to be a mental illness (see Box 16.1).

There are two major systems for classifying mental disorders. Each is periodically updated. The *Diagnostic and Statistical Manual of Mental Disorders* (**DSM**) of the American Psychiatric Association is the standard classification of mental disorders used by clinicians in the United States. It is widely used in clinical practice in many other countries, and in academic research. The current version is the *DSM-IV-TR* (APA, 2000).

The *International Statistical Classification of Diseases* (**ICD**) was developed by the World Health Organisation. It classifies all diseases, including psychological illnesses. The most recent version of this scheme is the *ICD-10* (WHO, 2004). For ease of use, the WHO has in addition produced a simplified classification of the mental disorders most commonly seen in

---

BOX 16.1   What is a mental illness?

Definitions of mental illnesses are not fixed. This is reflected in the need for regular revisions to diagnostic classification systems such as the *ICD* and *DSM*. Definitions of mental illnesses often reflect contemporary social issues.

For example, until 1973, homosexuality was included as a mental disorder in the American Psychological Association's classification of mental disorders. This was controversial because defining homosexuality as a disorder implied that it was something that should be cured, rather than a normal form of sexuality. Debate about pathologising homosexuality continued after 1973 because of the inclusion of a new disorder called 'Sexual Orientation Disturbance'.

Part of this debate focused on whether the psychological 'disturbance' observed in some homosexual people was a consequence of the sexual orientation itself, or a reflection of the discrimination and prejudice towards homosexual and bisexual people.

primary care (WHO, 1996). The WHO primary care guidelines include checklists and brief assessment activities for identifying symptoms and developing a management plan.

16.1.3 PSYCHIATRIC DISORDERS

Here we shall introduce four common psychiatric conditions that are likely to be seen in primary care because of their prevalence or their chronicity. These are mood disorders, anxiety disorders, schizophrenia, and personality disorders. We shall outline the key features, prevalence, treatment, and prognosis.

Mood disorders

We all have periods of feeling down or 'depressed' in response to losses or failures. We may also experience occasional brief periods of feeling very 'up' or 'manic'. When such changes in mood are long enough and intense enough to interfere with normal activities and relationships, they can be considered as mood disorders. The *DSM* and *ICD* distinguish between different manifestations of depression, mania, and combinations of **mania** and **depression** such as **bipolar disorder** (sometimes called manic depression). Depression not related to or associated with other conditions is sometimes called unipolar depression.

The key features of depressive disorders are a low mood, pessimism, a lack of energy, poor concentration, low self-esteem, poor sleep patterns, a reduced appetite, and a reduced libido. The key features of mania are an elevated mood, hyperactivity, impulsive behaviour, a lack of concentration, an increased appetite, and an increased libido. Bipolar disorder consists of alternating periods of mania and depression. The changes between mania and depression can be relatively rapid (within a few hours) but usually occur over a longer period.

The population prevalence of major depression is 2–3 per cent for men and 4–9 per cent for women, but approximately 10 per cent of men and 25 per cent of women will have a major depressive episode at some point in their lives. The population prevalence of bipolar disorder is less than 0.5 per cent. It has been estimated a primary care practitioner with a registered list of 2,000 patients may see 20-30 people per year with major depression, and one or two patients with an episode of mania (Gelder et al., 2005).

Mood disorders appear to result from a combination of genetic, physiological, and experiential factors. Twin studies suggest a genetic predisposition to depression and bipolar disorder (Sullivan et al., 2000). Studies of bipolar disorder have shown that changes in neurotransmitter levels correspond to changes from manic to depressive phases. Studies of major depression indicate the effect of reduced activity of the neurotransmitters dopamine, serotonin, and norepinephrine (Stahl, 2000). Endocrine disorders may be causally involved in some cases of depression (Plotsky et al., 1998).

Psychological factors are also important. Stressful experiences – particularly during key stages of neurobiological development – may help to explain how psychological responses to the environment affect the development of depression and bipolar disorder (Gutman and Nemeroff, 2003). Psychoanalytic explanations of depression view it as a response to a real or symbolic loss of a loved person or object: the individual feels worthless and hopeless and responsible for the loss. Beck's (1967) cognitive theory of depression and Seligman's (1975) theory of learned helplessness also highlight the importance of negative thinking in the onset and progression of depression (see Chapter 19).

Around half of all people who have one bout of depression will have a further depressive episode. Suicide attempts and completed suicide are considerably more common among depressed people. Various treatments for depression are available. Antidepressant drugs are the most widely available treatments. It is recommended that they be used only for moderate and major depression. For acute severe depression that has not responded to antidepressants, electroconvulsive therapy (ECT) may be used.

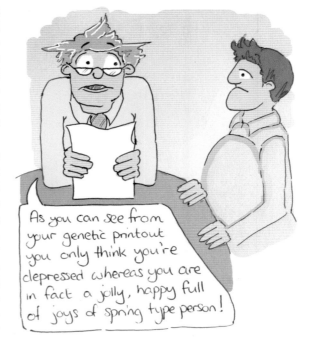

As you can see from your genetic printout you only think you're depressed whereas you are in fact a jolly, happy full of joys of spring type person!

Depression responds well to psychotherapy of various forms, particularly cognitive behavioural therapies (CBT) and interventions designed to enhance problem solving and social support. One approach to the treatment of moderate and severe depression may be to begin with antidepressants to alleviate immediate symptoms and then introduce psychological therapies.

People with bipolar disorder may have periods of illness separated by periods of several months of feeling well. Treatment may involve the use of an anti-depressant, an anti-psychotic, or a mood stabilising drug. Psychotherapies do not appear to be as successful in bipolar disorder as they are in unipolar depression.

Anxiety disorders

The term 'anxiety disorder' is an umbrella term which incorporates various different forms of abnormal and pathological fear and anxiety. An anxiety disorder may have a specific limited focus or it may be more diffuse.

A **Generalised Anxiety Disorder** (GAD) is characterised by excessive fearful anticipation and worrying thoughts. People with GAD may have interrupted sleep and difficulty in concentrating and may also feel depressed. Physical symptoms include agitation or excitation in the gastrointestinal, respiratory, cardiovascular, urinary, and muscular systems. Because GAD is continuous and not related to individual events or circumstances, it is separate from episodic anxiety such as phobia or panic disorder.

CASE STUDY 16.1 Depression

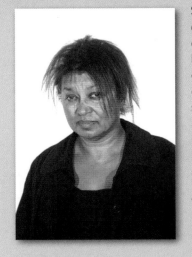

Sue is a 43 year old woman who was diagnosed with depression at age 16. Her account reflects a biopsychosocial model of mental illness: she believes that her depression was caused by a combination of a chemical imbalance and learned behaviours. Various childhood events may have resulted in her depression: she became very introverted after her parents separated and her best friend moved schools. During adolescence, Sue also began to have trouble sleeping, and lacked energy. She feels unlucky that the doctors she saw were not attentive to her psychological symptoms.

Sue's depression was diagnosed when she was 16. When she began taking anti-depressant medication, the initial side effects were unpleasant, including disrupted sleep and weight gain. However, these side effects reduced over time and she felt like she was *'given my life back'*. Sue feels that she can *'now be a normal person'*, and that antidepressants have *'totally changed'* her life. Diagnosis and treatment had other psychological benefits for Sue: the acknowledgement that her depressed mood was a result of serotonergic activity in her brain was a counter to people simply saying *'Cheer up! Why are you so miserable?'* and implying that depression was somehow her fault.

However, Sue realised that although antidepressant medication had *'sorted out my brain chemistry'* she was also aware that her depression was influenced by psychological factors: *'you have learnt all these negative ways of looking at things, and doing things ... from your parents at times.'* This realisation meant that Sue saw a need for long-term therapy to help her learn better ways of dealing with events in her life and try to change her *'total inferiority complex'*. Her experiences of hypnotherapy and counselling have helped her to develop a more positive approach to herself and her social interactions.

Adapted from www.healthtalkonline.org.uk © DIPEx.

Phobias are anxious reactions to particular situations or objects. The unpleasant physical and psychological experiences of GAD also accompany phobias, thus people may try to avoid the situations or objects which they fear. This may be possible for 'simple' phobias (e.g. a fear of blood or spiders), but avoidant responses can be quite debilitating when people have social phobias. **Panic disorders** are diagnosed when anxiety attacks occur unexpectedly and in the absence of an identifiable trigger for an anxious response.

In panic attacks the symptoms of anxiety rapidly escalate. Catastrophic thoughts are common – people may think 'I'm going mad' or 'I'm going to die'.

At any point, around 3 per cent of the general population have GAD, with the prevalence higher in women. Many people have phobias for which they do not seek treatment, but the prevalence of clinically significant simple phobias is around 5 per cent. Social phobia is present in around 3 per cent of people. Panic disorders are much less common – around 0.2 per cent of the population – but are more common among women.

Twin studies suggest that anxiety disorders have a genetic component (Hettema et al., 2001). There is some evidence of abnormal activity of the neurotransmitters GABA and serotonin (Coplan and Lydiard, 1998). Experiences are also important. Simple phobias often develop in childhood. Social phobia often arises from a discrete experience of anxiety in a public place. The aetiology of panic disorder is less clear, but it may result from a combination of serotonergic activity, excessive autonomic nervous system responses to stress, and excessive fearful responses to the resulting autonomic arousal (Gorman et al., 2000).

CASE STUDY 16.2   Generalised anxiety disorder

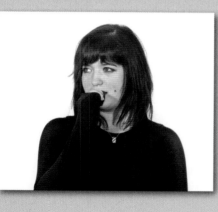

Ann is a 28 year old bank teller. In her early twenties she first developed the symptoms of a generalised anxiety disorder. There were no specific problems related to her work, personal life, or finances. She says:

I was just worried all the time about everything ... or anything. It didn't matter that there weren't any problems, I just got worried

The constant sense of worry began to make it hard for her to fall asleep at night. A lack of sleep led to fatigue, which combined with feelings of distraction at work, and resulted in her making 'silly little mistakes'.

Fatigue and a poor performance at work made Ann irritable and angry with her friends and family. She first sought help for her anxiety from her family doctor. To begin with, she used a benzodiazepine to reduce her physical symptoms and to help her sleep. However, her doctor also referred her to a therapist who dies experienced in treating anxiety disorders.

Through weekly hour-long sessions of CBT, Ann is learning more about her physiological responses to anxiety. She is also learning how her psychological responses to these physiological changes can be detrimental. She is developing plans for how better to deal with her anxiety when she feels it rising. She has also been keeping a 'diary' of the thoughts and emotions which accompany her physical symptoms of anxiety.

Without treatment, GAD will persist for several years in over 75 per cent of people. Phobias and panic disorders may continue for several years: phobias with a childhood onset may be particularly persistent. Medical treatments for anxiety disorders include anxiolytics (for short-term use) and antidepressants for patients with GAD or phobias involving depression. Psychological therapies include relaxation training, self-help methods, and CBT designed to change maladaptive thoughts about feared situations. Combinations of psychotherapy and pharmacotherapy are often more effective than either single treatment.

Schizophrenia

Schizophrenia is characterised by disorders of thought, mood, and anxiety. The key features of **schizophrenia** are psychotic symptoms such as delusions and hallucinations. Different subtypes of schizophrenia can be identified according to different combinations of 'positive' and 'negative' symptoms. The **positive symptoms** are additions to usual pre-existing functioning. They include thought disorders, hallucinations, and delusions. *Thought disorders* may take different forms, but all represent a variation from normal streams of thought. For example, there may be a lack of logical connections between different ideas. The most common *hallucinations* are auditory e.g. a person may imagine that they can hear the voice of another person commenting on their behaviour, or may experience a 'thought echo' in which they hear their thoughts spoken out loud. *Delusions* are false (often bizarre) beliefs which may be persecutory in nature. For example, a person may believe that the television is stealing their thoughts, or that their neighbours are spying on them for the government. The presence of such delusions without other symptoms of schizophrenia represents a delusional disorder.

The **negative symptoms** of schizophrenia are those which involve a loss of normal function. They are varied but tend to reflect impaired interpersonal and social functioning. Changes in mood may include a blunting of feeling, a reduced capacity to express emotions, and incongruous emotions (e.g. laughing in response to sad news). Reductions in attention and memory may accompany the thought disorders referred to above. Poverty of speech, depressed mood, and low motivation may combine with these emotional changes and lead to a withdrawal from normal social interactions.

The population prevalence of schizophrenia is around 0.5 per cent and the lifetime risk is around 1 per cent. It is twice as common among men as women. It has been estimated a primary care practitioner with a registered list of 2,000 patients may have eight patients with schizophrenia, but that this number will be substantially higher for doctors working in urban areas with large homeless populations (Gelder et al., 2005).

Schizophrenia results from a combination of genetic, physiological, and experiential factors. Twin studies indicate that some people have a genetic predisposition to this disorder (Sullivan et al., 2003). There is evidence that the lateral ventricles of the brain are enlarged in people with schizophrenia, that the hippocampal volume is reduced, and that dopamine and serotonin levels may be abnormal (Kapur and Remington, 1996; Nelson et al., 1998). Complications during pregnancy and birth increase the likelihood of schizophrenia (Cannon et al., 2002), as do negative childhood experiences such as neglect and abuse (Read et al., 2005). The onset of schizophrenia often follows distressing events or periods. Early or prolonged cannabis use also increases the risk of schizophrenia (Arsenault et al., 2004).

The prognosis for people with schizophrenia tends to be better if positive symptoms are intermittent rather than continuous and if negative symptoms are absent or do not worsen. Up to 10 per cent of people with schizophrenia will commit suicide. Antipsychotic medications can be effective for treating positive symptoms but do not affect the negative symptoms. A lack of adherence is often a problem in schizophrenia and may be influenced by medication side effects. Psychotherapy can be a useful adjunct to medication.

Personality disorders

Personality can be defined as the enduring characteristics of an individual expressed via behaviour in different settings. **Personality disorders** are difficult to define because personality itself is an elusive concept. Unlike other psychiatric disorders, personality disorders may have no clear time of onset. They consist of inflexible patterns of behaviour which deviate from social expectations and which causes distress, suffering, or harm to the individual or other people. The *DSM* divides personality disorders into three clusters:

- Odd/Eccentric – including paranoid and schizoid personality disorders.
- Dramatic/Emotional – including antisocial and borderline personality disorders.
- Anxious/Fearful – including obsessive-compulsive disorder.

Around 5–10 per cent of the population may have a personality disorder. Personality disorders are more common among younger people and among men. They appear to result from a combination of a genetic predisposition and experiential factors such as brain injury during a complicated birth or parent-child interactions.

Because personality is relatively stable, personality disorders tend not to be very responsive to treatment. Treatment often involves identifying ways to manage the person's behaviour in different social contexts, such as avoiding situations where the problem behaviour occurs and providing support to the immediate family. Comorbid psychological conditions or unhealthy patterns of alcohol and drug use should also be treated.

Summary

- Psychiatric disorders are the result of the interaction and combination of three Ps: predisposing, precipitating, and perpetuating factors.
- Medical and psychosocial factors may be as important as predisposing, precipitating, or perpetuating factors.

- The two major systems for classifying psychiatric disorders are the *Diagnostic and Statistical Manual of Mental Disorders* (DSM), and the *International Statistical Classification of Diseases and Related Health Problems* (ICD).
- The World Health Organisation has developed a simplified classification of the mental disorders most commonly seen in primary care.
- Psychiatric disorders differ from each other in terms of the presence, nature, and intensity of disorders of thought, mood, and anxiety.

16.2 DIAGNOSIS AND TREATMENT OF PSYCHIATRIC DISORDERS

16.2.1 PSYCHIATRIC ASSESSMENT

Diagnosing a psychiatric disorder may be straightforward in some cases. However, most psychiatric disorders are syndromes of symptoms and many of these symptoms may be aspects of different disorders. It is therefore important to conduct a thorough examination and assessment in order to evaluate differential diagnoses. A psychiatric interview involves taking a psychiatric history and conducting a mental state examination (Gelder et al., 2005; Stevens and Rodin, 2001). It is important to note that the nature of many psychiatric disorders may make the psychiatric interview more difficult than a standard clinical interview: patients may be apathetic, anxious, angry, deluded, or aggressive (see Chapter 18).

The psychiatric history should first attend to the presenting complaint and its history, including the patient's reports of the believed causes and subjective experiences. It is also important to gain information about the patient's pre-morbid personality. There may be a need to corroborate reports provided by a patient experiencing delusions or psychosis. The history should also gather information about the patient's psychiatric and medical history, including details of any medications and other treatments. Information relating to the patient's family history should identify the presence of any psychiatric disorders, drug/alcohol disorders, and causes of death.

An assessment of a patient's personal history should focus on (a) their early developmental experiences (including pregnancy and birth), (b) their educational and occupational history, (c) their current work and financial circumstances, and (d) their relationship history. It is also important to collect information about their use of alcohol, tobacco, other recreational drugs, and their forensic history. Risks to consider include (a) deliberate self harm and suicide, (b) aggressive behaviour directed toward others, (c) self-neglect (i.e. a lack of self care), and (d) neglect or exploitation by other people.

The **Mental State Examination** (Trzepacz and Baker, 1993) can aid psychiatric diagnoses. It provides a structured way of both observing and describing several aspects of psychological functioning. It uses the following schema:

- *Behaviour and Appearance* – The focus here includes the visible signs of physical health or injury and psychological wellbeing. It also includes the style and condition of clothing and self-presentation. Behaviours to look out for include excessive or reduced physical activity, including posture, speed of movement, restlessness, gait, etc.

- *Mood* (subjective and objective) – The patient's mood is their underlying emotional state. As well as seeking the patient's self-assessment of their mood, medical professionals should give their own assessment of this – euthymic ('normal'), dysthmic ('down'), or hyperthymic ('up').

- *Affect* – Affect is related to mood and consists of external manifestations of emotion. If there is no apparent abnormality, affect is described as reactive (appropriate to emotional cues). In psychiatric disorders, the affect may be blunted, irritable, changeable, suspicious, perplexed, or incongruous (i.e. not appropriate for the context).

- *Speech and Thought Form* – The tone, speed, and volume of speech may vary in different disorders e.g. lower, slower, and quieter speech in depression. Attend to whether the flow of ideas in speech is normal, or if it is disjointed, illogical, or repetitive.

- *Thought Content* – The content of thoughts expressed in speech is also important, because someone could present in a 'normal' voice a well-connected, flowing stream of bizarre ideas. Attention should also be given to whether the patient describes feelings of guilt, depression, anxiety, hopelessness, etc. The patient may also express feelings of depersonalisation (e.g. feeling unreal, detached, or empty), or derealisation (e.g. feeling like all the world is paper), and may give evidence of delusions (beliefs which are clearly unfounded but resistant to contrary evidence).

- *Perception* – Note any illusions i.e. mistaking one real object for another (e.g. a bush is mistaken for a person), as well as hallucinations i.e. perceiving something that is not present (e.g. hearing a non-existent voice or seeing a non-existent object).

- *Insight* – The focus here is on whether or not the patient thinks that they have a psychiatric disorder or any other impairment and whether they see any need for treatment.

- *Cognition* – Note whether or not there have been any changes from normal memory processes (short or long term) and capacities for problem solving and reasoning. The 'Mini-Mental State Examination' may be helpful here (Folstein et al., 1975).

CLINICAL NOTES 16.1

Psychiatric assessments

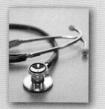

- It is helpful to think of psychiatric disorders as syndromes rather than simple discrete illnesses: this is because many psychiatric disorders present combinations of similar symptoms.

- Make sure you understand the various components of the Mental State Examination. This may help you detect a possible psychiatric morbidity in patients not presenting with psychiatric complaints.

(Cont'd)

- Brief assessments such as the Mini Mental State Examination and TYM (Test Your Memory) can be useful for identifying cognitive impairment. Make sure you are familiar with these assessments.
- When diagnosing and treating psychiatric disorders it is important to be aware of how predisposing, precipitating, and perpetuating factors can explain patients' current situations.
- Be aware of how psychiatric illnesses may affect patients' capacities to be involved in making decisions about their treatment.

16.2.2 MANAGEMENT AND TREATMENT OF PSYCHIATRIC DISORDERS

In treating any illness it is important to agree on a clear treatment plan with the patient and monitor their adherence and progress. Medical, psychological, and social interventions should be considered in every case. The different types of treatment are outlined below. Treatment should be planned in relation to immediate needs, short-term goals, and long-term goals.

Drug therapy

The drugs used in psychiatry can be divided into different categories (see Box 16.2). Some drugs can have more than one application e.g. benzodiazepines have anxiolytic and hypnotic effects. Many have marked side effects. This – along with patients' attitudes and beliefs about medication – may help to explain the low adherence rates among people with psychiatric disorders. Great care must be taken when considering prescribing psychotropic drugs to certain patient groups, including pregnant women (particularly during the first trimester), breastfeeding women, children, elderly patients, and patients with liver, kidney, or heart disorders. Care must also be taken when withdrawing or changing medication. More information about drug side-effects and contra-indications is available elsewhere (see Gelder et al., 2005).

As well as addressing the presenting psychiatric disorder, it is important to address problematic drug use. Use of tobacco, alcohol, and other recreational drugs is more common among people with psychiatric disorders than among the general population (Jané-Llopis and Matytsina, 2006). There is evidence of reciprocal causal associations between these behaviours. Some studies find that higher rates of smoking, drinking, and drug use can lead to increased risks of mental illness. Others find that increased use of cigarettes, alcohol, and other drugs are a consequence of psychiatric ill-health and proponents of the self-medication hypothesis would argue that such behaviour is used in an effort to manage psychiatric symptoms.

BOX 16.2   Major categories of psychotropic drugs

Type	Action	Indication	Class of drug
Anxiolytic (a.k.a. minor tranquiliser)	• reduce anxiety.	acute severe anxiety	benzodiazepine azapirone
Antipsychotic (a.k.a. major tranquiliser, neuroleptic)	• control delusions, hallucinations, and psychomotor excitement.	schizophrenia mania organic psychosis	phenothiazine butyrophenone substituted benzamide
Hypnotic	• promote sleep.	insomnia	benzodiazepine cyclopyrrolone zopiclone
Antidepressant	• relieve depression symptoms (but do not elevate mood in healthy people). • treat chronic anxiety, obsessive compulsive disorders.	depression	tricyclic SSRI – Specific Serotonin Reuptake Inhibitor SNRI – Serotonin and Noradrenaline Reuptake Inhibitor MAOI – Monoamine Oxidase Inhibitor
Psychostimulant	• treat hyperactivity in children. • elevate mood – but such use is avoided due to dependence.	narcolepsy hyperkinetic disorder in children	amphetamine
Mood stabiliser	• prevent recurrence of affective disorders.	bipolar disorder acute mood episodes	lithium carbamazepine valproate lamotrigine

Adapted from Gelder et al. (2005: 235)

Psychotherapy

Psychotherapy is an effective component of treatment for a variety of psychiatric disorders (Roth and Fonagy, 2004). As noted in Chapter 19, there are various types of 'talking cures'. Different therapies have different explanations for the causes of psychiatric ill-health. However, all share the belief that there is therapeutic value in helping patients to understand their past and present situation, manage their psychiatric symptoms, and develop more productive ways of thinking about themselves, their illness, and social interactions. There is substantial evidence of the efficacy of CBT for depression, anxiety disorders, phobias, and obsessive compulsive disorders. Indeed, in some cases of depression CBT may be more effective than antidepressant drugs (Butler et al., 2006). There is also evidence that psychodynamic and psychoanalytic therapies are effective for some psychiatric disorders (Anderson and Lambert, 1995; Leichsenring, 2005). In many cases, better outcomes result from a combination of medication and counselling. For example, in anxiety disorders anxiolytics may alleviate the immediate physical symptoms and thereby facilitate psychotherapy/counselling.

Electroconvulsive Therapy (ECT)

Severe depression may be treated safely and effectively using ECT (UK ECT Review Group, 2003). This procedure involves passing an electric current across the patient's brain to enhance monoamine function in the brain. In bilateral applications, electrodes are held on either temporal lobe to pass a current across the brain. In unilateral applications, the electrodes are placed over the non-dominant hemisphere. Although the bilateral process is more effective it has more side effects, particularly memory loss for events just before and just after treatment. ECT tends to be used for severe depression that has not responded to medication or which threatens the wellbeing of the patient or other people (e.g. mothers with severe post-natal depression, people with a high suicide risk).

Medical decision making in mental illness

Impaired cognitive functioning associated with some psychiatric disorders may hinder patients' capacities to be involved in decision making or to give informed consent to treatment. Those with thought disorders or impairments to memory and problem-solving capacities may find it hard to take in information or evaluate different treatment options. Patients who lack insight may not recognise that they are unwell and require treatment. The concept of a 'capacity' for decision-making is important, but there is debate as to how it should be defined (Wong et al., 1999).

In some cases, patients may be treated without obtaining their consent. For example, the UK Mental Health Act allows patients to be detained and treated without their consent if they pose a serious threat to the health and safety of themselves or other people. Issues of capacity and consent also arise in more common situations. Research Box 16.1 illustrates the complexities of the concept of 'consent' in mental health settings. Many of these issues also apply in the neuropsychiatric disorders described in the next section.

RESEARCH BOX 16.1   What does 'consent' mean in practice

Background

In principle, patients with the capacity to make an informed choice about treatment should be appropriately informed and free to give or deny their consent for treatment, without coercion. However, for patients detained in psychiatric hospitals, issues of consent are less straightforward.

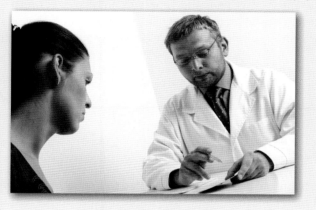

Methods and results

In-depth semi-structured interviews were conducted with five Responsible Medical Officers (RMOs) and seven consenting adult patients at a medium-secure psychiatric hospital.

One RMO neatly summed up the paradox of consent with detained patients:

There is no such thing as freely-given consent ... even with the patients that are consenting to take the medication, they're not really consenting patients because ... they know that taking medication regularly and in a compliant manner is likely to lead to their swift discharge from hospital.

One patient confirmed this:

I've learnt over the years to do as I'm told.

Discussions of consent focused on medication only; attendance at psychological treatment sessions was presumed to equate to consent. When RMOs talked about being 'cautious' when making decisions about treatment, they actually meant assuming a consent to treatment rather than a non-consent.

Significance

The concept of 'consent' in mental health settings is not always easy to define. Both patients and RMOs highlighted some of the challenges to the idea that treatment for patients with capacity should only be given with a patient's informed consent.

Photo © Endostock / Fotolia

Larkin, M. et al. (2009) Making sense of consent in a constrained environment, *International Journal of Law & Psychiatry*, 32, 176-183.

Summary

- A thorough psychiatric interview involves taking a psychiatric history and conducting a mental state examination.
- The mental state examination assesses: behaviour and appearance; mood and affect; speech and thought; perception; insight; and cognition.
- Many psychiatric disorders present as syndromes and symptoms are shared between many of these syndromes. This makes differential diagnosis important.
- When developing a treatment plan, medical, psychological, and social interventions should be considered.
- There is strong evidence that psychological therapies can be as effective as medication for many psychiatric disorders, in particular mood disorders.

16.3 NEUROLOGICAL DISORDERS

Degeneration or damage within the brain and nervous system can lead to a range of disorders. Their precise nature is determined by the location and extent of the impairment to normal functioning. Altered brain functioning can also be implicated in a range of psychiatric disorders. Because different brain regions have different functions (see Chapter 7), damage or disorders that are localised in specific brain regions tend to have specific outcomes. This section outlines a number of common neurological disorders, their psychological aspects and their treatment. It is followed by sections on neuropsychological assessment and rehabilitation.

Multiple Sclerosis (MS) is characterised by the inflammation and demyelination of the central nervous system. It may result in a loss of sensation or function in the limbs, incontinence, fatigue, pain, cognitive impairments, and mood disorders. In many countries, MS is the most common neurological disorder among young adults. It is believed to be an autoimmune disorder but the exact processes involved are not known and there is no cure. The unpredictable and variable nature of MS affects psychological wellbeing. Depression and anxiety appear to be more common among people with MS than in the general population or among people with similar levels of physical disability due to other causes (Mohr and Cox, 2001). In addition, learning, attention, and concentration may be impaired. Although there is no effective cure for MS, a recent synthesis of published research suggested that psychological interventions such as CBT can be effective for managing depression and helping people cope with the physical limitations arising from MS (Thomas et al., 2006).

Motor Neurone Disease (Amyotrophic Lateral Sclerosis) is a rare and terminal disorder which involves the progressive degeneration of motor neurons leading to progressive weakness in the skeletal muscles. The cause of the disease is not known and it is also not known why the sensory nerves, which have a similar structure, are not affected. Mood disorders are more common than cognitive impairments (Goldstein and Leigh, 1999). Anxiety and depression also appear to be correlated with the severity of functional impairment due to motor neurone disease. However, the relationship between functional impairment and overall quality of life appears to be moderated by the degree of social support that is available.

Disorders of the basal ganglia cause severe motor deficits (see Chapter 7). However, there are also important cognitive and emotional aspects of these disorders. Indeed, the symptoms of basal ganglia disorders have been referred to as the three Ds: dyskinesia, dementia, and depression (Rosenblatt and Leroi, 2000). **Parkinson's disease** is a severe motor disorder characterised by muscle stiffness, slowness of movement, an unstable posture, and muscle tremors (see Case Study 7.1). It is a progressive degenerative disorder resulting from a severe reduction in dopamine activity in the basal ganglia. There is no cure for Parkinson's disease. The standard treatment is the dopamine precursor L-Dopa, although promising advances have been made in stem-cell therapy (Xi and Zhang, 2008). Cognitive deficits are common and include impairments to memory and information processing. Depression, anxiety, lethargy, sleep disturbances, and pain are more common among people with Parkinson's disease than in the general population (Chaudhuri et al., 2006).

CASE STUDY 16.3   Social phobia in Parkinson's disease

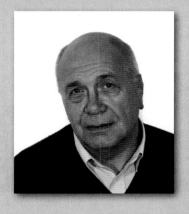

John is a 60 year old married man with three adult children. He first started to experience social phobia around five years ago – around the time that the physical symptoms of his Parkinson's disease first became evident. In addition to feeling anxious that tremors resulting from Parkinson's would make him look foolish, he also expressed concerns that seemed unrelated to the disease (e.g. worry about how his voice sounded on the phone and about saying 'the wrong things' to people).

During assessment, it emerged that John had been anxious in social situations since starting school. Once he began to experience the physical symptoms of Parkinson's disease, there was a marked increase in his social anxiety, starting with fears that others might notice his tremor and rapidly generalising this to other physical symptoms, such as his gait.

Treatment for John's social phobia consisted of 12 weekly group sessions of a cognitive-behavioural therapy called Self-Focused Exposure Therapy. In John's case, the first task was to identify the thoughts, emotions and physiological arousal that accompanied public speaking. Efforts were then made to replace catastrophic thoughts (e.g. *everyone will respond negatively to my tremors*) and overcome the desire to avoid social situations, because such thoughts and behaviour only made the problem worse.

(Cont'd)

Components of the intervention included 'in vivo' exposure (i.e. speaking in front of the group), and visual feedback using video and mirrors. These experiences helped John see that people did not make harsh negative judgements of either his tremors or his behaviour. Assessment using standardised measures revealed that the programme led to marked reductions in John's levels of anxiety and avoidance in social settings which were maintained after the treatment stopped.

Adapted from Heinrichs et al. (2001)

The basal ganglia disorder **Huntington's disease** is characterised by involuntary rapid, ceaseless movements or tics. Other symptoms include a loss of coordination and balance, slurred speech, and difficulties in swallowing. It is a genetically determined disorder caused by the progressive degeneration of neurons with receptors for the neurotransmitters GABA and Acetylcholine. There is no cure for Huntington's disease and death usually occurs 15–25 years after symptom onset. Treatment focuses on addressing the symptoms, preventing complications, and providing psychological support. Cognitive deficits are common and include impairments to memory retrieval, attention, and concentration. Compared to the general population, people with Huntington's disease are more likely to experience depression and suicidal behaviour (Paulsen et al., 2005).

Dementia, meaning 'deprived of mind', involves the progressive loss of cognitive function due to damage or disease in the brain. Dementia is not a single disorder but a syndrome, the symptoms of which vary between people depending on the location and cause of the disorder. Vascular dementias result from multiple small strokes which, in accumulation, produce a sufficient loss of neurons and accompanying changes in behaviour and cognition. As noted in Chapter 8, physical exercise may improve cognitive function in older people with or without dementia (Angevaren et al., 2008; Heyn et al., 2004).

Dementia of Alzheimer type (DAT or **Alzheimer's disease**) accounts for over half of all dementias. It involves the progressive loss of neurons and synapses in the cerebral cortex and particular subcortical regions. The cause of loss of neurons in DAT is not well understood, but is believed to be due to a combination of genetic factors and environmental influences. DAT is characterised by progressive impairments to memory, cognitive capacities, and social functioning which are commonly accompanied by confusion, irritability, and mood swings. People with DAT are more likely than the general population to experience anxiety (Teri et al., 1999). They may also experience psychosis – including delusions and hallucinations – especially if there is a rapid cognitive decline (Ropacki and Jeste, 2005). Among older people, it may be difficult to make a differential diagnosis between depression and the early stages of dementia because depressed people often experience impaired concentration and memory. Although depression and dementia often co-occur, it is unclear whether depression is a consequence of neural degeneration in the brain structures responsible for mood, or a reaction to an awareness of the onset of dementia (Rusted, 2007).

Neurological deficits often arise from a cerebrovascular accident or **stroke**: neural death occurs because of disruptions to the blood flow to the brain (see Chapter 12). The reduction of blood flow may be due to a blood vessel blockage (ischaemic stroke) or rupture (haemorrhagic stroke). The outcomes are determined by the size and location of the blood vessels involved. The brain regions affected by the disturbances to blood flow are unable to function properly, and this may result in impairments to voluntary movement, comprehension, and the production of speech or visual impairments. Depression and anxiety are more common in people who have experienced a stroke than in the general population. These disorders are important in their own right but they also inhibit the physical recovery from stroke (Chemerinski and Robinson, 2000). Other common psychological consequences of strokes are increased rates of irritability, agitation, eating disturbances, and apathy (Angelelli et al., 2004). There is, therefore, a need for physical, cognitive, and psychological rehabilitation.

Neurological impairment may be caused by a **traumatic brain injury** (TBI). TBIs commonly arise from blunt injuries to the head during 'closed head injuries' such as road traffic accidents, falls, assaults, or sporting injuries (Ponsford, 2004). In contrast, 'open head injuries' occur when a sharp object penetrates the skull and tend to result in more localised damage. Closed head injuries tend to result in a diffuse array of cognitive, behavioural, and emotional symptoms. Contusions occur when the brain is damaged by an impact with the skull (e.g. during car accidents). Such damage is particularly common in the basal forebrain, and frontal and temporal lobes. Shearing strains occur between tissues of different density (e.g. between white matter and grey matter) and can be as a result of rotational forces, such as landing a hook to one side of the head in boxing. Because multiple mechanisms may be involved in TBI, the resulting neural damage tends to be heterogeneous. Damage to the prefrontal cortex often leads to changes in personality, such as irritability and disinhibition. Rates of depression and anxiety are elevated following TBI, but the prevalence and severity of these psychological outcomes are influenced more by coping styles than the extent of the disability (Bowen et al., 1998; Ponsford, 2004). Emotional support and psychological interventions may, therefore, play an important role in rehabilitation.

Summary

- Neurological disorders may arise from progressive degenerative disease processes or acute events such as a stroke or traumatic brain injuries.
- The severity and impact of neurological disorders depends on the location and extent of the neurological damage involved.
- In addition to causing impairments to physical functioning, neurological disorders may also involve changes in mood and personality.

16.4 NEUROPSYCHOLOGICAL ASSESSMENT AND REHABILITATION

Neuropsychological rehabilitation focuses on treating the cognitive and emotional deficits arising from neural damage or degeneration. It may form part of a broader approach aimed at improving a person's physical, behavioural, and social functioning. An important part of rehabilitation programmes is a thorough neuropsychological assessment to establish the precise nature of any impairments and to enable the individualisation of rehabilitation programmes (Luria, (1963 [1948]).

16.4.1 NEUROPSYCHOLOGICAL ASSESSMENT

A neuropsychological assessment may be carried out for different purposes, including: (a) describing and measuring cognitive deficits; (b) a differential diagnosis (e.g. whether the cognitive deficits are part of another psychiatric disorder); and (c) monitoring the neuropsychological rehabilitation. A complete neuropsychological assessment involves the examination of all modes of sensation as well as memory and problem-solving capacities.

An important part of this process is an evaluation of a person's intellectual capacities. A useful tool is the **Mini Mental State Examination** (MMSE). The MMSE does not assess all the features assessed by the full Mental State Examination. Rather, it provides a brief (ten minute) standardised way of assessing someone's cognitive capacities (Folstein et al., 1975):

- Orientation e.g. the patient is asked to give the year, season, day, date, and month.
- Registration e.g. the patient is asked to repeat three unrelated objects named by the doctor.
- Attention and calculation e.g. the patient is asked to count backwards from 100 in 7s.
- Recall e.g. the patient is asked to give the names of the three objects named earlier.
- Language e.g. the patient is shown common objects and asked to name them; asked to repeat the sentence 'No ifs, ands, or buts'; follow some written instructions; write a sentence; copy a simple drawing.

The Addenbrooke's Cognitive Examination (ACE-R: Mioshi et al., 2006) covers similar ground. It is also possible to use paper and pencil tests of intelligence as part of this process. Recently, the brief self-administered Test Your Memory (TYM) was found to be just as effective as the longer MMSE and ACE-R for DAT and other dementias (Brown et al., 2009). Computer-administered tests are also available. For all such tests, standardised scores can be used to classify people as normal or with varying degrees of cognitive impairment.

CLINICAL NOTE 16.2

Neuropsychological rehabilitation and goal setting

- In designing rehabilitation for patients with neuropsychiatric disorders, it is important to set goals and targets that are relevant for each patient. This can increase their motivation and adherence. This general principle can be applied in other medical contexts.

- Goals should be SMART:
  - o **Specific** – stick to specific behaviours.
  - o **Measurable** – behaviour has to be measurable so progress can be recorded.
  - o **Achievable** – within their capabilities. This often means you need to start with very small goals.
  - o **Realistic** – goals need to be easily carried out and attained within the context of the patient's life.
  - o **Time** specific – give a time in which the goal must be achieved.
- An example of a SMART goal for a depressed and withdrawn patient might be to walk to the local shop every day for a week.

Physiological or neuroimaging assessments may also be made. Tests of cranial nerve function include assessments of:

- Scent perception, visual acuity, visual fields, and eye movement.
- Colour vision.
- Power of the jaw and facial muscles.
- Hearing.
- Head movements.

Tests of motor nerve function include an assessment of the reflexes and observations of any involuntary movements, weakness, or uncoordination. Sensation in the limbs can be assessed via the application of appropriate touch and temperature. Further investigation of the nervous system may include computerised tomography (**CT**), magnetic resonance imaging (**MRI**), and functional MRI (**fMRI**). Angiography and venography can provide information about blood flow within the brain. An analysis of cerebrospinal fluid can also give information about infections (e.g. meningitis, encephalitis) and some cancers.

16.4.2 NEUROPSYCHOLOGICAL REHABILITATION

The brain exhibits a certain amount of plasticity, and connections between neurons can change in response to experience (see Section 7.1.2). The prospects for a recovery from neural damage are influenced by the size and location of any damage, the state of the brain before injury (influenced by the person's age), and the person's personality and coping styles before the injury (Luria, 1963[1948]; Ponsford, 2004; Prigatano, 1999).

Key tasks for rehabilitation may include the rehabilitation of disorders of language, attention, memory, self-awareness, and behavioural problems. In all cases, it is important to address depression. Prospects for rehabilitation following TBI may be hampered if the brain injury means that the patient is unaware of the need for rehabilitation, or has experienced changes in attention and personality that make it harder for them to persist with rehabilitation tasks.

Recently there has been a trend toward community-based neuropsychological rehabilitation. Such programmes are designed to enhance the development of independence

(Ponsford, 2004; Prigatano, 1999). They often involve the provision of appropriate support services within the home and workplace. There has been increased use of technologies to aid memory, decision making, and the organisation of daily activities. Rather than being an exclusive relationship between patients and health professionals, rehabilitation has come to be seen as a partnership involving patients' families. All parties in this partnership must work to achieve optimal cognitive, physical, and social wellbeing.

Rehabilitation should be designed to achieve goals that are relevant to the person's lifestyle. This will make it more likely that the patient and their family will remain involved in goal setting and rehabilitation activities. The general principles of goal setting must apply here. Goals should be agreed with the patient and should be SMART: i.e., they should be:

Specific, Measurable, Achievable, Realistic, have Timelines for achievement.

The approaches used are influenced by the nature of the goals to be reached and the capabilities of the patient (Prigatano, 1999). They may entail learning new ways of performing tasks or interacting with people and coming to terms with limitations. This can be done by employing a range of techniques, including the use of external aids or tools. The techniques chosen should maximise the patient's attention to the immediate tasks (as well as the longer-term goals). This may be particularly important following TBI which results in impairments to attention, arousal, self-awareness, and executive function.

There is now much greater recognition of the need to address cognition, emotion, behaviour, and social functioning, and to acknowledge the links between these different aspects of patients' lives. This is the basis of the holistic approach. Rehabilitation must aim to improve cognitive functioning but also address any changes in mood and personality associated with the underlying neuropsychological impairment. It is now recognised that rehabilitation requires a broad theoretical base and that no single theoretical approach will be the most appropriate foundation for all patients.

Summary

- Neuropsychological rehabilitation focuses on addressing the cognitive and emotional deficits arising from neural damage or degeneration.
- Neuropsychological assessment can be used as part of a diagnosis, for planning rehabilitation, and for monitoring progress. It focuses on cognitive capacity and may also involve physiological or neuroimaging assessments.
- The prospects for rehabilitation in neurological disorders are influenced by the characteristics of the neurological impairment (nature, size, location, etc.) as well as the characteristics of the patient such as their coping style.
- Neuropsychological rehabilitation should be designed to meet the goals agreed by the patient. In addition to improving physical capacities, it is important to address any changes in mood and personality.

📖 FURTHER READING

Gelder, M., Mayou, R. & Geddes, J. (2005) *Psychiatry* (3rd edition). Oxford: Oxford University Press. A comprehensive, clear, and authoritative overview of psychiatry. A major limitation is that it contains no references. More detailed coverage is provided in the *Shorter Oxford Textbook of Psychiatry* (5th edition).

Prigatano, G.P. (1999) *Principles of Neuropsychological Rehabilitation*. Oxford: Oxford University Press. Provides a comprehensive coverage of neuropsychology and highlights the importance of considering the patient's subjective experience, including their premorbid state.

Stevens, L. & Rodin, I. (2001) *Psychiatry: An Illustrated Colour Text*. Edinburgh: Churchill Livingstone. Accessible brief chapters on a range of topics. Each two-page chapter gives a good introduction to each topic, which could be supplemented by further reading.

❓ REVISION QUESTIONS

1 Describe the 'three Ps' related to the onset and progression of psychiatric disorders.

2 Choose one psychiatric disorder. Outline its key features, causes, and treatment options.

3 What is assessed by the Mental State Examination? How is this done?

4 Briefly describe the applicability of drug therapy, psychotherapy, and electroconvulsive therapy for psychiatric disorders. Discuss the success rates of each.

5 Why are combinations of drug therapy and psychotherapy often more effective than either treatment mode in isolation?

6 Choose one neurological disorder. Outline its causes, physical and psychological symptoms, and prospects for treatment.

7 Why is a thorough neuropsychological assessment for rehabilitation necessary? What procedures are used in this assessment?

8 Outline the purposes and practices of neuropsychological rehabilitation.

HEALTHCARE PRACTICE

17 EVIDENCE-BASED MEDICINE

Figures

Research box

LEARNING OBJECTIVES

This chapter is designed to enable you to:

- Define evidence-based medicine.
- Identify the sources of information to be used when practising evidence-based medicine.
- Describe the factors which influence adherence to prescribed treatment.
- Discuss the importance of effective doctor-patient communication.

Ideally, all decisions about treatment would be based on sound evidence. This ideal lies behind the promotion of evidence-based practice. But what is meant by 'evidence-based medicine', and what counts as 'evidence'? This chapter begins with a description of evidence-based medicine, the second section focuses on evidence from research on adherence to treatment, and the third section describes research into doctor-patient communication. Chapter 18 builds on this last section and outlines the communication skills that have been shown to produce better patient outcomes.

17.1 EVIDENCE-BASED MEDICINE

17.1.1 WHAT IS EVIDENCE-BASED MEDICINE?

Evidence-based medicine (EBM) is based on the principal of 'integrating individual clinical expertise with the best available external clinical evidence from systematic research' (Sackett et al., 1996: 71). An important aspect of clinical expertise is taking into account the details of particular patients' predicaments, rights, and preferences. In their useful guide, Straus et al. (2005) state that to practise EBM we must:

1   Formulate an appropriate question. Questions must be phrased in a way that allows us to determine whether they have been answered. For example, if we want to know which of two possible treatments is better, then we need to define beforehand what we would consider to be a significant difference – we will then have a criterion to apply to our answers.

2 Find the best evidence to answer this question. The different sources of evidence will be discussed in more detail below.

3 Evaluate and appraise the evidence. Medical professionals must know how to distinguish between reliable and unreliable (or good and bad) evidence. Though evidence can aid decision making, the evidence itself does not make decisions.

4 Align our evaluation of the evidence with our own expertise and the details of the particular patient. We must understand how the evidence will apply to particular patients. As noted above, this means taking into account patients' rights and preferences and any contraindications for specific treatments.

5 Evaluate steps 1-4 in a process of continual feedback, refinement, and flexibility. It is important to evaluate not only the outcomes (i.e. whether the chosen treatment was successful) but also the processes of integrating the evidence with clinical judgement. Through such self-evaluation the process and practice of EBM should become more effective.

Ideally, steps 1 to 5 will form a feedback loop whereby our evaluation of the processes and outcomes of medical decision making informs the development of more appropriate question formulation, better evidence-gathering, better evaluation, and a better integration of evidence with clinical expertise (see Figure 17.1).

These five steps represent an ideal pattern, which may not be followed by all clinicians all of the time (Straus et al., 2005). Clinicians may shift between different modes of EBM depending on the nature of their work and the presenting condition. Often the third step may be skipped, with doctors preferring to use others' evaluations. However, all modes of EBM will involve formulating the right questions and integrating evidence with clinical expertise, patient characteristics, and circumstances.

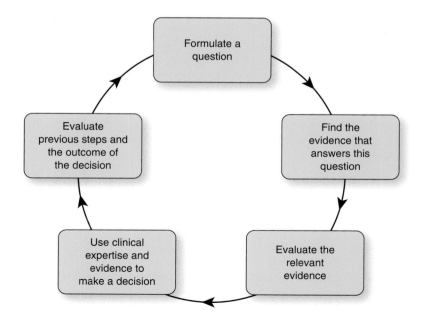

FIGURE 17.1 The cycle of activities in evidence-based medicine (based on Strauss et al., 2005)

17.1.2 A HIERARCHY OF EVIDENCE

In terms of finding the best evidence to answer appropriate treatment questions, Straus et al. (2005) identified a **hierarchy of evidence** for EBM. The components of this hierarchy are systems, synopses, syntheses, and studies. These will be described in an order of decreasing utility for practising EBM.

Systems

These are computerised decision-support systems which contain up-to-date information about different treatments and allow for the input of the details of particular patients to aid identification of the most appropriate treatment.

Synopses

These consist of brief up-to-date summaries of current best practice. Medical professionals may benefit from investing in evidence-based medicine journals and online resources (see Clinical notes 17.1).

CLINICAL NOTES 17.1

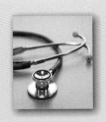

Finding up-to-date research evidence

- Use synopses of research such as the Database of Abstracts of Reviews of Effects (DARE), the journal *Evidence Based Medicine*, the American College of Physicians' *ACP Journal Club*, and *BMJ pico*.
- Look for recent meta analyses or systematic review papers.
- Use the Cochrane database to find up-to-date reviews of different treatments (www.cochrane.org).
- Be sure you know how to find the relevant primary research evidence using databases like PubMed (www.pubmed.gov) and develop the skills required to critically read such reports.
- Access Healthtalk online (www.healthtalkonline.org) for interesting case studies of patients' experiences of a range of illnesses and treatments.

Syntheses

Meta analyses and systematic reviews provide detailed descriptions of research findings through methodical searches of published literature to identify all relevant studies. **Meta analysis** is used to combine the results of similar studies for statistical data analysis (see Box

17.1). **Systematic reviews** provide summaries of published research but are not based on the statistical processes of meta analysis. In both cases there is usually an evaluation of the quality of studies, so that studies with weaker research designs have less influence than studies with more robust methodologies.

BOX 17.1   What is meta analysis?

Meta analysis is a statistical procedure used to combine the samples of several similar studies into one larger analysis. It is particularly useful for evaluating intervention studies because small sample sizes can affect the likelihood of finding statistically significant results.

The first step in meta analysis is to identify relevant studies – usually via a systematic searching of electronic databases. Once relevant papers have been identified, it is important to determine which studies are of a suitable quality for inclusion. Once suitable studies have been identified the combined data can be analysed to find the overall 'effect size' i.e. not only whether a treatment has a statistically significant effect on clinical outcomes, but also the magnitude of that effect.

Meta analysis can only be as good as the studies that are entered into it. Furthermore, meta analysis may be affected by the 'file drawer effect' where studies that do not find significant effects may never be published, and will instead languish in a filing cabinet. The real 'effect size' may therefore never be known.

Studies

These include individual studies and clinical trials as reported in peer-reviewed journals. One disadvantage of relying on single papers is that no single study will be perfect in terms of its design and execution. Even with good studies, the characteristics of the sample may not be the same as those of the patients to whom you are hoping to apply the findings. Thus, we would need to read and evaluate several papers in order to find the appropriate evidence to answer our questions. This is a difficult task: over 600,000 English-language records are added to the PubMed database each year. Finding the best and most relevant evidence therefore requires the development of good search skills and devoting a considerable amount of time to this endeavour. The hierarchy of evidence (Straus et al., 2005) suggests that individual research papers found via searches of databases such as PubMed have a low priority.

However, syntheses, synopses, and systems are all based, one way or another, on original research. Original research studies may employ one of several study designs. In a **randomised controlled trial (RCT)**, the efficacy of a treatment or intervention is assessed by comparing clinical outcomes in a group receiving the target treatment with a 'control group' which may receive routine care or a placebo. People are randomly allocated to treatment or control groups and statistical checks are made to ensure that the groups which will be compared at the end of a study do not differ at the start of the study. Methodological rigour is enhanced by ensuring that the patients and the researchers measuring clinical outcomes are 'blind' (unaware) of whether the patient received treatment or a placebo.

Other study designs include **case-control studies** – which compare people with a particular condition (cases) to a group of healthy people (controls) – and **cross-sectional surveys** – where standardised questionnaires are used with a group of patients or a sample of the general population. Increasingly, **qualitative interview methods** are being used to examine patients' experiences. Important information can also be gleaned from case series or **case reports**, but because these are based on small numbers of patients in specific contexts it may be inappropriate to apply their results to other clinical settings.

17.1.3 HOW TO READ A PAPER

It is important to know how to read and critically evaluate individual research papers. Medical research papers usually follow a set structure. The introduction should provide an accurate summary of current knowledge of the topic covered in the paper, give a rationale for the current study, and state clear research aims or hypotheses. The methods section should describe the study methods in sufficient detail that other researchers could replicate the study if they wanted to. The results section should present the results of any statistical analyses conducted to address the stated research questions or hypotheses. The discussion should give an accurate description of how the results of the study relate to existing knowledge and the implications for clinical practice.

Box 17.2 outlines several questions to ask when critically reading research papers. These questions cover all four sections of the research papers just described. This list is adapted from Greenhalgh's (2006) book, *How to Read a Paper*, which also gives useful tips for reading the different types of papers that appear in medical journals.

BOX 17.2   How to read a research paper

The following questions may be helpful for guiding critical reading of papers reporting original research. You may not be able to answer all of them at this stage of your education but you should aim to be able to.

- Where was the paper published?
  - journal esteem is a good first indicator of the quality of a study
- Was the study original?
  - does the introduction give thorough coverage of existing knowledge of the topic?
  - what does the study offer in terms of new information?

BOX 17.2 (Continued)

- Who were the participants/subjects/patients?
  - who was included/excluded?
  - was it a 'real life' study or an experimental study?
- Was the study design appropriate?
  - what was done and how was it measured?
- What was done to reduce bias?
  - was it necessary to have control group(s)?
  - were participants randomised to study groups?
- Was the treatment/intervention complete?
  - did all participants complete all requirements?
  - was there differential attrition (i.e. did drop outs differ from study completers)?
- Was the assessment/analysis blind?
  - did the researchers know who was getting which treatment?
- Were the preliminary statistical issues addressed?
  - was the sample size big enough?
  - was the duration of follow-up long enough to detect effects?
- Were appropriate analyses conducted?
  - were the appropriate statistical analyses conducted?
  - where necessary, was there adjustment for differential drop-outs?
- Were the conclusions supported by the analysis?
  - did the authors 'cherry pick' results that supported their argument?
  - were alternative explanations of the results considered?
  - was the influence of unmeasured explanatory factors considered?
- Were all conflicts of interest declared?
  - were all sources of funding and all researcher interests stated clearly?

(adapted from Greenhalgh, 2006)

Summary

- Evidence-based medicine (EBM) means integrating the best research evidence with a clinical judgement and knowledge of each patient.
- Different sources of information may be more or less useful for the practice of EBM. The availability of research syntheses may facilitate EBM.
- To practise EBM, medical professionals need to be able to assess the quality of individual research papers.

17.2 ADHERENCE TO TREATMENT

One important focus of EBM is an understanding of **adherence** to treatment. Better adherence results in better clinical outcomes (DiMatteo et al., 2002). It is therefore worrying that around 30 per cent of patients – across a range of medical conditions – do not take all of their medication as prescribed (DiMatteo, 2004a).

Most adherence research has focused on medication but the notion of non-adherence may also apply to other forms of medical treatment or therapy (e.g. exercise or physiotherapy) or behaviour modification (e.g. diet). The terms 'adherence' and 'compliance' are often used interchangeably. However, it has been argued that 'adherence' is preferable because it implies the active involvement of the patient in treatment processes, whereas 'compliance' implies that patients simply follow doctors' orders.

The relationship between adherence and non-adherence should be thought of not in binary terms but rather in terms of a continuum of 'more or less' adherence. This approach counters the idea that there is a 'non-compliant patient' type and acknowledges that adherence may not be perfect even in those who are strongly motivated to adhere. It also means we need to think of adherence in broad terms and consider the various ways in which patients may deviate from a prescribed treatment. They may deviate by:

- Taking too little of the prescribed treatment (e.g. too little of recommended exercise).
- Taking too much of the prescribed treatment (e.g. exceeding prescribed drug dosages).
- Not taking the treatment at the prescribed intervals (e.g. exercising too frequently or not as frequently as required).
- Not taking the treatment for the prescribed duration (e.g. ceasing antibiotic medication when one feels better).
- Taking other medication without the knowledge of the prescribing medical professional.

ACTIVITY 17.1

- Think back to the last time you were prescribed medication.
- Did you take all the doses? Did you take all of the doses at the prescribed times?
- If not, why not?

17.2.1 REASONS FOR NON-ADHERENCE: UNINTENTIONAL OR INTENTIONAL?

It is useful to distinguish between intentional and unintentional reasons for non-adherence (Myers and Midence, 1998). There may be various reasons for **unintentional non-adherence**. Patients may not understand the instructions for treatment or may forget the instructions. Non-adherence may occur because patients find it difficult to follow their regimen or simply forget to take doses. To reduce non-adherence we need to consider:

🐌 Patient understanding and recall of information.
🐌 Patient motivation.
🐌 The provision of resources to facilitate adherence.

Poor doctor-patient communication underlies much unintentional non-adherence (see Chapter 18).

Intentional non-adherence occurs when patients decide not to follow a treatment regimen. A useful model of behaviour in the domain of adherence is the **self-regulatory model** of illness representations (see Chapter 4). This model highlights the need to pay attention to a patient's understanding of their illness, including its cause and treatment. According to this model, there are three important aspects of self-regulatory processes. The first is rational planning of responses to illness; the second is emotional responses to illness and its treatment; the third component is the patient's monitoring and appraisal of their behaviour and of the progress of treatment. This model therefore emphasises the patient's ability to reflect on his/her actions and their consequences. It also highlights the constant interaction between the three components – beliefs, emotions, and appraisal. This model helps explain the various reasons for non-adherence, including defensive coping or denial of the threat posed by the illness, missing medication doses to avoid unpleasant side-effects, or stopping treatment early when symptoms subside.

17.2.2 REASONS FOR NON-ADHERENCE: MULTI-FACETED MODELS

Although the intentional/unintentional distinction discussed above is helpful, multifaceted models of adherence are probably more useful in prompting clinicians to identify and address a range of barriers to adherence. Recent reviews of research have identified several important characteristics of individuals, medical conditions and treatment regimens (DiMatteo, 2004a, 2004b; DiMatteo et al., 2000, 2007; Ingersoll and Cohen, 2008; Jin et al., 2008; Moore et al., 2004). These are illustrated in Figure 17.2 and Case Study 17.1.

Disease factors

Adherence tends to be better when patients experience symptoms of illness. This has clear implications for medical conditions with fluctuating symptoms (e.g. asthma) or no symptoms (e.g. hypertension). For less serious conditions, better adherence is found among patients with poorer health. For serious conditions, worse adherence is found among patients with poorer health. This difference may arise because people with more serious conditions have more physical, practical, and psychological barriers to adherence.

Treatment factors

Adherence falls as the complexity or burden of dosing regimens increases. It is generally easier for patients to adhere to single daily doses than multiple daily doses and their associated timing schedules. It is also easier to adhere to regimens that do not involve multiple medications, specific times, or dietary requirements. Adherence rates are lower when patients experience unpleasant medication side effects.

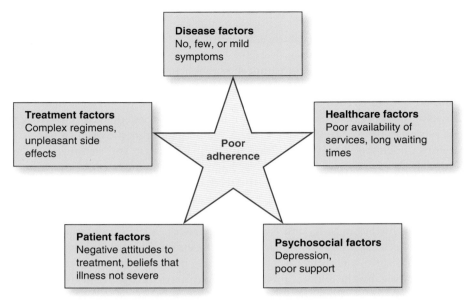

FIGURE 17.2   Multidimensional model of barriers to adherence

CASE STUDY 17.1   Barriers to adherence to antiretroviral medication for HIV

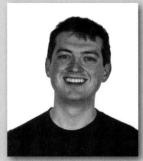

David is 36 and was diagnosed with HIV ten years ago. He has not been diagnosed with AIDS and his health has generally been good. He has been using combination antiretroviral therapy (ART) since his diagnosis. He has changed medication several times to make it easier to manage the timing and number of the doses of drugs. He is currently taking two antiretroviral medications – one of which is a combination of two drugs – in three doses. David finds this combination much easier to adhere to than earlier prescriptions:

It's so much easier having the combination pill. Before I started this I had to take three different drugs – one twice a day, one three times a day, and the other one once a day. I also had to try to have some on an empty stomach.

Like many people using ART, David has experienced unpleasant side effects such as nausea and headaches. When changing to his current medication, he initially developed a rash and experienced some insomnia. He has also experienced lipodystrophy – a redistribution of body fat caused by a disturbance in the fat metabolism – and his finger and toenails have become discoloured.

Obviously, I haven't been really sick yet, and I want to stay that way. Taking these drugs is probably the best way for me to stay healthy, but the side-effects do sometimes make me wonder ... I'm also worried about what all these drugs are doing to my liver.

Although David tries to maintain his adherence to his medication, and this has been helped by a simpler drug regimen, he does still sometimes miss doses:

Sometimes you go out and you meet someone, and one thing leads to another, and you end up going back to their house, and you don't take your medication. But that's usually only one or two doses. So, I hope that's not going to matter in the long run ... it doesn't seem to have so far.

This case study shows how adherence can be affected by a range of factors including a rational consideration of the potential benefits, concerns about the immediate and long-term side effects, and the difficulties of matching treatment regimens and lifestyles.

Patient factors

Adherence is not strongly influenced by demographic factors such as age, sex, or socioeconomic status. However, as noted in the discussion of intentional non-adherence, patients' beliefs exert an important influence on adherence. Better adherence is found when:

- Patients believe their condition is serious.
- They perceive more benefits from adherence.
- There are fewer barriers to adherence.
- Patients are more motivated.

Barriers to treatment include patients not agreeing with their diagnosis or treatment plan. They may also include concerns about side effects or the long-term effects of medication.

Psychosocial factors

Psychosocial factors are also important. Adherence tends to be poorer in patients who are depressed and have lower levels of social support. In addition to direct practical or emotional encouragement for treatment adherence, social support may have more general effects. For example, adherence is greater among people in families that are more cohesive and less conflict-ridden.

Healthcare factors

Practical issues such as accessibility of services and waiting times may affect adherence. One aspect of healthcare systems that has received much attention is **doctor-patient communication** and the doctor-patient relationship. A fuller consideration of the importance of doctor-patient communication is given in the next section of this chapter but poor communication

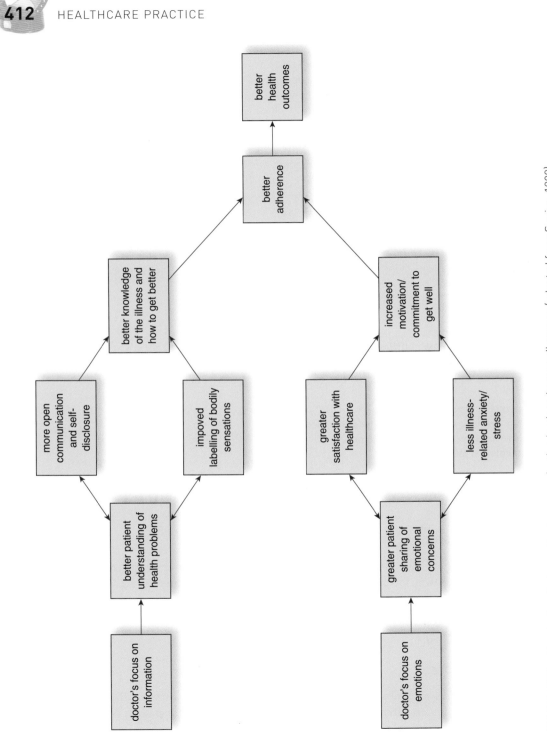

FIGURE 17.3 How better doctor-patient communication leads to better adherence (adapted from Squier, 1990)

may be a reason for non-adherence. Adherence tends to be better if patients have longer consultations and a trusting relationship with a doctor who expresses a genuine interest in their health. Better doctor-patient relationships lead to better adherence. Figure 17.3 displays the ways in which better doctor-patient communication can lead to better adherence and better patient outcomes.

Adherence is also influenced by the provision of information by the clinician and the efficient use of this information. The exchange of information should not just focus on facts about illness and its treatment but also on the emotional concerns of the patient (see Chapter 18). Good communication skills are required to elicit patients' beliefs, respond to them sensitively, and to include these when developing a treatment plan that will be most likely to be adhered to.

Adherence is better when patients are satisfied with the amount of information given and when they are able to understand and recall this information (see Clinical Notes 10.3). Patients need information to:

- Allow them to be adherent.
- Counter fears or misconceptions about their treatment.
- Counter feelings that they have not received adequate attention.

However, more information is not always a good thing. Too much information can hamper efficient decision making. Information about low treatment efficacy or side effects may lead to lower adherence rates.

CLINICAL NOTES 17.2

Agreeing treatment plans with patients

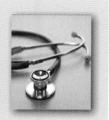

- Discuss the patient's beliefs, concerns, and intentions relating to treatment. Where possible, customise the regimen in accordance with the patient's wishes.
- Simplify the regimen as much as possible.
- Provide simple, clear instructions for taking medication.
- Elicit the patient's feelings about his or her ability to follow the regimen and discuss strategies for enhancing adherence.
- Consider the use of medication-taking systems, including electronic reminders.
- Emphasise the value of the prescribed regimen and the important of adherence for producing the best treatment outcomes.
- Obtain any necessary help from family members, friends, etc.

(Osterberg and Blaschke, 2005)

The value of written information is becoming more widely acknowledged, particularly for complex treatment regimens. Although written information such as instructions or leaflets may help to increase adherence, such information needs to be discussed with patients to ensure that they understand the content. Combinations of verbal and written information may be more effective than either in isolation. Combined approaches can repeat and reinforce information, as well as emphasise that the doctor is interested in the patient's understanding of the information and the importance of adherence. The benefits of written information can be further enhanced if that information can be customised or tailored to each patient (as opposed to generic letters or leaflets).

17.2.3 STRATEGIES FOR IMPROVING ADHERENCE

Various methods can be used to help patients follow through on their intentions to take medication. These include: specific action plans or implementation intentions, clear written or printed information, and the use of electronic reminders or monitors of medication use (Rosen et al., 2002).

A systematic review of interventions found that many are not successful and that many of those which are successful produce only modest improvements in adherence (McDonald et al., 2002). However, due to the complexity of interventions, it is difficult to determine the relative importance of various components. Nevertheless, the reviewers suggest that to increase adherence it may be important to: provide information, reminders, counselling, support, and reinforcement; discuss the severity of the patient's illness; and emphasise the importance of adherence before a treatment begins.

Adherence tends to be better when the doctor and patient are able to talk about it in a non-judgemental way (Noble, 1998). It is preferable that such discussions happen when treatment is being decided on rather than after the patient's non-adherence has occurred. It is also important to monitor adherence and to give appropriate feedback to patients (see Clinical Notes 17.3).

CLINICAL NOTES 17.3

Increasing adherence

- Monitor adherence. Watch for the markers of non-adherence such as missed appointments, missed refills, and a lack of response to medication.
- Express approval of adherence and encourage continued adherence. When appropriate, include objective measures of improvement due to treatment.
- Ask the patient about non-adherence and barriers to adherence in an understanding, non-confrontational way.
- If adherence appears unlikely, consider prescribing more 'forgiving' medications i.e. medications whose efficacy is less affected by missed doses. Options may include: medications with long half-lives, depot (extended-release) medications, or transdermal medication.

(Osterberg and Blaschke, 2005)

Summary

- Many patients find it difficult to adhere to treatment regimens.
- Poorer adherence is related to poorer health outcomes.
- A range of factors affect the likelihood of adherence to treatment regimens, including characteristics of the disease, treatment, and patient and healthcare factors.
- Adherence should be discussed at the time treatment is prescribed. Patients should also be given feedback on their adherence.

17.3 DOCTOR-PATIENT COMMUNICATION

In addition to helping improve adherence, doctors who communicate better with their patients are more likely to: detect emotional distress in their patients and respond to it appropriately; make accurate, comprehensive diagnoses; and have patients who are more satisfied with their care and less anxious about their health (Lloyd and Bor, 2004). Patients often receive less information than they desire from their doctors and doctors tend to overestimate the time they spend giving information and answering patient questions.

Information given to patients should be tailored to their needs and capacities. Doctors must pay attention to the complexity of their language and the speed of delivery. They should check that a patient understands the information they have been given. They should also attend to how a patient's emotions may affect their capacity to take in information and recall it after a consultation. (A fuller description of clinical interview skills is given in Chapter 18.)

To understand why doctor-patient communication is such a powerful phenomenon it is important to consider the purposes of medical communication, the communication behaviours doctors use, and the influence of communication skills on patient outcomes (Ong et al., 1995). Each of these aspects of communication is described below.

17.3.1 PURPOSES OF MEDICAL COMMUNICATION

Doctor-patient relationship

One purpose of medical communication is to develop a good doctor-patient relationship. Patients are more satisfied with doctors who take a partnership approach to treatment and decision making (e.g. Flocke et al., 2002). In psychotherapy, it is understood that a good therapeutic relationship is essential for successful interventions. Although Rogers' (1951) 'client-centred' approach was developed for psychotherapy, several of its principles also apply to doctor-patient relationships. Doctors should aim to be non-judgemental, respectful, and empathic by eliciting and responding sensitively to patients' concerns. Doctors should also be aware of the appropriate use of silence and non-verbal behaviour (see Chapter 18).

Doctors should also be attentive to what a patient is saying by paraphrasing or reflecting back to the patient what they have said. In addition, they need to be aware of what that patient is *un*able to say. Doctors who employ such techniques are more likely to detect underlying and undeclared emotional concerns (e.g. Girón et al., 1998). Doctors who attend to patients' emotional wellbeing are better able to reduce the anxiety or other heightened emotions which can impair attention being paid to medical information and the later recall of such information (see Chapter 10).

ACTIVITY 17.2

- Think back to the last time you consulted a doctor.
- How many of the behaviours just mentioned were displayed by your doctor?
- Was the doctor empathic? If so, how did they display their empathy?
- Which undesirable behaviours did they display?
- Reflecting on your own experiences as a patient can be used to improve your own communication skills as a doctor.

Exchanging information

The 'patient-centred' approach maintains that patients should feel able to express all of their reasons for consulting a doctor, whether these relate to symptoms or emotions. However, clinical interviews cannot be *completely* patient-centred: doctors do need to gather necessary information from the patient. The ideal medical interview, therefore, will integrate patient-centred and doctor-centred approaches (see Figure 18.1).

Just because a patient is given information there is no guarantee that there will be a transfer of knowledge or skills, or changes in behaviour. Any information given must be understood and used in positive and productive ways. Patients actively process information according to their pre-existing beliefs and understanding. As noted in Chapter 10 memory is an active process with a limited working capacity. Information provided to a patient may therefore not be remembered:

- If it is not understood in the first place.
- If there is too much information given.
- If it is not stored in memory (i.e. through repetition or rehearsal).

Much of the information given to patients does get forgotten or cannot be recalled accurately (Kessels, 2003). One way to increase the likelihood that information is understood in the first place is to ask patients to put into their own words what they have been told and to then correct any inaccuracies. However, this kind of checking for patient comprehension is rare (Braddock et al., 1997).

As noted elsewhere (see Chapter 10), it is also important to consider how strong emotions such as someone's fear and anxiety about their health can affect memory processes by limiting their attentional focus during consultations and thereby reducing the amount of information that they can recall (Kessels, 2003). Recall of information can be improved by developing and using recordings of important information and/or written materials prepared in a patient-friendly style (Watson and McKinstry, 2009). For example, one research review demonstrated that pictures which are relevant to written or verbal information can markedly increase the attention paid to, and the recall of, health information (Houts et al., 2006).

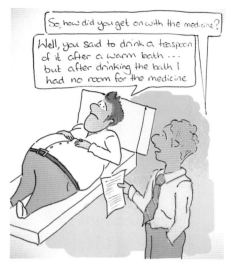

Medical decision making

In recent decades the paternalistic ideal of doctor-patient relationships where the doctor directs the care and makes decisions has been replaced by an ideal of **shared decision making**. This term should not be taken to imply a 50/50 share in decision making because patients may not feel capable of making decisions and may be worried about being responsible if they choose a treatment that is not effective. However, patients should be given as much information as they want about different treatment options before a final decision is made.

Charles et al. (1997) identified four characteristics of shared decision making:

- *Shared decision-making involves at least two participants*: the minimum requirement is that the doctor and patient are involved. Other parties may include relatives (e.g. parents), advocates, interpreters, or legal guardians. In some cases more than one doctor may be involved in decisions about treatment.
- *Both parties must share information*: The minimum requirement is that doctors give information about a treatment in order to gain informed consent. However, patients may bring important information about their circumstances and may have also gathered their own information about treatment options (some of which will be valid, some of which will not). Patients may want information for reassurance rather than to become involved in decision making.
- *Both parties must make an effort to be involved*: Although both doctor and patient should be involved in decision making, different patients may prefer different levels of involvement.
- *A decision must be made and both parties must agree to it*: It is important to consider both the process and outcome of shared decision making. Possible outcomes of shared decision making include no decision, disagreement between the doctor and patient, or agreement about a treatment plan.

Different patients will approach medical encounters in different ways so doctors must be adaptable when it comes to decision making. In adapting this model for primary care,

Murray et al. (2006) noted that shared decision making is not necessarily the 'optimal' mode of decision making. Many patients will not want to share the responsibility for this and will instead prefer an 'informed' model in which they are provided with as much information as they want but can leave the decisions to their physician. Because patients vary in their desire for an involvement in decision making, doctors must have the necessary skills, patient knowledge, and time to determine when and why patients wish to be involved (McKinstry, 2000). However, the research evidence suggests that the behaviour of many doctors precludes shared decision making (see Research Box 17.1). To some extent this reflects doctors' beliefs and behaviour, but structural factors such as the duration of consultations may also hamper them.

RESEARCH BOX 17.1   How common is shared decision making?

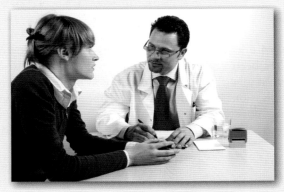

Background

Shared decision making is an important part of patient-centred care. This study was designed to determine how often shared decision making occurs and how it can be encouraged.

Methods and results

The primary data came from audio recordings of 62 primary care consultations. The researchers examined whether the Charles et al. (1997) criteria for shared decisionmaking had been met:

1 Both the patient and doctor are involved.
2 Both parties share information.
3 Both parties take steps to reach a consensus about the preferred treatment.
4 An agreement is reached about treatment.

Further data were derived from interviews with patients and doctors involved in these consultations.

The first two criteria – both patient and doctor being involved and sharing information – were not always met. In situations where these first two criteria are not met, it is highly unlikely that the last two criteria can be met. For example, dosage and side effects were not always discussed when new medication was prescribed. Furthermore, the fact that many doctors have no idea of their patients' views of medicine makes it harder to decide on the treatment that is most likely to be adhered to.

In interviews, physicians identified several barriers to shared decision making:

- Time pressures – one suggested it would take an hour to satisfy all four criteria.
- The assumption that patients merely wanted their problems solved and so doctors gave prescriptions without sharing the decision making.
- Doubt over patients' ability to understand medical terms and information.

One positive outcome was that many physicians appreciated the opportunity to consider how their consultation styles compared with models of shared decision making. Many were also interested in learning how to overcome barriers to shared decision making.

Significance

This study shows that more effort is needed to ensure that the sharing of information occurs so as to increase the likelihood of shared treatment decision making.

Photo © Endostock/Fotolia

Stevenson, F.A. et al. (2000) 'Doctor-patient communication about drugs: the evidence for shared decision making', *Social Science & Medicine, 50*: 829-840.

17.3.2 COMMUNICATION BEHAVIOURS IN MEDICAL SETTINGS

Analyses of doctor-patient communication indicate that asking questions is the second most common doctor behaviour after giving information and instructions (Bensing et al., 2003; Roter et al., 1988). However, such questions are most likely to be closed yes/no questions during the history-taking phase and are more likely to be **instrumental behaviour** (exchanges of facts) rather than **affective behaviour** (sharing emotions). Time pressures are often cited as a reason for a lack of attention to affective behaviours, as well as a barrier to shared decision making (see Research Box 17.1). However, longer consultations do not necessarily mean greater attention being paid to patients' emotions and concerns. One comparative study of US and Dutch physicians identified four different communication patterns which varied in their relative attention to affective and instrumental behaviours (Bensing et al., 2003). There was also variation between countries, suggesting medical training and professional cultures influence doctors' attention to affective issues.

Reviews of the research reveal important gender differences in doctor-patient communication (Hall and Roter, 2002; Roter and Hall, 2004). Female physicians are more likely to engage in patient-centred behaviours, whether this relates to shared decision making or affective behaviour. In turn, patients speak more in consultations with female physicians with the result that they share more biomedical/instrumental information and more emotional/affective information. However, the evidence suggested a reversal of these patterns in studies conducted in obstetric/gynaecological settings. Here male physicians engaged in more emotion-focused talk and elicited more affective information.

For both male and female doctors, communication skills can be enhanced by communication skills interventions and training (Rao et al., 2007). There is also evidence that interventions aimed at patients can improve doctor-patient communication. Although research has tended to focus on verbal behaviour, non-verbal behaviour is also very important – particularly for emotional communication (Ong et al., 1995). The full range of communication behaviours employed in medical consultations and their effects is covered in more detail in Chapter 18.

17.3.3 THE INFLUENCE OF COMMUNICATION SKILLS ON PATIENT OUTCOMES

Research reviews confirm that better doctor-patient communication results in a range of better patient outcomes, including better emotional wellbeing, the resolution of symptoms, improved functioning, better physiological measures, and better pain control (Teutsch, 2003). Verbal behaviours related to better patient outcomes include patient-centred questioning and empathic responses to patients, along with summarising and clarifying information given to, and received from, patients (Beck et al., 2002). Important non-verbal behaviours include adopting an open and direct posture, leaning towards the patient, and nodding where appropriate. Longer consultations and friendliness and courtesy on the part of doctors also tended to produce better outcomes.

Better doctor patient-communication appears to lead to better patient outcomes via several routes (Street et al., 2009). Better communication leads to better proximal outcomes including mutual understanding, patient satisfaction, trust, decision making, agreement about treatment, and patient motivation (Ong et al., 1995; Williams et al., 1998). Better intermediate outcomes include better adherence and self-care by patients, both of which lead to improved health outcomes (DiMatteo et al., 2002; Moore et al., 2004). These processes are reflected in Figure 17.3 which was introduced in the section on adherence. It has been suggested that better doctor-patient relationships may act as a form of social support (Ong et al., 1995). As a result it has been argued that for the best outcomes clinicians and patients should focus on the proximal and intermediate outcomes of respect, trust, and a commitment to adherence (Street et al., 2009).

17.3.4 COMMUNICATION ABOUT RISK

One important aspect of medical communication is the discussion of risk. However, there are many barriers to patients' understanding of risk. As noted earlier, people do not passively receive risk information: rather, they actively process it according to their pre-existing knowledge, beliefs and preferences (Leventhal et al., 2003; Marteau and Weinman, 2004).

Although many models of health behaviour are based on rational decision making (see Chapter 5) it is important to consider the emotional content of medical information. We must also consider whether people can understand risk information in the forms in which it is frequently communicated.

Understanding risk information

One difficulty in communicating risk information is that there are numerous ways to calculate and present risks. Information is often presented in the form of a **relative risk** – e.g. 'Smokers are five times more likely than non-smokers to develop lung cancer'. Such information is derived from population-based research which compares the relative likelihood of an outcome (e.g. lung cancer) in people exposed or not exposed to a risk factor such as smoking. Though such data are extremely useful at a population level, they do not always easily convert into numbers that apply to individuals.

Individuals are more likely to be persuaded by an **absolute risk** e.g. 'If you continue to smoke there is a 20 per cent chance you will develop lung cancer in the next ten years'. However, absolute risks may be difficult to calculate because you will need to incorporate a range of risk factors. Regardless of whether risk information is presented in relative or absolute terms, risk figures are always estimates which have margins of error – often given as **confidence intervals**. However, providing patients with risk estimates as well as confidence intervals may in fact hinder, rather than aid, comprehension. Simpler numerical information may be preferable because it is easier for patients to understand.

Many people have difficulty understanding health statistics and probabilities. The fact that many medical professionals also have difficulty understanding probabilities makes it even harder to convey this information accurately to patients (Gigerenzer et al., 2008). This difficulty with medical statistics is a specific aspect of a broader phenomenon. It could be argued that lotteries and the gambling industry rely on the fact that people do not understand probability and statistics! However, patients need to understand risk information so they can participate in shared decision making. To maximise patients' comprehension of numerical risk information it is recommended that doctors use 'real' numbers rather than probabilities (Gigerenzer et al., 2008: see also Box 17.3). Decision aids such as pictorial representations may also help patients to understand different event likelihoods (Edwards et al., 2002).

Emotional responses to risk information

Even when people understand statistical risks they do not necessarily apply these probabilities to themselves. Affective responses to risk information are an important influence on subsequent behaviour. People can often find exceptions to statistical risk information and apply these to their own preferred patterns of behaviour. For example, a heavy smoker who does not want to follow a recommendation to quit may say 'My grandmother smoked for all of her life, and she lived to 94'. A common phenomenon is **unrealistic optimism**

BOX 17.3   Recommendations for communicating risk information

	What to aim for ...	What to avoid ...
Use frequency statements instead of single-event probabilities	4 out of 10 patients taking this medication will experience insomnia.	There is a 40% likelihood of insomnia from taking this medication.
Use absolute risks instead of relative risks	Mammograms reduce the risk of dying from breast cancer from 5 in 1000 to 4 in 1000.	Mammograms reduce the risk of dying from breast cancer by 20%.
Use mortality rates instead of survival rates	There are 3 prostate cancer deaths per 1000 men in the USA, compared to 2 per 1000 men in the UK.	The 5-year survival rate for men with prostate cancer is 98% in the USA and 71% in the UK.

(adapted from Gigerenzer et al., 2008)

(Weinstein, 1987): that is, people often feel that they are less likely than other people to experience negative health outcomes and more likely to experience positive outcomes. Unrealistic optimism reduces the likelihood that people will engage in a healthy behaviour change, particularly when they believe they have some control over health outcomes (Klein and Helweg-Larsen, 2002).

To counter unrealistic optimism we must convince patients that the risks are real and serious (Floyd et al., 2000). Some health promotion campaigns use shocking graphic images in order to emphasise the seriousness of health risks and prompt behaviour changes (e.g. images of fatty deposits being squeezed from the arteries of deceased smokers, or graphic images of a motor vehicle accident). In one-to-one medical consultations techniques based on shock or fear may be employed (e.g. 'If you don't stop smoking you'll die before you're 60'). A paradox of risk communication is that a certain amount of anxiety may be necessary to motivate a behaviour, whereas too much anxiety can lead to inappropriate responses such as the denial of change real risks. If information or images are too shocking or frightening they may cause defensive avoidance of the issue i.e. people will stop thinking about their behaviour and its associated risks because they do not want to think about the feared outcome. Shocking images that appeal to the sense of fear are most likely to be successful when they are accompanied by clear information about what people can do to avoid undesirable outcomes and programmes designed to help them carry out healthy behaviours (Witte and Allen, 2000).

Summary

- Doctor-patient communication serves many purposes and is an important aspect of patient-centred care.
- If patients receive the information they need and are able to use this as part of the decision making about treatment, they are more likely to be satisfied with consultations, adhere to treatment, and experience positive outcomes.
- Better doctor-patient communication will result in improved doctor-patient relationships and exchanges of important information, better medical decision making, and more positive outcomes.
- Communication about risk is an important aspect of medical communication. However, many patients (and doctors) have difficulty in understanding the meaning of risk data. In addition, patients' emotional responses to risk information may help or hinder healthy behaviour.

FURTHER READING

Greenhalgh, T. (2006) *How to Read a Paper: The Basics of Evidence-Based Medicine* (3rd edition). Oxford: Blackwell. A useful guide on how to approach and make sense of research papers. Includes how to approach different kinds of papers, literature searches, and statistics.

Straus, S.E., Richardson, W.S., Glasziou, P. & Haynes, R.B. (2005) *Evidence-Based Medicine: How to Practice and Teach EBM*. London: Elsevier. This book is written mainly for experienced practitioners but does include some useful information that is suitable for students.

REVISION QUESTIONS

1   Give a definition of evidence-based medicine (EBM).

2   Why is it important for medical professionals to practise EBM?

3   What is meant by the hierarchy of evidence in EBM? What distinguishes sources of evidence higher in the hierarchy from those further down?

4   Describe the differences between intentional and unintentional non-adherence.

5   Outline the range of factors which influence adherence to a prescribed treatment.

6   Describe the different purposes of doctor-patient communication.

7   Describe the characteristics of shared decision making as identified by Charles et al. (1997).

8   Better doctor-patient communication leads to better patient outcomes. Outline the mechanisms that explain this link.

18 CLINICAL INTERVIEWING

LEARNING OBJECTIVES

This chapter is designed to enable you to:

- Describe different ways we communicate.
- Recognise the importance of the patient's agenda in clinical interviews.
- Outline communication skills for different stages of the clinical interview.
- Describe effective ways to deal with strong emotions in the clinical interview, such as anger, anxiety, and distress.
- Consider important factors when giving bad news to patients.

As we have seen in the previous chapter, how we communicate with patients is an important part of good medical practice. Good communication is associated with more accurate diagnoses, enhanced patient understanding, better adherence to treatment, greater patient satisfaction, and improved physical and emotional outcomes. Good communication also results in less iatrogenesis (i.e. adverse effects or complications), fewer complaints, and less litigation.

Communication in clinical settings requires particular skills. Communication skills training may involve mock clinical interviews, role-play, video recording, and feedback. Some students find this kind of training artificial but evidence shows it is an effective way to learn these skills. For example, one study evaluated third year medical students' performance in clinical exams (OSCEs) before and after communication skills training was introduced. Students who had communication skills training did better in their OSCEs. They were rated as more competent, having a better relationship with the patient, and better in terms of patient assessment, negotiation, and decision making. They also showed better organisation and time management during the consultation (Yedidia et al., 2003).

We shall start by examining how we communicate through verbal and non-verbal behaviour. The second section then looks at clinical interviewing, including different models of clinical interviews as well as specific skills and techniques to use in clinical interviews. The final section considers the communication skills required in difficult encounters, such as those with angry or distressed patients, or when giving bad news.

18.1 HOW WE COMMUNICATE

18.1.1 VERBAL COMMUNICATION

Verbal communication includes both *what* we say and *how* we say it. Speech is often surprisingly disjointed. The example below is a man talking about his sexual activity.

> Question: 'How important is it to be sexually active?'
>
> 'Sexually active is important. It is just now. Well … I've got – I don't treat women very well, I suppose. My mum always gets on my back for this, but I don't – I mean I cheat on them, and I deceive them, which is wrong, and I know it's wrong, but I think I'm kind of insecure in myself in that respect. Which is … I don't know why, but I just am. Yeah … I like to have sex quite a lot.'

A wide range of factors is used to interpret the meaning of what is said – including non-verbal behaviour and the social context. Consequently, even when *what* we say is very clear, people may still misinterpret it because of the influence of their expectations, beliefs, social context, the speech characteristics (e.g. our tone of voice), and non-verbal behaviour.

At a simple level, communication can be conceptualised as a messaging process like that shown in Box 18.1. It is possible for communication to break down at each of these stages. The message might be ambiguous (that is, difficulty may result from the way we *encode* the message), noise might make it difficult to hear (that is, there may be a difficulty concerning the *message transmission*), or the other person might misinterpret the message (that is, a difficulty may arise from the *decoding*).

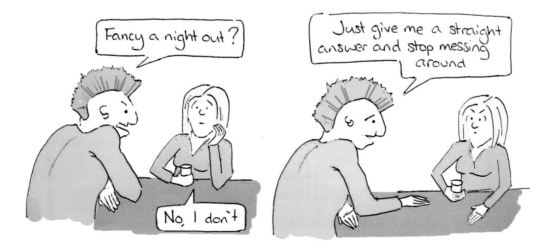

BOX 18.1   Communicating messages

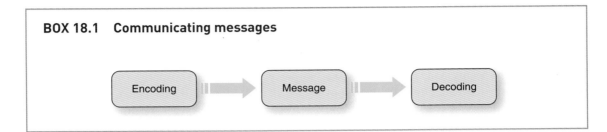

In medical practice, the words we use and the way we say things are both important. The way in which questions are asked can also influence how patients respond. **Closed questions,** which tend to start with words like *'did, is, have, can'*, require people to respond in fixed ways (typically, by saying *'yes'* or *'no'*). Such questions are useful for obtaining specific information or clarifying points, such as *'Have you taken any medication for this?'* or *'Is the pain sharp or dull?'* The disadvantage of closed questions is that very limited amounts of information are obtained. **Open questions,** on the other hand, encourage respondents to talk freely and tend to start with *'what, how, when, why'*, etc. Such questions are useful because they encourage the patient to express what is important in their own words e.g. *'What have you come to see me about today?'* or *'What does the pain feel like?'* The disadvantage is that they are less well suited for reaching definite goals or clarifying points.

Open and closed questions are both useful in clinical interviews. A common approach is the **'open-to-closed cone'** or **'funnel approach'** in which open questions predominate at the start of an interview and closed questions are used later. Open questions may be used first to obtain a broad picture of the problem from the patient's perspective. This provides an opportunity for the physician to listen to the patient and consider what other information might be important. The use of open questions at the beginning of an interview is extremely helpful in the exploration of problems: their power as an information-gathering tool cannot be over-emphasised. A common mistake in clinical interviews is to move to closed questions too quickly. As the interview moves on, however, using more specific open questions, probes, and closed questions can clarify information and find out more details than the patient may not mention otherwise.

There are some questioning styles that need to be avoided. These include multiple and leading questions. **Multiple questions** are those in which two or more questions are asked together e.g. *'Have you seen a doctor for this and what treatment did you have?'* Such questions will often result in people answering only one part of the question. **Leading questions** are those that imply a right answer e.g. *'You don't have any pain then?'* or *'No history of heart problems?'* Questions of this type impose our own assumptions on the patient and make it difficult for them to disagree. Research on forensic interviews has shown that even slight variations in wording can influence people's judgements. For example, assessing how fast a car was going when it hit a lorry will be influenced by the choice of verb used in the question (for example, 'smash' or 'hit'): people will say the car was going faster if the word *smashed* is used (Wright and Loftus, 2008). Therefore leading questions, or those using words that imply extent, may influence patients' responses and should be avoided.

Characteristics of speech also influence the interpretation of meaning. Features such as tone, pitch, pauses, sighs, and speed influence how speech is interpreted. These features may completely change the meaning of a sentence. For example, a sarcastic tone of voice may indicate that a person means the opposite of what they are actually saying. Speech characteristics may also be used as a guide to a person's mood. Fast, high-pitched speech usually indicates arousal, such as excitement or anxiety, whereas very slow speech can be characteristic of depression. This can be used in clinical practice to gauge and influence a patient's mood. For example, if you are talking to a patient who is angry or anxious, deliberately slowing your speech and using a lower pitch may help calm them.

In medical practice, the characteristics of our speech may reveal a good deal about our relationship with the patient. In one study, surgeons' consultations with patients were audiotaped and each surgeon's speech was rated for warmth, hostility, dominance, concern, and anxiety. For example, dominance was indicated if speech was moderately fast, loud, in a deep tone, and clearly articulated. Surgeons who were high on dominance and low on concern or anxiety were almost three times more likely to have been sued by patients (Ambady et al., 2002).

18.1.2 NON-VERBAL COMMUNICATION

Non-verbal communication plays a crucial part in communication. It includes facial expression, eye movements, spatial behaviour, posture, gestures, touch, and bodily contact. **Facial expression** is important in indicating mood or emotions, as shown in Chapter 2 (see Figure 2.1). **Eye movements** and eye contact help establish a rapport with another person. People look more at people they like and frequent or sustained eye contact is usually a sign of attentiveness. Conversely, reduced eye contact may signal avoidance or emotional problems, such as depression. It is important to get the balance of eye contact right. On the one hand, we want to appear attentive, so we need to have plenty of eye contact especially at the beginning of a consultation. On the other hand, prolonged eye contact can be interpreted as too intimate or aggressive: after all, long, and direct eye contact can be observed in courting couples, whilst boxers may try to intimidate their opponents by 'staring them down' before a fight.

Spatial behaviour is a form of non-verbal behaviour that may be either supportive or intimidating. It has been suggested that personal space can be divided into four zones (Hall, 1966):

1 Intimate zone (0–45cm/0"–18") – only lovers, close relatives, and very close friends are normally allowed into this zone.
2 Personal zone ranges (45–120cm/18"–4") – friends and family members are allowed into this zone.
3 Social zone (120–360cm/4"–12") – conversations with acquaintances and work colleagues usually take place in this zone.
4 Public zone (360–760cm/12"–25") – this is the zone that is often used when someone is giving a talk to an audience.

These distances apply to North American and Northern European cultures. However, there are large cultural differences in the demarcation of zones. For example, many Arab, Latin American, and Mediterranean cultures favour smaller distances in ordinary conversations. This variation in norms can create problems when people from different cultures meet because the person who is used to more space may feel uncomfortable, or that the other person is assuming a closer relationship than they have. There are also differences between certain patient groups. For example, people with schizophrenia need a larger personal space zone around them (Horowitz et al., 1969).

Cultures have implicit rules about the use of space which affect everything from which seat we take in a lecture theatre to where we put our towels on a beach. If someone's personal space is invaded they will usually withdraw. If this is not possible, people may use other non-verbal behaviour to diffuse the situation. For example, if we are forced to stand close to strangers we are able to tolerate it better if eye contact is reduced (Yoshida and Hori, 1989). This probably explains why commuters on tube trains do not look at each other!

ACTIVITY 18.1

Next time you are on public transport or in a cinema, pay attention to where people sit. Usually, as long as the space is not completely full, people will try to keep a certain distance from people they do not know.

Spatial behaviour has a number of implications for clinical practice. First, we must be careful how we position ourselves in relation to patients. We must not be so close that we invade their personal space, or so far away that we signal this is a formal 'public zone' encounter. The traditional consultation room set-up, where the doctor sits behind a desk, is not conducive to a good rapport. If a desk is necessary it is far better to position ourselves at the corner so that there is no barrier between us and the patient.

Second, physical examinations and procedures need to be performed with a lot of care because we are entering a person's intimate zone. Uncaring remarks or even a lack of acknowledgement of the person during this time can have a particularly negative impact because they have allowed us into their intimate space. Finally, personal space varies between individuals, so we should not assume we know what is appropriate. Instead, we should watch for non-verbal cues that a patient might not be comfortable with our proximity.

Posture is an indicator of attentiveness, interest, a social relationship, and someone's attitude towards us. Closed postures, where people have their arms and legs crossed and/ or are hunched, indicate a lack of engagement or defensiveness. Good postures for clinical interviewing include:

- An open posture (nothing crossed).
- Body facing towards the patient.
- Attentive (leaning forward).
- Relaxed (sends the message 'I am relaxed; I have time for you').

Patients rate clinicians who use such postures as having more empathy and a better rapport (Harrigan et al., 1985).

In social situations posture also indicates personal alliances. When people like each other, they often mirror each other's posture. Research shows that mirroring strengthens the rapport with patients in clinical interviews (Sharpley et al., 2001), though it needs to be used judiciously. It is obviously not appropriate to mirror the posture of a highly anxious patient who has crossed their arms and legs and is huddled over. Mirroring is best used after the initial session, as there is some evidence it can have a negative effect if used in the first encounter (LaFrance and Ickes, 1981).

Finally, **touch** can be a very powerful, human response, particularly when someone is distressed. Touch must always be used appropriately, with due regard to the sensitivities of the patients and professional codes of conduct. People vary greatly on what they consider acceptable touching and there are strong cultural differences.

Clinical examinations involve touch – sometimes of very intimate areas. This will be accepted by most people because of the social roles of patient and doctor. A professional medical touch is associated with improved patient outcomes (Field et al., 2007; Kiernan, 2002). Four factors are important if we are to use touch positively (Gelb, 1982):

1 The therapeutic encounter must have clear boundaries.
2 The touch must be appropriate to the circumstances.
3 The patient should feel they have control over physical contact.
4 The touch must be for the patient's benefit not the therapist's.

Guidelines for physical examinations are given in the Clinical Notes 18.1.

CLINICAL NOTES 18.1

Physical examinations

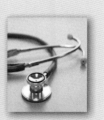

When carrying out clinical examinations it is basic good practice to:

- Explain what you are going to do.
- Ask the person's permission.
- Ask if they have any concerns.
- Respect their modesty.
- Never comment on their anatomy or state whilst carrying out the examination.
- Watch the person's body language for any signs of discomfort.

Summary

- We communicate through verbal and non-verbal behaviour.
- Verbal communication includes both what we say and how we say it.
- Communication can break down at the stages of (a) encoding, (b) message transmission, or (c) decoding.
- How we say things can override the meaning of what we say (e.g. sarcasm) and are good indicators of mood.
- Non-verbal behaviours include facial expression, eye movements, spatial behaviour, posture, and touch.
- Good clinical interview skills include a relaxed, open posture, good eye contact, and appropriate use of space and touch.

18.2 CLINICAL INTERVIEWING

Models of the clinical interview have been developed to help physicians understand the processes involved and improve their communication and interview skills. In this section we shall concentrate on two models. The first outlines the different perspectives of doctors and patients and encourages a more patient-centred approach to interviewing (the doctor-patient model). The second outlines the various stages of a clinical interview and considers which communication skills and techniques may be useful for each stage (the Calgary-Cambridge model; see Kurtz and Silverman, 1996).

18.2.1 THE DOCTOR-PATIENT MODEL

The doctor-patient model is shown in Figure 18.1 (sometimes referred to as the disease-illness model). This model raises the importance of considering different agendas during the clinical interview. The first is the **doctor's agenda**: the doctor needs to explore and identify any underlying disease. For this reason they need to ask about symptoms, carry out investigations, and consider differential diagnoses. The second is the **patient's agenda**: this arises from the patient's concern with their illness (e.g. their experience of sickness). As we have already seen in Chapter 4, patients have ideas and beliefs about what is wrong and they may have concerns about the illness and the impact it will have on them.

One strength of this model is the equal emphasis placed on the two agendas. Substantial evidence confirms the importance of considering the patient's agenda and using patient-centred clinical interviews. For example, consideration of a patient's beliefs and concerns in a consultation has been shown to lead to fewer follow-up appointments, investigations, referrals (Stewart et al., 1997), complaints, and malpractice claims (see Research Box 18.1). Patients are also more likely to discuss difficult issues like a prognosis in cancer and to report more satisfaction (Shields et al., 2009).

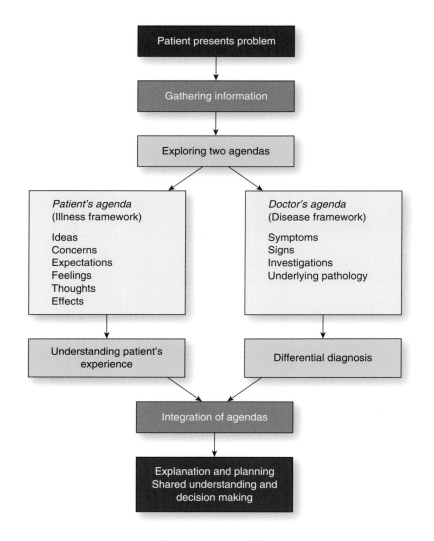

FIGURE 18.1 Doctor-patient agenda (McWhinney, 1989)

Another strength of this model is the focus on collaboration between the doctor and patient. The model specifies that, after a consideration of the different agendas, there should be an integration of agendas and shared planning and decision making about the treatment. Evidence confirms that collaborative approaches to treatment are more effective. For example, a review of 48 studies found that consultations with a collaborative relationship where the patients' perspective was considered led to better adherence in pediatric and adult samples, as well as in primary and secondary care (Arbuthnott and Sharpe, 2009).

RESEARCH BOX 18.1   Patient-centred interviewing and malpractice claims

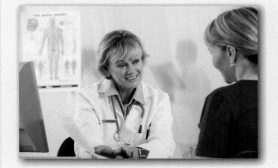

Method

Ten routine consultations for each of 115 primary care physicians were videotaped to enable a detailed examination of their communication skills. Doctors were divided into those who had no previous law suits or claims for malpractice against them and those who had had two or more claims.

Results

Doctors who did not have claims for malpractice against them:

- Used more statements of orientation e.g. telling patients what to expect and signposting what would happen during a consultation.
- Laughed and used humour more.
- Solicited patients' opinions.
- Checked for patient understanding.
- Encouraged patients to talk.

Ironically, doctors who had a history of malpractice claims spent longer in consultations (18 minutes) than doctors who did not have a history of malpractice claims.

Significance

This study and other studies demonstrate quite clearly that good communication skills and considering the patient's agenda result in better and more efficient practice.

Photo © Carlosseller/Fotolia

Levinson, W. et al. (1997) Physician-patient communication, *JAMA, 277*: 553–559.

18.2.2 THE CALGARY-CAMBRIDGE MODEL

The Calgary-Cambridge model of clinical interviewing is shown in Figure 18.2. This model is different to the previous one in that it focuses on the structure of the interview and indicates what skills may be relevant to each stage of the clinical interview. It provides a clear structure that is useful for medical education because it helps us to concentrate on the learning skills that are relevant to each stage. Students can thus build up their skills as they become competent at each stage.

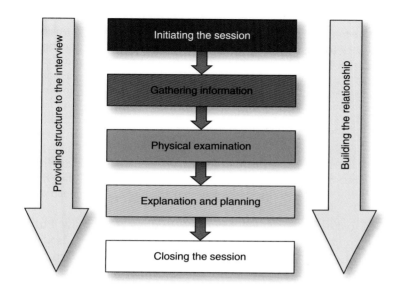

FIGURE 18.2   Calgary-Cambridge model of clinical interviewing

Initiating the session involves starting to establish a rapport with the patient and identifying the reason for the consultation. The skills that the Calgary-Cambridge guide lists as important at this stage are shown in Box 18.2. It is vital, especially in hospital settings, to get your introduction right and not to assume the patient knows either who you are or what the interview will involve.

BOX 18.2   Initiating the clinical interview

Establish an initial rapport

- Greet the patient and ask for or check their name.
- Introduce yourself and tell the patient what your role is.
- Show interest and respect for the patient.
- Maintain good eye contact and body posture.

Identify the reasons for the consultation

- Use open questions to find out about the problems the patient would like to discuss.
- Listen carefully to what the patient says and do not interrupt.
- Check whether there is anything else the patient wants to discuss (e.g. 'so you've come about these headaches, is there anything else you'd like to discuss today?')

Adapted from Silverman et al. (1997)

Using open questions at the beginning of the consultation is a very good way to obtain maximum information from the patient – providing we then listen to what they say! A classic research study in the 1980s found that doctors interrupted a patient after an average of 18 seconds (Beckman and Frankel, 1984). Yet contrary to popular belief, the more a doctor interrupts, the longer a clinical interview will typically take (Menz and Al-Roubaie, 2008). Interruptions disrupt the patient's concentration and lead them to expect they will only have a few seconds to say what they want to say. Attentive listening is therefore as important as asking the right kind of questions.

Active or attentive listening is a skilled process that involves listening, facilitating responses, and picking up on patient cues. A number of skills can be used to help the patient tell their 'story' or expand on their situation. These include:

- **Encouragement:** non-verbal and verbal encouragement, such as *'uh-huh'*, *'go on'*, or *'I see'* signal that the patient should go on with their story. This involves only minimal interruption and gives the patient the necessary confidence to keep going. Facilitative comments should be **neutral** e.g. not using words like *'right'* or *'good'* which could be misinterpreted as meaning that what the patient is saying is correct.
- **Silence:** Verbal facilitation is ineffective unless it is followed by an attentive silence, yet most of us find such silences uncomfortable and tend to leap in quickly if a response is not forthcoming. A useful skill therefore is to leave a slightly longer pause after the patient has finished speaking before you start speaking. A lot of multiple questions arise from our discomfort with silence.

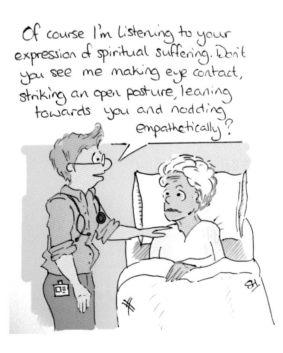

- **Reflection (echoing):** Reflecting back or echoing the last few words the patient has said may encourage them to expand or continue talking. Students sometimes worry that echoing will sound unnatural but it is remarkably well accepted by patients. Repetition encourages the patient to continue with their last phrase so is more directive than encouragement or silence.
- **Paraphrasing:** Paraphrasing involves restating in your own words the content or feelings behind the patient's message. It is not quite the same as summarising or checking because it is intended to sharpen rather than just confirm your understanding. Paraphrasing checks whether your *interpretation* of what the patient means is correct.

Gathering information is the second stage of the clinical interview and involves exploring the problem further, understanding the patient's perspective, and providing structure to the consultation. The communication skills that the Calgary-Cambridge guide identifies as important for this stage are shown in Box 18.3.

BOX 18.3   Gathering information

Explore the problem further

- Facilitate and clarify the patient's story of the problem.
- Use open and closed questions.
- Use active listening.
- Summarise the patient's points from time to time to check your understanding.
- Use clear, concise questions or comments and avoid jargon.

Understand the patient's perspective

- Explore and acknowledge the patient's ideas and concerns about the problem.
- Determine how it affects the patient's life.
- Explore patient goals and expectations.
- Encourage the patient to express feelings and thoughts.
- Pick up on the patient's verbal and non-verbal cues and check and acknowledge as appropriate.

Provide a structure to the consultation

- Summarise the patient's points at the end of a line of enquiry to check for understanding before progressing.
- Signpost moving from one section to another (e.g. 'We'll come back to that in a minute, but first I would like to ask you a few questions about your family history').
- Sequence the interview logically.
- Use appropriate timing to keep the interview on task.

Adapted from Silverman et al. (1997)

Explanation and planning involves the aspects covered in Chapter 17. These include: providing the correct amount and type of information; aiding accurate recall and understanding; achieving a shared understanding that incorporates the patient's perspective; and shared decision making. The communication skills that the Calgary-Cambridge guide lists as important for this stage are shown in Box 18.4.

The final stage of the interview consists of **closing the interview**. This stage can have a disproportionate effect on what patients take away from the interview (see primacy and recency effect in Chapter10]). Providing a summary of what has been discussed and agreed gives an opportunity to check that understanding has been shared and that the patient is happy with the agreed treatment. In addition, **safety netting** – where we tell the patient what to do if the treatment plan does not work or if other symptoms arise – may prevent future difficulties. Simple things such as asking whether there is anything else the patient wants to discuss and saying goodbye properly can make a big difference to the patient's experience of the consultation. The communication skills that the Calgary-Cambridge guide identifies as important for this stage are shown in Box 18.5.

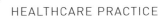

BOX 18.4   Explanation and planning

Provide the correct amount and type of information

- Establish what the patient knows already.
- Give information in manageable chunks.
- Check for understanding.
- Ask what other information might be helpful.
- Make sure information is given at appropriate times.

Aid accurate recall and understanding

- Organise information into logical, discrete sections.
- Use explicit categorisation or chunks e.g. 'There are three things that are important …'
- Repeat and summarise information.
- Use concise statements that are easily understood and avoid jargon.
- Check patient understanding at the end and clarify where necessary.

Achieve a shared understanding

- Link explanations to the patient's agenda.
- Encourage the patient to contribute.
- Pick up on verbal and non-verbal patient cues.
- Elicit patient's beliefs, reactions, and feelings about the information given.

Shared planning and decision making

- Share your own thoughts, ideas, and dilemmas as appropriate.
- Involve the patient by offering suggestions rather than orders and giving the patient a choice.
- Negotiate a mutually acceptable plan.
- Check with the patient if the plan is acceptable and whether they have any concerns.

Adapted from Silverman et al. (1997)

BOX 18.5   Closing the clinical interview

- Briefly summarise the session and agreed treatment plan.
- Lay out and agree with the patient the next steps both for you and them.
- Provide a safety net: explain any possible unexpected outcomes and what to do if the plan doesn't work – as well as how and when to seek help.
- Make a final check that the patient agrees and is comfortable with the plan.
- Ask if there are any questions or other items to discuss.

Adapted from Silverman et al. (1997)

In approximately one in five consultations patients raise a new problem in this final stage of the interview (White et al., 1994). Often this will be the problem the patient is most worried about. One way to avoid the problem being raised only at the end of the interview is to gather information as skilfully as possible earlier on. Research confirms that physicians who ask about patients' beliefs, who are responsive to patients, give plentiful information, and discuss treatments with patients are less likely to find such new problems being raised during the closing stage of interviews (White et al., 1994).

Summary

- The doctor-patient model indicates the importance of considering the patient's agenda.
- The Calgary-Cambridge model is a useful guide to the communication skills that are important at different stages of the clinical interview.
- Good clinical skills include thorough introductions that encompass an explanation of who you are, what the interview is about, and consent.
- Gathering information is best achieved using a funnel of open-to-closed questions.
- Physical examinations should involve an explanation, respect, and a sensitivity to patient cues.
- Explanation and planning involves providing the right amount and type of information in a way that achieves a shared understanding and a treatment plan.
- Closing the interview should include a summary, a check of understanding and agreement, and safety netting.

18.3 DIFFICULT INTERVIEWS

In medicine we work with patients from cradle to grave. Medical care therefore often involves extreme emotions in response to birth, challenging events or illnesses, life-threatening events, and death. Some of the most difficult interviews for healthcare professionals are those that involve high levels of negative emotions such as anger, distress, grief, anxiety, or fear. Such emotion raises challenges for the doctor in an interview. It is hard to discuss, and make decisions, about treatment with a patient who is highly emotional. It is important to acknowledge and deal with patients' emotions because these will influence their thoughts, actions, and ultimately their wellbeing (see Chapter 2).

In this section we shall focus on the communication skills doctors need to help patients who are angry, anxious, or distressed. Then, in the final section of the chapter, we shall look at how to give sad or bad news.

18.3.1 COMMUNICATING WITH ANGRY PATIENTS

Though anger and aggression are linked, they are not the same. Anger is an emotion, whereas aggression is a behavioural response involving some form of attack on an object or person. The link between anger and aggression means that when we are confronted with an angry person it is normal to feel under attack, particularly if the anger is directed at us. However, the true cause of the anger may be something different – for example, illness, a disability, or frustration.

It has been suggested that, when confronted with an angry patient, doctors typically respond in one of three ways (Lipp, 1986): they may try to ignore the anger and keep going with the interview as 'normal'; they might get angry back; or they may try to pacify the patient. Each of these strategies may make the anger worse. Ignoring someone's anger rarely diffuses it and consequently the consultation is likely to go badly. Though getting angry back is an understandable human response, it merely escalates the situation. In addition, trying to pacify the patient (e.g. by telling them to calm down) may potentially inflame the situation.

As we saw in Chapter 2, anger has a range of effects on us. It is associated with strong physiological arousal and a narrowed focus on what provoked the anger. Until the anger has dissipated, it will be hard for the patient to think about or deal with anything else. Common underlying reasons for anger may include:

- Feeling hurt or let down: If people are emotionally hurt they will often protect themselves by getting angry about it. In this case the anger will usually be directed at a particular person or group. Expressing this type of anger may lead to crying.
- Broken rules: Cognitive theory suggests we all have our own 'rules' about how both we and other people should behave (see Chapter 19). If people break our rules we may get angry. For example, I might have a rule that 'I must always be there for people when they need me'. If a doctor is then not there for me when I need them (e.g. cancels an appointment or keeps me waiting for a long time) I might get angry.
- Goal frustration: If we are prevented from doing things or reaching goals that are important to us, then it is common to feel frustration and anger (see Chapter 9). Injury and illness often prevent people from attaining their goals so anger and frustration may be common.

ACTIVITY 18.2

- Think back to the last time you were really angry with someone.
- Why was this?
- Were you hurt or had they broken one of your rules?
- What could they have done that would have stopped you feeling angry?

Like all strong emotions, anger needs to be expressed and diffused before an interview can continue. The following points can be helpful when trying to achieve this:

- **Check your own emotional response:** If you feel angry, anxious, or upset it will be harder for you to calm the patient. Remind yourself that anger is an emotion and not necessarily an attack and that the source of their anger could be the illness or hurt and so is not necessarily about you.
- **Acknowledge the anger:** Recognise that the person is angry and that it is important to deal with this. For example, you may say, '*I can see you're angry and I think it's important we talk about this first*'.
- **Find out the source of the anger:** Let the patient talk! Giving them space to verbalise and vent what they are angry about is the first step towards diffusing that anger. People cannot remain angry forever – especially when they are with a sympathetic person.
- **Empathise:** The most effective way to tackle anger is to empathise or understand. You do not have to agree with the patient to be able to understand why they might be angry. Simple statements such as '*I can see why you're angry*' may prove very effective.
- **Disarm:** Many patients who are angry say all they want is for the other person to understand and apologise. Some healthcare professionals worry that an apology means they are admitting fault or liability, but it is possible to express regret without agreeing the person is right by saying something like '*I'm sorry if that upset you*'. In addition, in some circumstances it may be appropriate to give a clear apology.

18.3.2 COMMUNICATING WITH ANXIOUS PATIENTS

Anxiety and fear are a normal response to the perceived threat of illness or injury and thus are common in healthcare settings. People differ in their anxiety levels and responses. Those with the personality trait of neuroticism will have higher levels of anxiety (see Chapter 2).

Anxiety makes people hypervigilant for signs of threat. Consequently, they are likely to react strongly to unexpected events, symptoms, or negative news. Anxiety also makes people less flexible in their coping strategies, so specific strategies become more rigidly applied. Anxious people may need to know exactly what will happen next so that the additional threat of unexpected events is reduced. Mere reassurance does not often work with anxious people – in fact it can backfire because they may feel that you do not understand. In dealing with an anxious patient the following may help:

- **Use your body language and speech:** As we saw at the beginning of this chapter, characteristics of speech and non-verbal communication can help someone calm down. Adopt a relaxed and open body posture (non-threatening), lower the tone of your voice slightly, and slow your speech down.
- **Acknowledge the anxiety:** As with anger, recognise the person's anxiety (e.g. '*You seem quite worried*').
- **Find out the main source of the anxiety:** Anxiety can become generalised, so asking someone why they are anxious may elicit only a general or defensive response. Use a more focused question such as '*Are you worried about anything in particular?*', '*What is it you are particularly worried/anxious about?*' or '*What was it that brought this anxiety on?*'
- **Empathise:** As with anger, empathy and understanding can be very helpful responses to strong emotion. In cases of terminal illness, where the threat of death is inevitable, empathy is crucial. In these cases we cannot 'fix' anxiety or any other strong emotion – we can only empathise and provide support.

- **Minimise the threat:** Anxiety is based on a perceived threat. Therefore, one way to lower anxiety is to reduce or remove that threat. This is best done by providing information as opposed to mere reassurance. For example, a pregnant woman might be anxious about her baby dying. In this instance, finding out why she believes this will happen and giving her information about the actual risk of it happening (or not) will be more effective than telling her not to worry. If there is a high risk, then involve patients in planning screening or treatment so that the risk of adverse consequences is minimised.
- **Increase feelings of safety:** A related technique is to increase feelings of safety through information. For example, you might tell patients about monitoring or other procedures that can prevent complications developing.

Fear and panic are extreme forms of anxiety and require a different approach. They invoke very strong physical and behavioural responses such as fight, flight, freezing, or turning to the group (see Chapter 4). Soothing responses in these circumstances are similar to those we might use with a frightened animal. Our body language and voice can be used to calm the person. Offer support and empathy and, if something triggered their fear or panic, remove them from that situation or stop the procedure. Strong fear or panic rarely lasts long so this should subside after a few minutes at most. Be prepared to stay with the person and remain calm while their fear or panic reduces. Distraction can be useful, when it is sensitively timed, because this can help the patient refocus away from the threat.

18.3.3 DEALING WITH DISTRESS

Distress is a very general term. It is used here to describe situations where patients break down and cannot stop crying. Distress can result from anger, anxiety, or fear and so dealing with this draws on similar principles to dealing with those emotions. Two particular points should be borne in mind:

- Though it is natural to want to stop someone crying, it is not helpful to tell the patient to stop. Even if you say this empathically, the underlying message is that you think they should not be upset or crying.
- Though empathy and understanding are important, too much empathy can *increase* someone's distress. If they are really distressed they will be consumed by their feelings: in these circumstances empathy may serve to keep them focused on these feelings. In such cases it is more useful to try to get them focused on specific events or facts which will lower their distress. This is not to say you need to be completely unempathic, only that you need to help them focus. For example, you might say *'I can see it's really upsetting – is there anyone I can call at home to come and be with you?'*

ACTIVITY 18.3

- Think about a time when you were really upset about something important.
- When someone was sympathetic did it make you more or less upset?

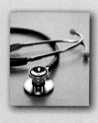

CLINICAL NOTES 18.2

Dealing with strong emotions

- If strong emotions are ignored the consultation will be difficult and ineffective.
- Anger is associated with aggression/attack but these are not the same.
- People can express anger safely if helped.
- Useful techniques include acknowledging the emotion, identifying the reason for the emotion, empathising/understanding, and disarming.
- Anxiety is the result of a perceived threat and is associated with hypervigilance and inflexible coping.
- Anxiety can be helped by reducing the perceived threat and increasing feelings of safety.
- High levels of distress will reduce if the person has to focus on specific events or facts.

18.4 GIVING BAD NEWS

One of the hardest tasks in medicine is to give bad news to patients or relatives. This can range from diagnosing a chronic illness to giving news about a death or disability. However, any news that brings with it some restriction or potential loss can be sad or bad news. A sprained ankle will be bad news for an athlete; an infectious illness will be bad news if diagnosed the day before someone planned to go away on the holiday of a lifetime.

Reviews of research in this area have identified three important factors. First, people appreciate it if the clinician is kind, confident, sensitive, and caring. People also prefer clinicians to show concern and distress rather than being aloof and detached. Second, people appreciate it more if the news is given clearly, using simple terms, and if they have time to talk about it with the clinician and ask questions. Third, people appreciate a quiet and private setting (Joekes, 2007).

Many different guidelines for how to give bad news have been proposed, though these have been based more on consensus than research evidence. The principles in these guidelines overlap a good deal. Here, a six-step approach (or SPIKES) is outlined (Baile et al., 2000; Buckman, 1992).

1 **Setting up:** Prepare thoroughly for the interview. Make sure you have all the relevant information. Locate the interview somewhere private, where you will not be interrupted. Allow yourself the time to give the news and then deal with people's responses and questions.
2 **Patient's perception:** Start by checking how much the person already knows and understands so you can tailor the bad news appropriately. Use an open question here such as, *'What have you been told so far?'*

3 **Information needed:** Ask the person how much they want to know about the diagnosis, prognosis, and treatment. This helps tailor the type and amount of information you give in this session to what the person wants and is able to cope with.

4 **Knowledge given:** Impart knowledge of the bad news. It can help to pre-warn the person by saying something like, *'It's not the good news we hoped for'* and then pausing. This allows the person a short time to prepare for the bad news. Give the bad news clearly and in simple language. Ambiguous statements should be avoided (for example, saying a test was *'positive'*, which means the opposite in pathology to lay language). Give the information in small, manageable chunks.

5 **Emotional response:** A range of emotional responses may arise when giving bad news including shock, disbelief, fear, anxiety, distress, grief, and anger. As discussed in the previous section, the best way to deal with emotional responses is to recognise them and empathise. With very bad news there is little you can do but offer empathy and support. Evidence suggests that people will appreciate this.

6 **Summarising and strategy:** Towards the end of the interview the clinician should summarise the main points or outcomes of the interview and consider or agree a future strategy such as curative or palliative treatment. This helps focus the person on the next steps, gives some certainty, provides a known support structure, and where possible may provide hope.

CASE STUDY 18.1   Giving bad news

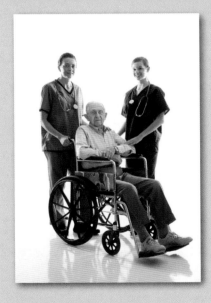

Jack is a 70 year old man who has been diagnosed with secondary progressive multiple sclerosis.

'When I was first diagnosed in the hospital, a consultant, who I'm glad to say has now retired, said to me, "Oh, we've got your diagnosis. I'm sorry, you've got a, an incurable disease and we can't treat it"

Now that was true, but I think the [other] doctor, the ward doctor, came back to me and when he explained it to me in detail and in drawings, I felt much happier.'

Interviewer: Can you tell me how you would have preferred to have been told?

'As the [other] doctor did, he sat on the side of the bed, he had a pad of plain paper and a pencil and he drew the spinal column, right, and he showed the scarring as much, as near as he could, my particular scarring.

He explained how messages travelled and he said, "The trouble is when they hit a scar they're delayed, they go to the next scar and they're delayed a bit further, and further and further and further." If you've only got slight scarring or very little scarring that's when it's MS. But unfortunately I've got quite severe scarring, and so the messages are delayed quite a bit.'

Interviewer: How do you think that information should be given?

'Well, I think it should be given in the way that my present consultant has given me other news. He sits you down and he smiles at you and first of all you realise that he's on your side, he's with you and he understands you and he understands you as a person, and when he tells you or gives you news – like when he gave me the final diagnosis – it was done in a way that, in fact he held my hand, you know, and he told me first of all, he built up to it, he didn't just blurt it out.'

Interviewer: You were talking about how you feel information like that should be given?

'Gently, but factually, I mean when, certainly people like to know the facts and I'm one of them, but if they're going to be pretty dramatic then I think it's only right that they should be given to you in a very sympathetic, that's the word I think, in a sympathetic way and that you realise, as the patient, that the person giving you that information understands that you're going to have to take that, take it on board and, and come to terms with that, which for me has been very difficult because of other reasons, not that, I think it's very important the way that these things are broken.

It doesn't really matter how brave you are or how not brave you are, if you're going to have bad news of any sort, any sort of bad news, I'm sure there must be a way of, of easing it so that you can make it as gentle as you can to the person that's going to have to receive it.'

(Adapted from www.healthtalkonline.org.uk © DIPEx. Photo © iofoto/Fotolia)

CLINICAL NOTES 18.3

Giving bad news

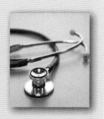

- Give bad news in a private setting.
- Give the news clearly and make sure there is enough time to talk about it.
- Be kind and caring – it is OK to show your own distress (within reason).
- **SPIKES** is a useful mnemonic to remember the **S**etting, **P**atient perception (what do they know), **I**nformation needed (what do they want to know), **K**nowledge giving, **E**motional response, **S**ummarising and strategy.

CONCLUSION

In this chapter we have looked at the different ways in which we communicate and how these may be used in clinical practice to be more effective. The doctor-patient model of the clinical interview reminds us that the patient's agenda is as important as the doctor's agenda and that the relationship should be collaborative. The Calgary-Cambridge model provides a useful framework to think about the different stages of a clinical interview and which skills are relevant to each.

This chapter has also covered a variety of techniques and skills that can be useful in both routine and difficult clinical interviews. However, skills need to be practised in order to learn them. They may feel awkward and demanding initially, but with practice they will feel more easy and natural. Usually with learning skills we move from (a) unconscious incompetence to (b) conscious incompetence to (c) conscious competence to (d) unconscious competence. Clinical skills are a good example of this, so the more you practise the more quickly you will reach unconscious competence!

FURTHER READING

Ayers, S. et al. (2007) *The Cambridge Handbook of Psychology, Health and Medicine* (2nd edition). Cambridge: Cambridge University Press. Includes short chapters on communicating risk, healthcare professional-patient communication, breaking bad news, medical interviewing, written communication and teaching communication skills.

Coulehan, J.L. et al. (2001) "Let me see if I have this right ...": Words that help build empathy, *Annals of Internal Medicine, 135:* 221–227. This is a useful article on how to be empathic in clinical situations.

Platt, F.W. and Gordon, G.A. (1999) *The Field Guide to the Difficult Patient Interview.* A pocket guide to communication skills for difficult clinical interviews. An easy, accessible book with useful tips.

Silverman, J., Kurtz, S. and Draper, J. (1998) *Skills for Communicating with Patients.* Oxford: Radcliff Medical Press. Describes the Calgary-Cambridge approach to communication skills in detail and is written in an accessible style.

REVISION QUESTIONS

1 Describe three types of non-verbal behaviour and discuss how these are relevant to clinical practice.

2 How do our characteristics of speech influence communication?

3 Describe the doctor-patient model of the clinical interview.

4 Discuss the evidence that doctor-patient communication affects patient outcomes.

5 Outline the Calgary-Cambridge model of clinical interviewing and illustrate it with the communication skills that are relevant to the different stages of the interview.

6 Describe the key communication skills for effective information gathering in clinical interviews.

7 Outline the six main points for good clinical practice when conducting a physical examination.

8 What communication skills are useful for diffusing anger in clinical settings?

9 Discuss the key communication skills for closing a clinical interview.

10 Outline the SPIKES model for giving bad news.

19 PSYCHOLOGICAL INTERVENTION

LEARNING OBJECTIVES

This chapter is designed to enable you to:

- Outline various psychological specialties and their applications to medical settings.
- Understand the theoretical bases of various psychological therapies.
- Describe cognitive behaviour therapy, psychodynamic therapy, and counselling.
- Understand the use of psychotherapeutic techniques in clinical practice.

Mental illness is surprisingly common and affects up to one in six adults. A recent report showed that mental illness is responsible for 40 per cent of disability and labelled it '*Britain's biggest social problem*' (Layard, 2006). Less severe problems, such as a depressed mood, will be experienced by most people at some point in their lives. Psychological interventions therefore have the potential to make a huge difference to individuals and society and are likely to play an increasing role in clinical practice.

However, the range of psychological professionals and interventions can be confusing. Many professions are involved in psychotherapy – for example, psychiatrists, psychologists, counsellors, mental health nurses, and psychotherapists. It is not always clear who does what. As with medicine, psychology includes many specialisms. These encompass: health psychology; clinical psychology; counselling psychology; occupational psychology; forensic psychology; neuropsychology; educational psychology; research; and teaching psychology. Box 19.1 summarises a range of psychological specialties. In practice, an individual's work may span two or three specialisms: for example, a clinical psychologist may also teach in a university.

In most Western countries psychology is regulated by organisations such as the British Psychological Society, the Health Professions Council, and the American Psychological Association. These organisations monitor and regulate the content of psychological degrees and training in the same way that medicine is regulated by the General Medical Council (UK) or the Liaison Committee on Medical Education (USA). Psychologists need to be registered with the relevant organisation and apply for professional status in order to practise.

BOX 19.1   Psychology specialties

Speciality	What do they do?	Where do they work?	Training (UK)
Clinical psychologist	Assess and treat mental health problems such as depression, schizophrenia, and personality disorders.	Health and social care settings like hospitals, community mental health teams, and health centres.	Clinical doctoral degree including work placements in mental health settings.
Counselling psychologist	Assess and treat moderate mental health problems such as depression and anxiety.	Wide variety of places such as hospitals, prison services, education, and industry.	Undergraduate degree plus specialist diploma or doctorate.
Health psychologist	Health promotion, health services research, treats health problems such as obesity, smoking cessation, and pain management.	Health and social care settings like hospitals, health centres, and other health-related organisations.	Health psychology Master's degree and doctoral degree.
Forensic psychologist	Work in legal processes, criminal behaviour, and investigations, including rehabilitation work with offenders.	Prison services, secure hospitals and rehabilitation, police and probation services.	Forensic psychology Master's degree and diploma, including two years work placement in forensic settings.
Educational psychologist	Assess and provide remedial work for children with behavioural or learning difficulties.	Schools, education departments, and local authorities.	Educational doctoral or Master's degree plus one year work placement in educational settings.
Occupational psychologist	Work with individuals and organisations to increase effectiveness of employees and organisations.	Industry, commerce, and other large organisations.	Occupational psychology Master's degree plus two years working in occupational settings.
Neuropsychologist	Assess and rehabilitate people with brain injury or disorders.	Healthcare settings such as hospitals and neurological and community rehabilitation services.	Doctoral degree (usually clinical, educational or health) plus diploma in neuropsychology.
Sport and exercise psychologist	Work with athletes, sports people, and	Health services, employment and	Three year training including sport and

(Continued)

Speciality	What do they do?	Where do they work?	Training (UK)
	teams to enhance performance.	psychiatric contexts; work with professional sports teams and national governing bodies.	exercise doctoral degree, or five years working in sport and exercise psychology.
Teaching/research psychologist	Teach psychology in schools or higher education. University teachers also carry out research	Schools, further education colleges, and universities.	Doctoral degree plus teaching qualification in many instances.

(Continued)

(adapted from the British Psychological Society http://www.bps.org.uk/careers/areas/areas_home.cfm)

CLINICAL NOTES 19.1

Finding a psychologist or psychological services

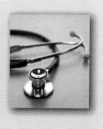

To find an individual psychologist search the directories at the following websites:

- British Psychological Society www.bps.org.uk
- Health Professions Council www.hpc-uk.org
- American Psychological Society www.apa.org (USA)
- For accredited CBT therapists www.babcp.com

To find an NHS psychology service go to:

- NHS Choices www.nhs.uk/ServiceDirectories and search on Psychological Therapy services for your area.

This chapter focuses on the use of psychotherapy in healthcare settings. First it explains the main types of psychotherapy used to treat various mental health problems. Then it looks more specifically at interventions for physical health problems, such as motivational interviewing to help people change their behaviour and the provision of support groups for cancer patients.

19.1 WHAT IS PSYCHOTHERAPY?

Here we shall use the term 'psychotherapy' very broadly to mean any form of therapy that involves talking and exploring psychological issues. The aim of **psychotherapy** is to resolve mental health problems. Psychotherapy usually involves one-to-one sessions in which patients talk through their problems. However, there are different types of psychotherapy, each with its own theoretical foundations. As a consequence, the forms of psychotherapy differ hugely. They may include writing, drawing, imagery work, role-play, and homework.

The shortage of psychotherapists and the high cost of treatment mean other forms of treatment, such as group therapy or computerised therapy, are becoming more common. Computerised therapy can be used alone by the patient or in conjunction with a therapist or specialist nurse who oversees their progress. Evidence suggests computerised programs are an effective treatment for less severe affective disorders such as depression or anxiety. For example, *Beating the Blues* is a program developed for moderate depression or anxiety. It has been utilised in many primary care settings and involves patients watching an introductory videotape and then carrying out up to 15 sessions of one hour each with homework between each session. At the end of each session a printed summary of the session is given to the patient and doctor. Patients do not have additional personal sessions but can meet with their doctor to check on their progress and medication if this is needed. Evidence suggests this program is more effective than GP treatment alone at reducing moderate anxiety and depression, facilitating social adjustment and a return to work (Proudfoot et al., 2003, 2004).

The theories on which psychotherapies are based include Freudian theory, humanistic and existential theory, behaviourism, and cognitive theory. Figure 19.1 shows how these theories have resulted in different approaches to psychotherapy, each with their own philosophical assumptions and techniques. For example, **humanism** assumes (a) that humans are essentially good, (b) that we strive for personal growth and development, and (c) that we have free will and can therefore make choices. The humanistic approach to therapy, which was very popular in the 1960s and 1970s, is founded on the principle that the therapist provides an **unconditional positive regard**: whatever a person has done will be understandable given that person's experience. The focus in humanistic therapy is on the person's unique experience, needs, and personal growth. The humanistic approach continues to be used in therapy today and is also evident in patient-centred medicine.

Modern psychotherapy draws on a range of theoretical approaches including cognitive behaviour therapy (CBT), psychodynamic therapies, counselling, and systemic therapies.

CLINICAL NOTES 19.2

Computerised and online psychotherapy

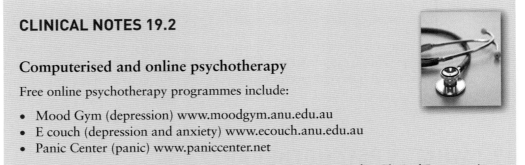

Free online psychotherapy programmes include:

- Mood Gym (depression) www.moodgym.anu.edu.au
- E couch (depression and anxiety) www.ecouch.anu.edu.au
- Panic Center (panic) www.paniccenter.net

For a wide range of free self-help resources, see the Centre for Clinical Interventions resources at www.cci.health.wa.gov.au

Commercial packages include:

- Beating the Blues* (depression) www.ultrasis.com
- Fear fighter* (anxiety and panic) www.fearfighter.com
- Overcoming bulimia (bulimia) www.overcomingbulimiaonline.com
- Overcoming anorexia (for carers) www.overc="">overcominganorexiaonline.com
- Living life to the full (life skills) www.livinglifetothefull.com
- ThinkWell (stress, mild anxiety/depression) www.thinkwell.co.uk

  * In the UK these are available in some GP practices

Psychotherapies often overlap with each other and thus are not easy to classify. For example, cognitive analytic therapy (CAT) combines CBT and psychoanalytic principles in therapy. Interpersonal therapy focuses on relationship processes in depression and draws on psychodynamic principles, CBT techniques, and brief crisis intervention. Eye-movement desensitisation and reprocessing is a specific therapy used to treat post-traumatic stress disorder (PTSD), which is referred to as integrative but incorporates a lot of CBT principles. The next section will look in more detail at the most widely used psychotherapies in healthcare settings, namely CBT, psychodynamic therapy, and counselling.

19.1.1 COGNITIVE BEHAVIOUR THERAPY

CBT is founded on behaviourism and cognitivism. There have been two waves of CBT (Hayes, 2004). The first derived from **behaviourism**, which focuses on people's behaviour and how it is learned and shaped by events. Behaviourism describes the processes through which people's behaviour is shaped, including classical conditioning, operant conditioning, and modelling, which are outlined in Chapter 10. Behavioural therapy involves changing maladaptive behavioural responses and substituting these with new responses. For example, phobias are often conditioned responses to an object that is associated with fear because of a negative or traumatic experience in the past. Typical behavioural techniques used in therapy include monitoring behaviour through activity charts, rehearsing positive behavioural responses, setting graded task assignments, and using goal-setting to encourage or reinforce new behaviours.

Behaviourism emphasises scientific, or empirical, testing. Behavioural therapy therefore includes carrying out **behavioural experiments** in which people test their views of what will happen under certain circumstances. Consider, for example, the case of a patient who has a social phobia and who avoids social situations because they get highly anxious, assume everyone notices, and thinks they are odd. This can lead to a vicious cycle where social situations are avoided. The more they are avoided the more anxious the person will become about attending them. The person's assumptions are not challenged or disproved because there is no opportunity for them to have a good experience of a social situation. This combination of negative assumptions and avoiding social events (avoidance behaviour) creates a negative cycle that perpetuates the phobia. In these circumstances, a behavioural experiment might be for the patient to attend a social situation, monitor their anxiety (which should reduce over time), monitor how they act, and also notice how other people respond to

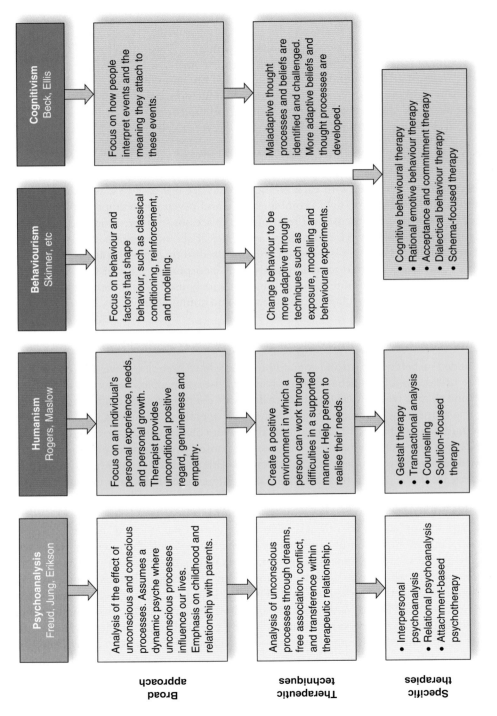

FIGURE 19.1 Main approaches to psychotherapy

them – whether positively or negatively. Another possibility might be to ask other people how they feel in social situations and whether they ever get anxious. This can normalise a certain degree of social anxiety. Behavioural experiments reduce anxiety in many ways: they increase the exposure to social situations which reduces anxiety, challenges negative beliefs, and breaks the negative cycle. We once heard of a therapist who went out and acted in bizarre ways in an attempt to show a patient how *little* other people would notice!

It can be seen that behavioural experiments will affect a person's thoughts as well as their behaviour. From a cognitive viewpoint, behavioural experiments encourage people to become aware of underlying assumptions, specify and test them, and then revise their thoughts and behaviour. There is ongoing debate about whether or not behavioural experiments work mainly through behavioural or cognitive means (Salkovskis et al., 2006). Regardless of how they work, however, behavioural experiments are powerful tools of change and are particularly effective for treating anxiety disorders. They are also useful when treating people with low cognitive ability, such as young children or people with learning difficulties. Case Study 19.1 gives an example of how cognitive and behavioural methods were used to treat a woman with PTSD after a difficult birth.

CASE STUDY 19.1   CBT for postnatal PTSD

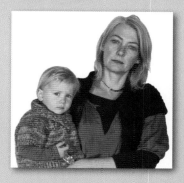

Sarah is 35 years old, married, and has a 14 month old daughter. Sarah had a termination of a pregnancy when she was 19 years old, which she kept a secret for 16 years because she thought people would judge her negatively.

Sarah's labour was induced and there was confusion over when it would happen. Sarah panicked because she was unprepared and her husband was not there. The midwife was not sympathetic to Sarah's high levels of anxiety. After a painful internal examination during which Sarah cried and asked the midwife to stop, the midwife said 'If you think that's painful, what are you going to be like giving birth?' From this point onwards Sarah's labour and delivery were characterised by pain, extreme distress, and fear of the midwife.

Sarah's daughter was delivered by emergency caesarean section after a long labour during which Sarah thought she might die. Sarah started to feel the surgery half way through and was given morphine. She reported dissociating (feeling detached from herself and like the labour was unreal) and cannot remember anything for 12 hours after the delivery. She said the first few months after the birth 'are a blur' and it took her a year to bond with her daughter. The main themes of Sarah's birth seemed to be feeling terrified, vulnerable and out of control; high levels of confusion and dissociation; and confirmation of her belief that others will judge her and hurt her through her experience with the midwife.

(Cont'd)

After the birth Sarah suffered from postnatal depression, was prescribed antidepressants, and attended a support group. Sarah first attended CBT 14 months after giving birth. She was highly distressed, appeared to be reliving the birth experience, was crying and shaking. She had the full range of PTSD symptoms including flashbacks, nightmares, and strong physical and emotional reactions to reminders of birth, feeling emotionally numb yet crying all the time. Her flashbacks were of seeing herself lying in the delivery room feeling helpless and terrified as the midwife came into the room.

Therapy consisted of various cognitive and behavioural techniques. Techniques used in treatment included:

1 *A behavioural experiment* where an anonymous survey was carried out of people's opinions of Sarah's abortion to challenge her belief that others would judge her. The survey described the circumstances in which Sarah fell pregnant and had the abortion and asked people what they would think of her. People who did not know Sarah completed the survey and responses included pro-life and pro-abortion views. This dramatically changed Sarah's beliefs about herself, the abortion, what others would think of her and the importance she placed on others' views.

2 *Mild exposure in the form of reliving exercises.* Sarah was asked to imagine the birth as if it were currently happening and talk through the events in detail.

3 *Stronger exposure* through visiting the labour ward with the therapist to help Sarah overcome her fear and avoidance.

4 *Cognitive exercises* to change Sarah's appraisals of difficult events in the birth, such as using a role-play to act out confronting the midwife and reducing Sarah's fear.

5 *Visualisation exercises* to rewrite her flashbacks. For example, she imagined the anaesthetist in the delivery room who she felt comfortable and safe with, as opposed to the frightening midwife.

6 *Positive reformulation* to consolidate these changes in Sarah's beliefs.

After ten sessions of CBT Sarah's PTSD symptoms disappeared and her maladaptive beliefs about herself and others changed.

(Ayers et al., 2007)

The second wave of CBT derived from cognitivism which views thoughts as being central to how we feel and behave. This is now the dominant view in psychology and the importance of cognition is apparent in many of the theories and research outlined in this book. The main cognitive theory of mental illness was proposed by Aaron Beck (1967), who argued that appraisal and the personal meaning of events are central in the development and maintenance of psychopathology. According to Beck, early experiences lead to sets of **core beliefs or schema** about ourselves, the world, and others. These beliefs are not necessarily rational because most of them are formed in childhood without the benefit of adult logic. Core beliefs can lead to **maladaptive assumptions** – sometimes referred to as 'rules for living' (Fennell, 1998).

Beck was particularly interested in depression. He argued that people become depressed when they have a depressogenic triad of beliefs that:

1   As a person they are deficient in some way.
2   Their future is hopeless.
3   Their experiences confirm (to them) that they are a failure.

Evidence largely supports the existence of this depressive style of thinking, which is present during depression but not after a person recovers.

CBT is used to treat a wide range of psychological problems, not only depression. In fact the underlying theory can be applied to most of us, even when we are functioning well. Consider, for example, a person whose core beliefs include the following:

1   'I am unlovable'.
2   'Other people will judge me'.

These beliefs could stem from having overly judgemental or unloving parents. This person might compensate for these core beliefs by having rules for living such as 'If I do everything perfectly then people will love me', 'If I do things well people will not criticise me' or 'I must not show negative emotions or people will judge me'. These rules can help the person to function well and feel good about themselves as long as they adhere to these high standards. However, keeping up these standards will put them under considerable strain and make them vulnerable if something happens to make them think they've failed, such as not doing well in an exam or being made redundant. Under

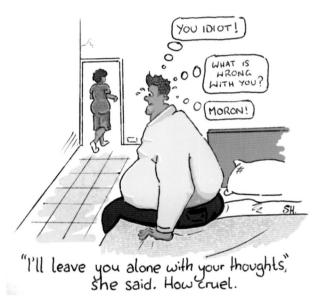

"I'll leave you alone with your thoughts," she said. How cruel.

these circumstances it is possible they will develop depression because they have violated their rules and so activated their underlying belief that they are unlovable.

A difficulty in therapy is that people are not usually consciously aware of their own core beliefs and rules for living. However, these beliefs are usually reflected in the moment-to-moment **automatic thoughts** we have, especially in difficult situations. Thus CBT involves monitoring automatic thoughts to help uncover a person's rules and beliefs. These are put together in a formulation, which can be written or diagrammatic. The formulation is then used as a guide for the therapist and patient to understand the problem and work out ways to test and challenge existing beliefs and build new, more adaptive beliefs. Testing beliefs can be done using cognitive and behavioural methods. Cognitive methods include guided discovery or Socratic questioning, where the therapist helps the patient examine and question their existing beliefs by considering evidence of whether or not they are correct. Case Study 19.1 illustrates the testing of beliefs using cognitive and behavioural methods. The formulation for the woman featured in this case study is shown in Figure 19.2.

ACTIVITY 19.1

Think about the last time you felt upset or angry and write down the following:

- What was the situation or trigger?
- What thoughts went through your mind (automatic thoughts)?
- How did these thoughts influence how you felt?
- Can you identify any of your rules (assumptions) that might have been broken?

The defining features of CBT are given in Box 19.2. CBT is now being applied to an increasing range of mental and physical disorders and is also expanding to include newer techniques. Cognitive theories have been developed for specific psychological disorders such as

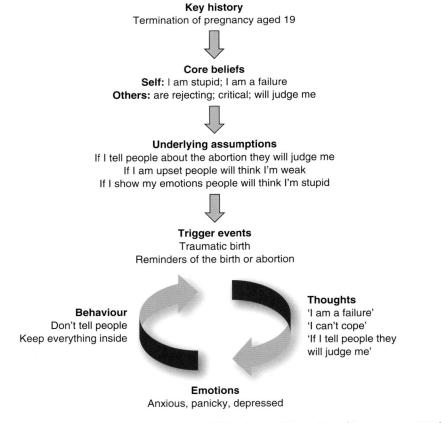

Key history
Termination of pregnancy aged 19

Core beliefs
Self: I am stupid; I am a failure
Others: are rejecting; critical; will judge me

Underlying assumptions
If I tell people about the abortion they will judge me
If I am upset people will think I'm weak
If I show my emotions people will think I'm stupid

Trigger events
Traumatic birth
Reminders of the birth or abortion

Behaviour
Don't tell people
Keep everything inside

Thoughts
'I am a failure'
'I can't cope'
'If I tell people they
will judge me'

Emotions
Anxious, panicky, depressed

FIGURE 19.2   Case formulation of woman with PTSD after a difficult birth (Ayers et al., 2007)

depression (Beck, 1967), panic (Clark, 1986), anxiety (Wells, 1997), PTSD (Ehlers and Clark, 2000), and personality disorders (Young et al., 2004). These theories have led to CBT treatment protocols for different disorders.

BOX 19.2 Core features of CBT

1 Collaborative relationship between therapist and client.
2 Education of the client about CBT approach so that they can become their own 'therapist'.
3 Focus on the present problem – 'here and now'.
4 Structured sessions with content (agenda) agreed between the therapist and client at the beginning of each session.
5 Goal directed with aims for therapy stated at the beginning and work in therapy is directed towards achieving these aims.
6 Short-term therapy, typically between 6 and 24 sessions.
7 Examination of maladaptive beliefs.
8 Cognitive challenging of maladaptive beliefs through Socratic questioning.
9 Use of behavioural experiments to test maladaptive beliefs (empirical approach).
10 Use of general and specific formulations to guide understanding and change.

The most recent developments in CBT have been referred to, collectively, as CBT's third wave (Hayes, 2004). These focus less on challenging the content of thoughts and more on the *relationship* that we have with thoughts and emotions. Techniques such as acceptance (Hayes et al., 1999), mindfulness (Segal et al., 2002) and developing a compassionate mind (Gilbert, 2000) can encourage a person to accept their thoughts and emotional responses and not see them as all-defining or permanent. This prevents psychological symptoms being made worse by negative appraisals.

There is little doubt that CBT is gaining in popularity. It is now the recommended treatment for many psychological and physical disorders, including depression, PTSD, anxiety disorders, eating disorders, chronic fatigue, and chronic pain (Department of Health, 2001). The increasing use of CBT is based on evidence that it is an effective treatment for these disorders. A review of CBT treatment for generalised anxiety disorder found it was as effective as pharmacological treatment in reducing anxiety, depression, and increasing quality of life. In addition, CBT achieved a lower drop-out rate than pharmacological treatment (Mitte, 2005).

Increasingly, CBT has been used as an adjunct to treatments of chronic illnesses. Reviews of randomised controlled trials have generally found positive effects of CBT treatment for illnesses as diverse as chronic fatigue (Price and Couper, 2000), tinnitus (Martinez Devesa et al., 2007), traumatic brain injury (Soo and Tate, 2007), sleep problems (Montgomery and Dennis, 2002), and asthma (Yorke et al., 2004). However, the effects of CBT are often limited to psychological outcomes, such as quality of life and measures of distress, rather than to physical functioning.

The rising popularity of CBT means it is now in danger of being applied in a blanket fashion to areas where there is little or inconsistent evidence of its efficacy. For example, there are instances where CBT appears helpful but does not result in clinically significant change, such as with child sexual abuse (MacDonald et al., 2006) or domestically abusive men (Smedslund et al., 2007). There is also evidence that other therapies can be just as effective as CBT or more so, such as interpersonal therapy for depression (Department of Health, 2001). A more considered view might be to recognise that CBT works very well for *some* disorders where it can lead to an improvement in *some* outcomes, but that it is by no means providing a panacea.

19.1.2 PSYCHODYNAMIC THERAPY

Psychodynamic therapy is based on Freud's theory of the psyche and psychopathology. The central idea is that we have a dynamic unconscious – hence the term psycho*dynamic* therapy. This dynamic unconscious involves a continuous conflict between drives and impulses on the one hand, and our ego and social constraints on the other hand. Conflict, suppression, and a building up of psychological defences then influence our behaviour, thoughts, and feelings which can lead to psychopathology.

Psychodynamic theory has been extensively developed and refined and there are now many different types of psychodynamic therapy. These include interpersonal psychoanalysis, relational psychoanalysis, and attachment-based psychotherapy. Carlyle (2007) outlines three common principles in psychodynamic therapies. The first is the importance of early childhood experience. Modern psychodynamic theory incorporates work on **early attachments** (Bowlby, 1958) which indicates that the relationship a child has with their primary caregiver between the ages of six months and three years of age is fundamental in forming a person's early experience and their expectations of social relationships (see Chapter 8). Attachment is not the only important early experience. Research suggests playing helps children to learn about the rules for appropriate behaviour and social roles. It also helps them to test their own abilities and regulate their emotions. For example, a child play-fighting with a parent will learn about acceptable and unacceptable levels of aggression.

Psychodynamic theory puts forward two processes by which early experiences affect development. The first is **introjection**, where the child internalises aspects of their parents or other significant people into themselves. The second process is **projection**, where people project aspects of their own internal world onto others. The most well known example of projection is when you view another person negatively because they do something or represent something you dislike about yourself. For example, a father may react angrily when his son does not achieve top grades at school because the father is frustrated by his own lack of achievement and success. The father is therefore projecting a part of himself that he dislikes onto his son and reacting strongly because of this.

Psychopathology in adults is therefore thought to result from early experiences being negative in some way, such as having neglectful or over-intrusive parents or a childhood that involved trauma, loss, or separation. The negative experience then results in adults who have difficulties coping with life or relationships. As a result, psychodynamic therapies stress the importance of the **therapeutic relationship**. The therapeutic relationship is thought of as a regular, contained, space for patients to work through and understand their difficulties. This means psychodynamic therapy is regular and intensive – often happening once or twice a week for more than a year – to provide the patient with a frequent and predictable time in their life to deal with their difficulties.

Through regular contact, the therapist starts to symbolise a parent for the patient. The therapeutic relationship therefore becomes a 'stage' on which interpersonal difficulties are played out. This is known as **transference** where the way the patient views and relates to the therapist is thought to represent their underlying issues or interpersonal difficulties with parents or other significant people. A psychodynamic therapist therefore remains as neutral as possible and is not supposed to bring their own characteristics or feelings into therapy. This aspect of psychodynamic therapy is summed up by the stereotype of the therapist who says nothing whilst the patient lies on the couch and talks. This, however, is an extreme stereotype, which may not apply in practice.

The third common principle in psychodynamic therapies is the importance of personal **defences** which are the ways in which people avoid difficult or painful thoughts. There are many different types of defences, including denial, repression, humour, rationalisation, escapism, and regression. Like coping strategies, defences are not necessarily maladaptive. For example, a person who has to have complicated surgery may well deny or repress thoughts of possible complications or a painful recovery, which will minimise the threat of surgery and reduce their anxiety beforehand. The defining features of psychodynamic therapy are given in Box 19.3 and Case Study 19.2 shows the psychodynamic treatment of sexual dysfunction.

BOX 19.3   Core features of psychodynamic therapy

1 Therapist remains neutral so transference can occur and the underlying issues can be explored.
2 Assumption of dynamic unconscious.
3 Focus on the past, particularly early childhood experience and conflict, and the suppression or psychological defences that have resulted.
4 Focus on interpersonal relationships and how these are influenced by childhood experience, subsequent defences, projection, etc.
5 Exploration of maladaptive personal defences.
6 Intensive therapy, typically comprising of one or more sessions a week for at least a year.

The emphasis on unconscious processes means psychodynamic theory is difficult to test scientifically and it has been widely criticised for this. Many would argue that psychodynamic therapy remains a matter of faith (Tallis, 1996), although advances in neuroimaging studies, such as fMRI, have demonstrated that unconscious neural activity in the brain often pre-empts our voluntary action (Wegner, 2003). Because of these criticisms and the lack of consistent evidence, psychodynamic therapy is rarely recommended in guidelines for the treatment of mental health disorders and is expressly recommended *against* in some instances, such as for PTSD (NICE, 2005).

CASE STUDY 19.2   Psychodynamic therapy for sexual dysfunction

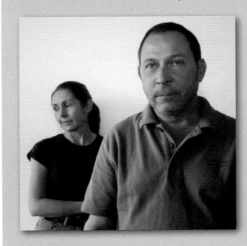

Laura is 38 and suffers from dyspareunia (pain on intercourse) and an inability to have sexual intercourse. Dan suffers from dyspepsia (indigestion) and backache. His mother died when he was five.

Laura and Dan had a son who died at 15 months of a hereditary brain disorder. When he died Laura was pregnant and this baby also died of the same disorder when ten months old. The following year Laura had an ectopic pregnancy and chose to be sterilised.

At the funeral of their first child Laura said she felt 'numb' and her family sent her shopping to distract her. Laura and Dan went on to foster and adopt two children. Their sexual dysfunction started after the death of their first child.

Psychodynamic therapy

Laura and Dan's symptoms were interpreted as physical manifestations of the distress caused by the loss of their children and fertility. Their problems were therefore thought to be due to unresolved loss and bereavement. Dan and Laura were seen individually and as a couple by the same therapist for a year.

The therapist described Laura as 'wooden and lifeless' when discussing her experiences. This was interpreted as a defence mechanism where Laura was no longer in touch with her feelings but projected them onto others so that they felt distress. The fostering, adoption and work with disabled children was her way of escaping from the pain of bereavement.

The therapist explored Dan's relationship with his mother who died when he was five. The therapist suggested his marriage was an attempt to replace the relationship he had with his mother. Dan therefore felt rivalry with his own children whilst they were alive because they took away Laura's attention. When the babies died he felt responsible and guilty so reacted very negatively to Laura's distress because it reminded him of this. Laura's dyspareunia and frigidity may therefore have been an angry attempt at retribution because he did not allow her to grieve.

Following this insight the couple were able to have intercourse again. After Laura had an orgasm she broke down and said it was as if she was 'crying from the deepest depths of herself'. She reported recovering mental images of her babies when they were dead, whereas previously she could only picture them alive. By the end of therapy Dan's symptoms had disappeared and Laura's dyspareunia was intermittent but tolerable. The couple were sexually active and reported that their marriage had improved greatly.

(adapted from Lewis and Casement, 1986)

Proponents of the psychodynamic approach argue this dismissal of psychoanalysis by treatment guidelines is premature and unjustified (Smith, 2007). Reviews of the research looking at the effectiveness of psychoanalysis for disorders such as personality disorders, anxiety, and depression have shown conflicting results. Some find that psychodynamic therapy is ineffective (Roth and Fonagy, 2004) while others conclude it is effective (Leichsenring, 2005). A Cochrane review of high quality evidence recently concluded that there is evidence for 'modest to moderate gains' for common disorders such as anxiety, depression, and interpersonal problems (Abbass et al., 2006).

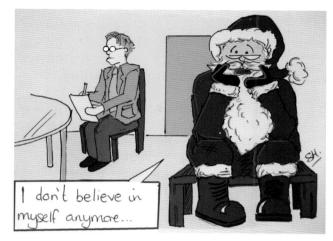

19.1.3 COUNSELLING

Counselling is an integrative approach that draws on psychodynamic, existential, humanistic, systemic, and CBT principles. How these approaches are integrated will depend upon the counsellor's training and experience. As a result, there is considerable variety which makes counselling difficult to summarise. However, there are three core principles. The first is that it is **client-focused**. The needs of the client are put first and the aim of counselling is to increase or protect the person's psychological wellbeing (Farsides, 2009).

The second principle is that counselling aims to provide a safe and accepting environment in which the patient can explore and reflect on their difficulties. This is partly based on the principle of providing people with **unconditional positive regard** to facilitate self-acceptance and feelings of self-worth. For example, parents and society place expectations on us about performance, achievement, and what is seen as successful or worthwhile. This means we only feel worthwhile if we reach expectations and perform well in these areas. A counsellor might explore this with a patient whilst at the same time accepting them regardless of their achievements or failures. This provides the person with an insight into their behaviour and feelings at the same time as allowing them to experience a relationship where they are liked and accepted for who they are.

The third core principle is that counselling is **non-directive** and the emphasis is on the patient exploring, clarifying, and solving their problems. The role of the counsellor is to facilitate this process (Bor and Allen, 2007).

Counselling tends to be used with mild or moderate anxiety and depression, or with people who are in difficult circumstances or crises. Counselling is also being increasingly used in healthcare settings to help patients adjust to difficult events such as a diagnosis of HIV, cancer, a late miscarriage or stillbirth, or to help patients make difficult decisions such as during infertility treatment or genetic testing. In the UK, counsellors are often employed in primary care settings so that GPs can refer their patients immediately to psychotherapy, without having to refer to secondary care teams in hospitals or community mental health teams. The defining features of counselling are given in Box 19.4.

BOX 19.4   Core features of counselling

1 Therapist provides unconditional positive regard and accepts client for the person they are.
2 Therapist is non-judgemental and provides a safe space in which the client can work through their problems.
3 Needs of the client are primary.
4 The client explores their problems and solutions and the therapist facilitates this.
5 Sessions are directed towards the overall aim of improving a client's psychological wellbeing.
6 An integrative or eclectic approach is taken towards therapeutic techniques. These are drawn from various psychotherapeutic approaches such as CBT and psychodynamic therapy.
7 A short-term therapy, typically consisting of between 6 and 16 sessions.

Currently, evidence for the efficacy of counselling is limited. This is partly because it is difficult to define a 'standard' approach to counselling so research has focused on evaluating more clearly outlined therapies like CBT. Research into counselling is often limited by factors such as counselling being poorly defined or not compared to other forms of therapy. However, where evidence is available it is promising. For example, a review of counselling in primary care settings for psychological and psychosocial problems concluded that this was more effective than physician care in the short term, but that over the long term they are equally effective (Bower and Rowland, 2006). Similarly, a study of counselling or CBT for chronic fatigue syndrome found they were equally effective in reducing fatigue, anxiety, depression, and social adjustment, with 47 per cent of patients recovering (Ridsdale et al., 2001).

19.2 WHICH THERAPY IS BEST?

The issue of whether one type of therapy is better than another is contentious. There is a good deal of evidence to suggest that CBT and some interpersonal therapies are effective treatments for depression and anxiety disorders. Though psychodynamic therapy is widely practised, there is a lack of evidence to support it. Richardson (2006) argues that 'where one therapy appears to have an advantage over others in terms of empirical research this is usually because the others have failed to accumulate the relevant evidence'. It may be that different therapies are equally effective for some disorders and there is emerging evidence this may be the case. For example, a recent study of more than 1,300 patients who had had CBT, interpersonal, or psychodynamic psychotherapy found that all three therapies had resulted in an improvement and had been equally effective (Stiles et al., 2006).

    This finding suggests that non-specific factors like the therapeutic relationship or placebo effect may play an important role in the effectiveness of psychotherapy. The importance of a good relationship between the patient and therapist is well established, and evidence shows that it leads to better outcomes, regardless of the type of psychotherapy (Department of Health, 2001). Whether therapy also works through a placebo effect is less widely considered, though Kirsch (2007) has suggested that this is the case because psychotherapy involves no active physiological substances and instead relies on a patient's expectations, experience of therapy, and beliefs about therapy to treat illness.

So what can we conclude from this? There is little doubt that psychotherapy is effective in the treatment of mental health. Which type of psychotherapy is best is likely to vary for different psychological problems and individuals. Although the current guidelines favour CBT, this position may change as the evidence accumulates for counselling and psychodynamic approaches. It would be nice to think that in the future psychotherapy will move away from a 'winner takes all' mentality where one type of therapy has to prove itself as being better than all the others and will start to integrate those approaches and techniques shown to be effective under different circumstances. This is already evident in counselling, which draws on techniques from many different approaches to therapy.

Summary

- There are many different types of psychotherapy.
- Therapies have developed from theories of psychoanalysis, humanism, behaviourism, and cognitivism.
- Dominant approaches to therapy at present are CBT, psychodynamic therapy, and counselling.
- CBT is a structured, short-term therapy that focuses on the present problem and changes maladaptive beliefs and behaviour.
- Psychodynamic therapy is an intensive, long-term therapy that focuses on a person's early childhood experience, interpersonal relationships, and unconscious conflicts.
- Counselling is a short-term therapy that can consist of one approach to therapy, such as psychoanalysis, but is often more integrative or eclectic.
- Evidence shows CBT is an effective treatment for disorders such as anxiety and depression.
- There is some indication that different types of therapy may be equally effective for some disorders. This may be due to the importance of non-specific factors such as the therapeutic relationship or a placebo effect.

19.3 PSYCHOLOGICAL INTERVENTIONS IN MEDICAL SETTINGS

Psychological interventions in medical settings extend beyond psychotherapy in that they do not purely aim to resolve mental health problems but also include any intervention to promote physical or mental health in medical settings. This includes interventions such as health promotion, pain management, self-management in chronic illnesses, crisis intervention, stress management, and support groups. Descriptions of some of these interventions are given in Box 19.5. Examples and case studies of these interventions can be found throughout this book as indicated in Box 19.5.

BOX 19.5 Psychological interventions in medical settings

Psychological Intervention	Aims	What it consists of	Use	See example
Assessment	Assess an individual's psychosocial needs.	Interview and questionnaires to assess patient's needs and mental state.	For severe or chronic illnesses that require multidisciplinary management.	
Pain management	Help patients manage their pain to increase activity levels and wellbeing.	Education about pain, CBT techniques such as monitoring activity and pain, setting goals, empowering the patient.	For chronic pain of any kind e.g. back pain, pelvic pain, arthritis etc	Chapter 4
Motivational interviewing	Help people to change risky health behaviours.	Exploring and understanding a person's current beliefs & behaviour. Facilitating change through developing the discrepancy between person's values and current behaviour. Build confidence that change is possible.	For smoking, alcohol use, other drug addictions, eating disorders and depression.	Chapter 2
Self-management	Help people manage their illness or recovery. Includes adherence to medication, rehabilitation and facilitating psychological wellbeing.	Examining beliefs about illness, illness behaviour and emotions. Facilitating change to promote good self-management of illness.	For chronic illnesses e.g. multiple sclerosis, diabetes, heart disease, asthma, irritable bowel syndrome, arthritis etc.	Chapter 4

(Cont'd)

Psychological Intervention	Aims	What it consists of	Use	See example
Health promotion	Promote health and positive health behaviours. Reduce risky health behaviours.	Education and promotion of health through information and interventions to reduce risky behaviours.	With the normal population e.g. people attending primary care, antenatal clinics, sexual health clinics and smoking cessation.	Chapter 5
Crisis intervention	Support people in times of crisis and help them adjust and cope.	Supporting patients to work through what has happened and encourage positive adjustment.	After a diagnosis of a serious illness such as cancer, heart disease, multiple sclerosis etc; in palliative care.	Chapters 6, 11 & 12
Stress management	Help people to manage stress effectively.	Education about stress; understanding and breaking down stress, appraisal processes and responses. Exploring more adaptive ways to cope.	When stress may exacerbate conditions such as heart disease, premenstrual tension. Healthcare professionals in high stress jobs.	Chapter 3
Support groups	Encourage contact with, and support from, other people in similar circumstances.	Groups of 6–12 people with similar problems. Usually facilitated by a healthcare professional.	With groups such as people with cancer, heart disease or following stillbirth.	Chapter 11
Bereavement counselling	Help people cope with and come to terms with their loss.	Individual or couple counselling to help people mourn their loss and find ways to cope.	For the loss or bereavement of a significant other e.g. a stillbirth, relatives of dying patients.	Chapter 6
Neuropsychological rehabilitation	Assess, treat and rehabilitate people with a brain injury to reduce disability and increase quality of life.	Examination of cognitive, behavioural, emotional, and social function. Rehabilitation through various techniques e.g. goal setting, skill training, and increasing awareness.	Following brain injury or neurodegenerative diseases such as dementia.	Chapter 16

There is general support for the effectiveness of psychological interventions for promoting health and wellbeing, although this varies according to the type of intervention and target group. Interventions can be broadly grouped into:

- Those that aim to change health behaviours.
- Those that aim to help people cope with difficult or stressful circumstances.
- Those that target particular symptoms or illnesses, such as pain management.

19.3.1 INTERVENTIONS FOR CHANGING BEHAVIOUR

Interventions to change health behaviours include health education, health promotion, and motivational interviewing. **Health promotion** is a broad area, ranging from national advertising campaigns to group interventions with patients who have a particular illness. Its effectiveness varies according to the method chosen and the people targeted. Providing blanket information to everyone is less effective than targeting information. Evidence has clearly shown that educational interventions are more effective if they are relevant to the people they target, are individualised, can provide feedback on people's learning, facilitate change by providing ways in which people can take action, and reinforce the desired behaviour (Kok, 2007). This has informed health promotion and there are many advertising campaigns targeting specific groups, such as those in Figure 19.3.

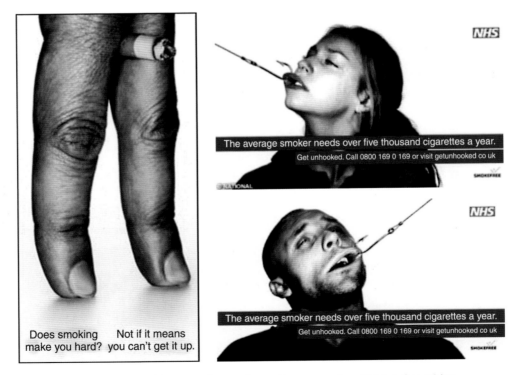

FIGURE 19.3 Targeted health promotion: anti-smoking campaign. © Nick Georghiou.

Motivational interviewing is used to change risky behaviour and promote healthy behaviour. Motivational interviewing was developed as a treatment for substance abuse, where people often have positive and negative attitudes towards the problem behaviour. It is a form of directive counselling that helps patients explore their reasons for a behaviour and their ambivalence towards a problem behaviour and try to resolve it. Motivational interviewing is more focused and goal-directed than normal counselling, although the emphasis here is not on *persuading* someone to change but on *helping* them to develop their own motivation to change. This is done through (a) empathising with the situation the person is in, (b) avoiding argumentation or persuasion, (c) examining the discrepancy between what the person wants to do and what they are actually doing, (d) examining resistance and (e) bolstering the person's self-efficacy (Miller, 1995). An example of motivational interviewing is given in Chapter 2 (see Case Study 2.2).

Evidence shows that motivational interviewing can be highly effective (see Research Box 19.1). A recent review of 72 clinical trials of using motivational interviewing across a wide range of behaviours showed it is very effective in the short term. In the long term, change was most likely when motivational interviewing was used in addition to a standard treatment (Hettama et al., 2005). It is therefore a useful approach for healthcare practitioners to use to help people change behaviours such as substance abuse and non-adherence to treatments.

RESEARCH BOX 19.1 Promoting safe sex for people with HIV in South Africa

Background and method

South Africa has a very high rate of HIV with almost 19 per cent of the population infected. Cultural norms mean that unsafe sex is common practice. This study evaluated a brief 15 minute intervention to reduce unsafe sex in patients with HIV. The intervention was based on motivational interviewing principles and was an 8-step programme as follows:

1 Introduce a discussion of safe sex.
2 Assess the patient's risk behaviour.
3 Determine how important it is to the patient to change the risk behaviour.
4 Determine how confident the patient is that they can change.
5 Identify the information, motivation, behavioural skills and other barriers to practising safe sex.
6 Discuss specific strategies for overcoming these barriers.
7 Negotiate a risk reduction goal or action plan.
8 Write the agreed goal on a 'prescription' form and give this to the patient.

152 patients were randomly allocated on a 2:1 basis to receive the intervention (n=103) or normal care (n=49). The intervention was delivered by lay HIV counsellors who had had at least 10 hours of training and weekly supervision from a professional.

(Cont'd)

Findings

55 per cent of patients were sexually active and 27 per cent of these reported having unsafe sex.

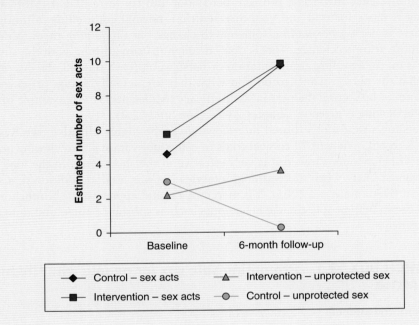

Over six months all patients became more sexually active. However, patients who received the intervention had significantly less unprotected sex than before the intervention. In contrast, patients who did not have the intervention had more unprotected sex.

Significance

This shows that a brief intervention using lay counsellors was very effective at reducing unsafe sex in HIV patients and hence reducing the spread of HIV and AIDS. Another important finding is that patients without the intervention had *more* unsafe sex over time so there is a real cost to doing nothing.

Cornman, D.H. et al. (2008) Clinic-based intervention reduces unprotected sexual behaviour among HIV-infected patients in KwaZulu Natal, South Africa: Results of a pilot study, *Journal of Aquired Immune Deficiency Syndromes, 48* (5): 553–560.

19.3.2 INTERVENTIONS FOR DIFFICULT CIRCUMSTANCES

Interventions to help people cope with stressful or difficult circumstances include stress management, critical incident debriefing, crisis intervention, bereavement counselling, and support groups. **Stress management** has been used with occupational groups, patient groups, and health professionals. It is based on our understanding of the processes of stress and coping (see Chapter 3) and helps patients identify the factors contributing to their stress and to find more adaptive ways to cope. In healthcare settings, stress management has most often been provided for patients with cancer or heart disease. In this context stress management reduces anxiety, depression, perceived pain, and increases quality of life for patients. However, there is little evidence that it has any effect on the course of illness or morbidity (Kenny, 2007).

Critical incident debriefing was initially developed to help emergency service workers cope with the traumatic events they attended, such as disasters, homicide, or road traffic accidents. Debriefing was carried out in groups and this approach was rapidly applied to a range of traumatic situations. However, evidence has shown that debriefing is *not* effective and in some cases can make people worse. As a result, many of the guidelines recommend against using it. Despite this, debriefing is still used in some settings in varying forms. For example, 78 per cent of hospitals in the UK offer some form of midwife-led debriefing to women after difficult or traumatic birth experiences (Ayers et al., 2006).

ACTIVITY 19.2

Think of a time you found really stressful or difficult.

- How did you cope with it?
- What did you find most helpful?

Debriefing shares some similarities with **crisis intervention** and bereavement intervention in that all of these try to ameliorate a situation rather than prevent it happening in the first place. Crisis intervention is used in situations where there has been threat of harm or violence, such as terrorist attacks, violent crime, domestic violence, or suicide attempts. It draws on a range of psychological theories and techniques to support people through a critical period (Roberts, 2005). Evidence for crisis intervention with medical patients suggests it reduces anxiety and PTSD, but is less effective for reducing depression (Stapleton et al., 2006). In addition, crisis intervention is more effective when it involves more than one session and is carried out by an experienced therapist (Stapleton et al., 2006).

Bereavement intervention is used following the death of a significant other, such as a spouse, parent, or child. Bereavement interventions will vary according to which theoretical view is taken of bereavement. The psychodynamic view focuses on unresolved conflicts or issues with the deceased. Stage theories of bereavement emphasise the different stages a person needs to go through, such as numbness, yearning, despair, and recovery (Payne et al., 1999). Stress theories of bereavement emphasise the stress of bereavement and the loss of resources to cope. Support theories emphasise the loss of social support and the disruption of support networks.

In a review of bereavement intervention, Kato and Mann (1999) considered the different theoretical viewpoints and whether these can account for the evidence that:

1 Men are more affected by the death of a spouse than women – they are more likely to get depressed or die in the year after their wife dies.
2 How the person dies affects the nature of grief – an unexpected death is likely to result in more severe grief than an expected death.

They concluded that these facts were best accounted for by stress or support theories of bereavement. However, their review of the evidence found that bereavement interventions as a whole had little effect on depression or grief and only a small effect on reducing physical symptoms. More recent evidence shows that bereavement interventions are only really effective for high risk individuals – for example, in cases where the death was unexpected, where there was a high level of dependency in the relationship, and where the person had a history of psychological problems (Jordan and Neimeyer, 2003).

CLINICAL NOTES 19.3

Psychotherapy techniques and clinical practice

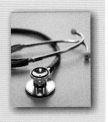

- Recognise that individuals come to you with their own emotional baggage, core beliefs, past experience, and relationship history.
- Do not underestimate the effects of a good doctor-patient relationship and placebo.
- Give patients an unconditional positive regard to improve the doctor-patient relationship and the person's psychological wellbeing.
- Be on the patient's side, understand their experience, and work with them to encourage change.
- Remember that helping people to 'face their fear' is essentially a form of exposure and so can be an effective treatment for anxiety.
- Help people to distance themselves from negative thoughts e.g. to accept the thoughts and think of them as a wave that will just wash over them and recede.

19.3.3 INTERVENTIONS FOR SPECIFIC ILLNESSES OR SYMPTOMS

Interventions targeted at specific illnesses or symptoms are wide ranging and include self-management interventions, support groups for patients with particular problems or illnesses, pain management, and neuropsychological rehabilitation.

Self-management interventions draw on a number of the theories outlined in Chapters 4 and 5 to help people manage their illness or rehabilitation effectively, with the aim of improving their psychological and physical wellbeing. Specific self-management interventions have been designed for many illnesses such as arthritis, asthma, diabetes, hypertension, chronic obstructive pulmonary disease, headache, and back pain (Mulligan and Newman, 2007). Generic self-management programmes for chronic disease have also been developed (Lorig et al., 2001).

Evidence shows self-management interventions are effective in the short term and can improve health behaviours and the management of an illness, such as adherence to medication. Self-management interventions can also lead to improved physical and emotional wellbeing. However, these effects are not always maintained over the long term (Mulligan and Newman, 2007). An example of a self-management intervention for MI is given in Chapter 4 (see Research Box 4.3).

Support group interventions are based on the large body of evidence that social support is associated with health and wellbeing and that, conversely, social isolation is a risk for many illnesses. Support interventions usually consist of a group of up to 12 people with similar problems or circumstances who meet eight to ten times. Groups can either consist of patients only or be facilitated by a health professional. Support groups aim to increase the support available to people, increase education and the sharing of knowledge about relevant circumstances, and hopefully increase the sharing and modelling of positive coping strategies.

The popularity of support groups for patients was boosted by a study that showed women with breast cancer who attended a support group lived on average 18 months longer than those who did not attend a support group (Spiegel et al., 1989). Since then the evidence has been less consistent and, although support groups usually improve psychological wellbeing and quality of life, they do not have a consistent impact on morbidity or mortality (Gottlieb, 2007). It is possible this is because they work better for some people than others. For example, if a person has a poor social network and does not express their emotions or cope particularly well, then a support group could be very helpful by increasing their social network, helping them talk about their feelings, and letting them see other group members modelling better ways of coping. Conversely, a person with many close friends and family members supporting them might not benefit from a support group.

There are many other interventions for specific illnesses. Pain is discussed in detail in Chapter 4 and evidence shows **pain management** programmes based on education and CBT can reduce pain, negative mood, negative coping, and abnormal pain behaviour, and improve social functioning (Morley et al., 1999). **Neuropsychological rehabilitation** uses a wide range of psychological theory to treat and rehabilitate people with neuropsychological problems, such as brain injury (see Chapter 16). Families are usually highly involved in this process. Technologies, such as computerised reminders and memory aids, are rapidly being developed to help patients adapt and function in the community (Wilson, 2007). Research into the effectiveness of neuropsychological rehabilitation has focused on specific techniques. For example, there is evidence that memory rehabilitation and specific attention skills training can be effective but that general attention training is not (Park and Ingles, 2000).

Summary

- Psychological interventions in medical settings include health promotion, interventions for difficult circumstances, and interventions for specific illnesses or patient groups.
- These interventions are wide ranging and draw on a range of psychological theories and techniques.
- Evidence shows psychological interventions in healthcare settings are effective. In particular health promotion, motivational interviewing, self-management, pain management, and neuropsychological rehabilitation.
- However, the effect of many of these interventions is limited to psychosocial outcomes.
- Critical incident stress debriefing is the only intervention where there is evidence that it should *not* be used.
- Bereavement interventions are largely ineffective, except with high-risk individuals.

📖 FURTHER READING

Bramber, M.R. (2006) *CBT for Occupational Stress in Health Professionals*. Hove: Routledge. Outlines the use of CBT to help cope with problems like performance anxiety, health anxiety, perfectionism, and burnout.

Rollnick, S., Miller, W.R. & Butler, C.C. (2008) *Motivational Interviewing in Health Care: Helping Patients Change Behavior*. New York: The Guilford Press. Outlines the basic principles and core skills required for motivational interviewing.

White, C.A. (2001) *Cognitive Behaviour Therapy for Chronic Medical Problems*. Chichester: Wiley. Provides an introduction to using CBT with a wide range of medical problems including surgical, cardiac, dermatological, cancer, pain, and diabetes.

? REVISION QUESTIONS

1 Describe two theories that are based on different types of psychotherapy.

2 Describe the core features of Cognitive Behaviour Therapy.

3 Outline the cognitive theory of depression and discuss the role of the depressogenic triad of negative beliefs.

4 Briefly compare and contrast behavioural and cognitive techniques for treating psychological problems.

5 What is a formulation and what is its role in psychotherapy?

6 Briefly outline three core principles of psychodynamic therapy.

7 Describe five core features of counselling.

8 Outline three psychological interventions used in medical settings and discuss whether these are effective.

9 What is unconditional positive regard and which theory or theories does it originate from?

10 Outline three psychological specialties and discuss their potential application to healthcare.

BIBLIOGRAPHY

Abbass, A.A., Hancock, J.T., Henderson, J. & Kisely, S. (2006) Short-term psychodynamic psychotherapies for common mental disorders, *Cochrane Database of Systematic Reviews, 4* (Art. CD004687).

Abraham, C. & Sheeran, P. (2007) The health belief model, in S. Ayers et al. (eds), *Cambridge Handbook of Psychology, Health and Medicine* (2nd edition). Cambridge: Cambridge University Press. pp. 97–102.

Adams, J.A. (1971) A closed loop theory of motor control, *Journal of Motor Behaviour, 3:* 111–150.

Adamson, S.J., Sellman, J.D. & Frampton, C.M.A. (2009) Patient predictors of alcohol treatment outcome: A systematic review, *Journal of Substance Abuse Treatment, 36:* 75–86.

Ader, R. (2003) Conditioned immunomodulation: Research needs and directions, *Brain, Behavior and Immunity, 17* (suppl. 1): s51–s57.

Ainsworth, M.D.S., Blehar, M.C., Waters, E. & Wall, S. (1978) *Patterns of Attachment: A Psychological Study of the Strange Situation.* Hillsdale, NJ: Erlbaum.

Ajzen, I. (1988) *Attitudes, Personality, and Behavior.* Buckingham: Open University Press.

Akobeng, A.K., Ramanan, A.V., Buchan, I. & Heller, R.F. (2006) Effect of breast feeding on risk of coeliac disease: A systematic review and meta-analysis of observational studies, *Archives of Disease in Childhood, 91:* 39–43.

Albarracín, D. et al. (2001) Theories of reasoned action and planned behavior as models of condom use, *Psychological Bulletin, 127:* 142–161.

Albarracín, D. et al. (2003) Persuasive communications to change actions: An analysis of behavioral and cognitive impact in HIV prevention, *Health Psychology, 22:* 166–177.

Alder, J., Fink, N., Bitzer, J., Hösli, I. & Holzgreve, W. (2007) Depression and anxiety during pregnancy: A risk factor for obstetric, fetal and neonatal outcome? A critical review of the literature, *Journal of Maternal-Fetal and Neonatal Medicine, 20:* 189–209.

Allan, R., Scheidt, S. & Smith, C. (2007) Coronary heart disease: Cardiac psychology, in S. Ayers et al. (eds), *Cambridge Handbook of Psychology, Health and Medicine* (2nd edition). Cambridge: Cambridge University Press. pp. 648–653.

Allen, K., Blascovich, J. & Mendes, W.B. (2002) Cardiovascular reactivity and the presence of pets, friends, and spouses: The truth about cats and dogs, *Psychosomatic Medicine, 64:* 727–739.

Alsaker, F.D. (1992) Pubertal timing, overweight, and psychological adjustment, *Journal of Early Adolescence, 12:* 396–419.

Alvarez, G.G. & Ayas, N.T. (2004) The impact of daily sleep duration on health: A review of the literature, *Progress in Cardiovascular Nursing, 19*: 56–59.

Ambady, N., LaPlante, D., Nguyen, T., Rosenthal, R., Chaumeton, N. & Levinson, W. (2002) Surgeons' tone of voice: A clue to malpractice history, *Surgery, 132*: 5–9.

American Psychiatric Association (2000) *Diagnostic and Statistical Manual of Mental Disorders, 4th Edition*. Washington, DC: APA.

American Psychiatric Association (2004) *Diagnostic and Statistical Manual of Mental Disorders, 4th Edition*. Washington, DC: APA.

Amsel, E. & Renninger, K.A. (eds) (1997) *Change and Development: Issues of Theory, Method and Application*. Mahwah, NJ: Lawrence Erlbaum.

Anderson, C.A. (2004) An update on the effects of playing violent video games, *Journal of Adolescence, 27*: 113–122.

Anderson, E.M. & Lambert, M.J. (1995) Short-term dynamically oriented psychotherapy: A review and meta-analysis, *Clinical Psychology Review, 15*: 503–514.

Andrade, J., Deeprose, C. & Barker, I. (2008) Awareness and memory function during paediatric anaesthesia, *British Journal of Anaesthesia, 100*: 389–396.

Angelelli, P. et al. (2004) Development of neuropsychiatric symptoms in poststroke patients: A cross-sectional study, *Acta Psychiatrica Scandinavica, 110*: 55–63.

Angevaren, M., Aufdemkampe, G., Verhaar, H.J., Aleman, A. & Vanhees, L. (2008) Physical activity and enhanced fitness to improve cognitive function in older people without known cognitive impairment, *Cochrane Database of Systematic Reviews, 3* (Art. CD005381).

Anstey, K.J. & Luszcz, M.A. (2002) Mortality risk varies according to gender and change in depressive status in very old adults, *Psychosomatic Medicine, 64*: 880–888.

Antoni, M.H. et al. (2006) Randomized clinical trial of cognitive behavioral stress management on Human Immunodeficiency Virus viral load in gay men treated with highly active antiretroviral therapy, *Psychosomatic Medicine, 68*: 143–151.

Antonovsky, A. (1987) *Unraveling the Mystery of Health: How People Manage Stress and Stay Well*. San Francisco, CA: Jossey-Bass.

Arbuthnott, A. & Sharpe, D. (2009) The effect of physician-patient collaboration on patient adherence in non-psychiatric medicine, *Patient Education and Counseling, 77*: 60–67.

Arden-Close, E., Gidron, Y. & Moss-Morris, R. (2008) Psychological distress and its correlates in ovarian cancer: A systematic review, *Psycho-Oncology, 17*: 1061–1072.

Arnett, J.J. (2004) *Emerging Adulthood: The Winding Road from Late Teens through the Twenties*. Oxford: Oxford University Press.

Arnold, R., Ranchor, A., Sanderman, R., Kempen, G., Ormel, J. & Suurmeijer, T. (2004) The relative contribution of domains of quality of life to overall quality of life for different chronic diseases, *Quality of Life Research, 13*: 883–896.

Arseneault, L., Cannon, M., Witton, J. & Murray, R.M. (2004) Causal association between cannabis and psychosis: Examination of the evidence, *British Journal of Psychiatry, 184*: 110–117.

Asch, S.E. (1956) Studies of independence and conformity: A minority of one against a unanimous majority, *Psychological Monographs: General and Applied, 70*: 1–70.

Asher, R. (1949) Myxoedematous madness, *British Medical Journal, 2*: 555–562.

Ashley, W.R., Harper, R.S. & Runyon, D.L. (1951) The perceived size of coins in normal and hypnotically induced economic states, *American Journal of Psychology, 64*: 564–572.

Ashworth, M., Godfrey, E., Harvey, K. & Darbishire, L. (2003) Perceptions of psychological content in the GP consultation: The role of practice, personal and prescribing attributes, *Family Practice*, 20: 373–375.

Ayers, S. & Ford, E. (2009) Birth trauma: Widening our Knowledge of postnatal mental health. *European Health Psychologist*, *11* (2), 16–19.

Ayers, S., Claypool, J. & Eagle, A. (2006) What happens after a difficult birth? Postnatal debriefing services, *British Journal of Midwifery*, 14: 157–161.

Ayers, S., Copland, C. & Dunmore, E. (2009) A preliminary study of negative appraisals and dysfunctional coping associated with post-traumatic stress disorder symptoms following myocardial infarction, *British Journal of Health Psychology, 14*: 459–471.

Ayers, S., Joseph, S., McKenzie-McHarg, K., Slade, P. & Wijma, K. (2008) Post-traumatic stress disorder following childbirth: Current issues and recommendations for research, *Journal of Psychosomatic Obstetrics & Gynaecology*, 29: 240–250.

Ayers, S., McKenzie-McHarg, K. & Eagle, A. (2007) Cognitive behaviour therapy for postnatal post-traumatic stress disorder: Case studies, *Journal of Psychosomatic Obstetrics & Gynaecology, 28*: 177–184.

Bachen, E., Cohen, S. & Marsland, A.L. (2007) Psychoneuroimmunology, in S. Ayers et al. (eds), *Cambridge Handbook of Psychology, Health and Medicine* (2nd edition). Cambridge: Cambridge University Press. pp. 167–172.

Bae, J.-M., Lee, E.J. & Guyatt, G. (2008) Citrus fruit intake and stomach cancer risk: A quantitative systematic review, *Gastric Cancer*, 11: 23–32.

Bagnardi, V., Zatonski, W., Scotti, L., La Vecchia, C. & Corrao, G. (2008) Does drinking pattern modify the effect of alcohol on the risk of coronary heart disease? Evidence from a meta-analysis, *Journal of Epidemiology and Community Health, 62*: 615–619.

Bahrke, M.S., Yesalis, C.E. & Brower, K.J. (1998) Anabolic-androgenic steroid abuse and performance-enhancing drugs among adolescents, *Child & Adolescent Psychiatric Clinics of North America*, 7: 821–838.

Baile, W.F. et al. (2000) SPIKES – a six-step protocol for delivering bad news: Application to the patient with cancer, *The Oncologist, 5*: 302–311.

Baker, F.C. & Driver, H.S. (2004) Self-reported sleep across the menstrual cycle in young, healthy women, *Journal of Psychosomatic Research, 56*: 239–243.

Balsa, A.I. & McGuire, T.G. (2003) Prejudice, clinical uncertainty and stereotyping as sources of health disparities, *Journal of Health Economics*, 22: 89–116.

Bandura, A., Ross, D. & Ross, S.A. (1961) Transmission of aggression through imitation of aggressive models, *Journal of Abnormal and Social Psychology*, 63: 575–582.

Barak, Y. (2006) The immune system and happiness, *Autoimmunity Reviews*, 5: 523–527.

Bar-Haim, Y., Lamy, D., Pergamin, L., Bakerman-Kranenburg, M.J. & van Ijzendoorn, M.H. (2007) Threat-related attentional bias in anxious and non-anxious individuals: A meta-analytic study, *Psychological Bulletin, 133*: 1–24.

Batson, C.D., Duncan, B., Ackerman, P., Buckley, T. & Birch, K. (1981) Is empathic emotion a source of altruistic motivation?, *Journal of Personality & Social Psychology*, 40: 290–302.

Baumeister, R.F., Campbell, J.D., Krueger, J.I. & Vohs, K.D. (2003) Does high self-esteem cause better performance, interpersonal success, happiness, or healthier lifestyles?, *Psychological Science in the Public Interest*, 4: 1–44.

Beck, A.T. (1967) *Depression: Clinical, Experimental and Theoretical Aspects*. New York: Harper & Row.

Beck, R.S., Daughtridge, R. & Sloane, P.D. (2002) Physician-patient communication in the primary care office: A systematic review, *Journal of the American Board of Family Practice, 15*: 25–38.

Beckman, H.B. & Frankel, R.M. (1984) The effect of physician behaviour on the collection of data, *Annals of Internal Medicine, 101*: 692–696.

Beer, J.S. & Lombardo, M.V. (2007) Insights into emotion regulation from neuropsychology, in J.J. Gross (ed.), *Handbook of Emotion Regulation*. New York: Guilford. pp. 69–86.

Beer-Borst, S. et al. (2000) Dietary patterns in six European populations: Results from EURALIM, a collaborative European data harmonization and information campaign, *European Journal of Clinical Nutrition, 54*: 253–262.

Bellisle, F., Monneuse, M.O., Steptoe, A. & Wardle, J. (1995) Weight concerns and eating patterns: A survey of university students in Europe, *International Journal of Obesity and Related Metabolic Disorders, 19*: 723–730.

Belloc, N.B. (1973) Relationship of health practices and mortality, *Preventative Medicine, 2*: 67–81.

Benarroch, E.E. (2007) Enteric nervous system: Functional organization and neurologic implications, *Neurology, 69*: 1953–1957.

Bennett, D.S. (1994) Depression among children with chronic medical problems: A meta-analysis, *Journal of Pediatric Psychology, 19*: 149–169.

Bennett, P. (2007a) Coronary heart disease: Impact, in S. Ayers et al. (eds), *Cambridge Handbook of Psychology, Health and Medicine* (2nd edition). Cambridge: Cambridge University Press. pp. 644–647.

Bennett, P. (2007b) Inflammatory bowel disease, in S. Ayers et al. (eds), *Cambridge Handbook of Psychology, Health and Medicine* (2nd edition). Cambridge: Cambridge University Press. pp. 759–760.

Bensing, J.M., Roter, D.L. & Hulsman, R.L. (2003) Communication patterns of primary care physicians in the United States and the Netherlands, *Journal of General Internal Medicine, 18*: 335–342.

Berk, L.S., Felten, D.L., Tan, S.A., Bittman, B.B. & Westengard, J. (2001) Modulation of neuroimmune parameters during the eustress of humor-associated mirthful laughter, *Alternative Therapies in Health & Medicine, 7*: 62–76.

Berkman, L.F. et al. (2003) Effects of treating depression and low perceived social support on clinical events after myocardial infarction, *Journal of the American Medical Association, 289*: 3106–3116.

Berkowitz, L. (1989) Frustration-aggression hypothesis: Examination and reformulation, *Psychological Bulletin, 106*: 59–73.

Bernal, M. et al. (2007) Risk factors for suicidality in Europe: Results from the ESEMED study, *Journal of Affective Disorders, 101*: 27–34.

Berry, L.M., Andrade, J. & May, J. (2007) Hunger-related intrusive thoughts reflect increased accessibility of food items, *Cognition and Emotion, 21*: 865–878.

Beswick, A.D. et al. (2004) Provision, uptake and cost of cardiac rehabilitation programmes: Improving services to under-represented groups, *Health Technology Assessment, 8* (41).

Bibace, R. & Walsh, M.E. (1980) Development of children's concepts of illness, *Pediatrics*, 66: 912–917.

Bischofberger, J. (2007) Young and excitable: New neurons in memory networks, *Nature Neuroscience*, 10: 273–275.

Bisson, J.I., Jenkins, P.L., Alexander, J. & Bannister, C. (1997) Randomised controlled trial of psychological debriefing for victims of acute burn trauma, *British Journal of Psychiatry*, 171: 78–81.

Blaxter, M. (1990) *Health and Lifestyles*. London: Routledge.

Blyth, F.M., March, L.M., Brnabic, A.J., Jorm, L.R., Williamson, M. & Cousins, M.J. (2001) Chronic pain in Australia: A prevalence study, *Pain*, 89: 127–134.

Bodley-Tickell, A.T. et al. (2008) Trends in sexually transmitted infections (other than HIV) in older people: Analysis of data from an enhanced surveillance system, *Sexually Transmitted Infections*, 84: 312–317.

Bogart, L.M., Bird, S.T., Walt, L.C., Delahanty, D.L. & Figler, J.L. (2004) Association of stereotypes about physicians to health care satisfaction, help-seeking behavior, and adherence to treatment, *Social Science & Medicine*, 58: 1049–1058.

Bolling, K., Grant, C., Hamlyn, B. & Thornton, A. (2007) *Infant Feeding Survey, 2005*. London: The Information Centre.

Bonanno, G.A. & Kaltman, S. (2001) The varieties of grief experience, *Clinical Psychology Review*, 21: 1–30.

Bor, R. & Allen, J. (2007) Counselling, in S. Ayers et al. (eds), *Cambridge Handbook of Psychology, Health and Medicine* (2nd edition). Cambridge: Cambridge University Press.pp. 348–351.

Borg, V. & Kristensen, T.S. (2000) Social class and self-rated health: Can the gradient be explained by differences in life style or work environment?, *Social Science & Medicine*, 51: 1019–1030.

Borrell-Carrio, F., Suchman, A.L. & Epstein, R.M. (2004) The biopsychosocial model 25 years later: Principles, practice and scientific enquiry, *Annals of Family Medicine*, 2: 576–582.

Boudreau, F. & Godin, G. (2007) Using the theory of planned behaviour to predict exercise intention in obese adults, *Canadian Journal of Nursing Research*, 39: 112–125.

Bowen, A., Neumann, V., Conner, M. & Tennant, A. (1998) Mood disorders following traumatic brain injury: Identifying the extent of the problem and the people at risk, *Brain Injury*, 12: 177–190.

Bower, P. & Rowland, N. (2006) Effectiveness and cost effectiveness of counselling in primary care, *Cochrane Database of Systematic Reviews*, 3 (Art. CD001025).

Bowlby, J. (1958) The nature of the child's tie to his mother, *The International Journal of Psycho-Analysis*, 39: 350–371.

Bowlby, J. (1969) *Attachment and Loss: Vol. 1. Attachment*. New York: Basic Books.

Bowlby, J. (1973) *Attachment and Loss: Vol. 2. Separation: Anxiety and Anger*. New York: Basic Books.

Braddock, C.H., Fihn, S.D., Levinson, W., Jonsen, A.R. & Pearlman, R.A. (1997) How doctors and patients discuss routine clinical decisions. Informed decision-making in the outpatient setting, *Journal of General Internal Medicine*, 12: 339–345.

Bramley, N. & Eatough, V. (2005) The experience of living with Parkinson's disease: An interpretative phenomenological analysis case study, *Psychology & Health*, 20: 223–235.

Bray, G.A. (2000) Reciprocal relation of food intake and sympathetic activity: Experimental observations and clinical implications, *International Journal of Obesity Related Metabolic Disorders*, 24: s8–s17.

Brewin, C.R., Andrews, B. & Valentine, J.D. (2000) Meta-analysis of risk factors for posttraumatic stress disorder in trauma-exposed adults, *Journal of Consulting and Clinical Psychology*, 68: 748–766.

Brewster, K.L. & Rindfuss, R.R. (2000) Fertility and women's employment in industrialized nations, *Annual Review of Sociology*, 26: 271–296.

Broadbent, E. & Petrie, K.J. (2007) Symptom perception, in S. Ayers et al. (eds), *Cambridge Handbook of Psychology, Health and Medicine* (2nd edition). Cambridge: Cambridge University Press. pp. 219–223.

Brooks-Gunn, J. & Paikof, R.L. (1992) Changes in self feelings during the transition towards adolescence, in H. McGurk (ed.), *Childhood Social Development*. Hove: Laurence Erlbaum. pp. 63–97.

Broom, A. & Tovey, P. (eds) (2009) *Men's Health*. New York: Wiley.

Brown, H. & Randle, J. (2005) Living with a stoma: A review of the literature, *Journal of Clinical Nursing*, 14: 74–81.

Brown, J., Pengas, G., Dawson, K., Brown, L.A. & Clatworthy, P. (2009) Self administered cognitive screening test (TYM) for detection of Alzheimer's disease, *British Medical Journal, 338*: 1423–1430.

Bruinsma, F. et al. (2006) Concern about tall stature during adolescence and depression in later life, *Journal of Affective Disorders*, 91: 145–152.

Brummett, B.H. et al. (2001) Characteristics of socially isolated patients with coronary artery disease who are at elevated risk for mortality, *Psychosomatic Medicine, 63*: 267–272.

Buckman, R. (1992) *How to Break Bad News*. UK: Papermac.

Bulik, C.M., Berkman, N.D., Brownley, K.A., Sedway, J.A. & Lohr, K.N. (2007) Anorexia nervosa treatment: A systematic review of randomized controlled trials, *International Journal of Eating Disorders, 40*: 310–320.

Burger, J.M. (1999) The foot-in-the-door compliance procedure: A multiple-process analysis and review, *Personality and Social Psychology Review*, 3: 303–325.

Burgess, H., Sharkey, K. & Eastman, C. (2002) Bright light, dark and melatonin can promote circadian adaptation in night shift workers, *Sleep Medicine Reviews*, 6: 407–420.

Buske-Kirschbaum, A., von Auer, K., Kreiger, S., Weis, S., Rauh, W. & Hellhammer, D. (2003) Blunted cortisol responses to psychosocial stress in asthmatic children: A general feature of atopic disease?, *Psychosomatic Medicine, 65*: 806–810.

Busse, J.W., Montori, V.M., Krasnik, C., Patelis-Siotis, I. & Guyatt, G.H. (2008) Psychological intervention for premenstrual syndrome: A meta-analysis of randomized controlled trials, *Psychotherapy and Psychosomatics, 78*: 6–15.

Butler, A.C., Chapman, J.E., Forman, E.M. & Beck, A.T. (2006) The empirical status of Cognitive-Behavioural Therapy: A review of meta-analyses, *Clinical Psychology Review*, 26: 17–31.

Cameron, L.D. & Moss-Morris, R. (2004) Illness-related cognition and behaviour, in A.A. Kaptein & J.A. Weinman (eds), *Health Psychology: An Introduction*. Oxford: Blackwell. pp. 84–110.

Cameron, L.D., Leventhal, E.A. & Leventhal, H. (1993) Symptom representations and affect as determinants of care seeking in a community-dwelling, adult sample population, *Health Psychology, 12*: 171–179.

Campbell, S.M. & Rowland, M.O. (1996) Why do people consult the doctor?, *Family Practice, 13*: 75–83.

Cancer Research UK (2008) Latest UK Cancer Incidence and Mortality Summary – Rates, Available at http://publications.cancerresearchuk.org/WebRoot/crukstoredb/CRUK_PDFs/mortality/IncidenceMortalitySummaryRates.pdf (last accessed 22 July 2009).

Cancer Research UK (2010) *Diet and Cancer: The Evidence*. Available at http://info.cancerresearchuk.org/healthyliving/dietandhealthyeating/howdoweknow/diet-and-cancer-the-evidence (last accessed 2 January 2010).

Cannon, M., Jones, P.B. & Murray, R.M. (2002) Obstetric complications and schizophrenia: Historical and meta-analytic review, *American Journal of Psychiatry*, 159: 1080–1092.

Capellino, S. & Straub, R.H. (2008) Neuroendocrine immune pathways in chronic arthritis, *Best Practice and Research: Clinical Rheumatology*, 22: 285–297.

Capitanio, J.P., Mendoza, S.P., Lerche, N.W. & Mason, W.A. (1998) Social stress results in altered glucocorticoid regulation and shorter survival in simian acquired immune deficiency syndrome, *Procedings of the National Academies of Science*, 95: 4714–4719.

Carey, M. et al. (2000) Using information, motivational enhancement, and skills training to reduce the risk of HIV infection, *Health Psychology*, 19: 3–11.

Carlson, N.R. (2007) *Physiology of Behavior* (9th edition) Boston, MA: Allyn & Bacon.

Carlyle, J. (2007) Psychodynamic psychotherapy, in S. Ayers et al. (eds), *Cambridge Handbook of Psychology, Health and Medicine* (2nd edition). Cambridge: Cambridge University Press. pp. 379–383.

Carrico, A.W. & Antoni, M.H. (2008) Effects of psychological interventions on neuroendocrine hormone regulation and immune status in HIV-positive persons: A review of randomized controlled trials, *Psychosomatic Medicine*, 70: 575–584.

Carroll, D., Ebrahim, S., Tilling, K., Macleod, J. & Smith, G.D. (2002) Admissions for myocardial infarction and World Cup football: Database survey, *British Medical Journal*, 325: 1439–1442.

Cash, T.F. & Deagle, E.A. (1998) The nature and extent of body-image disturbances in anorexia nervosa and bulimia nervosa: A meta-analysis, *International Journal of Eating Disorders*, 22: 107–126.

Caso, J.R., Leza, J.C. & Menchen, L. (2008) The effects of physical and psychological stress on the gastrointestinal tract, *Current Molecular Medicine*, 8: 299–312.

Centers for Disease Control and Prevention (CDC) S (2008) State-specific prevalence of obesity among adults - United States, 2007, *Morbidity & Mortality Weekly Report*, 57: 765–768.

Champagne, F. & Meaney, M.J. (2001) Like mother, like daughter: Evidence for non-genomic transmission of parental behaviour and stress responsivity, *Progress in Brain Research*, 133: 287–302.

Chan, A.O.O. et al. (2005) Differing coping mechanisms, stress level and anorectal physiology in patients with functional constipation, *World Journal of Gastroenterology*, 11: 5362–5366.

Chapillon, P., Patin, V., Roy, V., Vincent, A. & Caston, J. (2002) Effects of pre- and postnatal stimulation on developmental, emotional, and cognitive aspects in rodents: A review, *Developmental Psychobiology*, 41: 373–387.

Charles, C., Gafni, A. & Whelan, T. (1997) Shared decision-making in the medical encounter: What does it mean? (Or it takes a least two to tango), *Social Science & Medicine*, 44: 681–692.

Chartrand, T.L, Van Baaren, R.B. & Bargh, J.A. (2006) Linking automatic evaluation to mood and information processing style: Consequences for experienced affect, impression formation, and stereotyping, *Journal of Experimental Psychology: General, 135*: 70–77.

Charuvastra, A. & Cloitre, M. (2008) Social bonds and posttraumatic stress disorder, *Annual Review of Psychology, 59*: 301–328.

Chase, W. G. & Ericsson, K. A. (1982) Skill and working memory, in G.H. Bower (ed.), *The Psychology of Learning and Motivation, Vol. 16*. New York: Academic Press. pp. 1–58.

Chaudhuri, K.R., Healy, D.G. & Schapira, A.H. (2006) Non-motor symptoms of Parkinson's disease: Diagnosis and management, *Lancet Neurology, 5*: 235–245.

Chemerinski, E. & Robinson, R.G. (2000) The neuropsychiatry of stroke, *Psychosomatics, 41*: 5–14.

Chen, R., Cohen, L.G. & Hallett, M. (2002) Nervous system reorganization following injury. *Neuroscience, 111*: 761–773.

Cherry, D., Burt, C. & Woodwell, D. (2001) National ambulatory medical care survey: 1999 summary, *Division of Healthcare Statistics, 204*: 322.

Chida, Y. & Steptoe, A. (2008) Positive psychological well-being and mortality: A quantitative review of prospective observational studies, *Psychosomatic Medicine, 70*: 741–756.

Chida, Y. & Steptoe, A. (2009) The association of anger and hostility with future coronary heart disease, *Journal of the American College of Cardiology, 53*: 936–946.

Chomsky, N. (1965) *Aspects of the Theory of Syntax*. Cambridge, MA: MIT Press.

Christenfeld, N. & Gerin, W. (2000) Social support and cardiovascular reactivity, *Biomedicine & Pharmacotherapy, 54*: 251–257.

Christensen, A.J. & Ehlers, S.L. (2002) Psychological factors in end-stage renal disease: An emerging context for behavioral medicine research, *Journal of Consulting & Clinical Psychology, 70*: 712–724.

Christensen, A.J. et al. (2002) Effect of a behavioral self-regulation intervention on patient adherence in hemodialysis, *Health Psychology, 21*: 393–397.

Christian, L.M., Graham, J.M., Padgett, D.A., Glaser, R. & Kiecolt-Glaser, J.K. (2007) Stress and wound healing, *NeuroImmunoModulation, 13*: 337–346.

Church, K. & Mayhew, S.H. (2009) Integration of STI and HIV prevention, care, and treatment into family planning services: A review of the literature, *Studies in Family Planning, 40*:171–186.

Cialdini, R.B., Schaller, M., Houlihan, D., Arps, K., Fultz, J. & Beaman, A.L. (1987) Empathy-based helping: Is it selflessly or selfishly motivated?, *Journal of Personality & Social Psychology, 52*: 749–758.

Ciechanowski, P.S., Katon, W.J. & Russo, J.E. (2000) Depression and diabetes: Impact of depressive symptoms on adherence, function, and costs, *Archives of Internal Medicine, 160*: 3278–3285.

Ciesla, J.A. & Roberts, J.E. (2001) Meta-analysis of the relationship between HIV infection and risk for depressive disorders, *American Journal of Psychiatry, 158*: 725– 730.

Clark, D. & Seymour, J. (1999) *Reflections on Palliative Care*. Buckingham: Open University Press.

Clark, D.M. (1986) A cognitive approach to panic disorder, *Behaviour Research and Therapy, 24*: 461–470.

Clark, K.M. et al. (2006) Breastfeeding and mental and motor development at 5½ years, *Ambulatory Pediatrics*, 6: 65–71.

Clarke, D.M. & Currie, K.C. (2009) Depression, anxiety and their relationship with chronic diseases: A review of the epidemiology, risk and treatment evidence, *Medical Journal of Australia*, 190: s54–s60.

Cohen, R.D. (2002) The quality of life in patients with Crohn's disease, *Alimentary Pharmacology & Therapeutics*, 16: 1603–1609.

Cohen, S. (2005) The Pittsburgh common cold studies: Psychosocial predictors of susceptibility to respiratory infectious illness, *International Journal of Behavioral Medicine*, 12: 123–131.

Cohen, S., Frank, E., Doyle, W.J., Skoner, D.P., Rabin, B.S. & Gwaltney, J.M. (1998) Types of stressors that increase susceptibility to the common cold in healthy adults, *Health Psychology*, 17: 214–223.

Cohen, S., Kamarck, T. & Mermelstein, R. (1983) A global measure of perceived stress, *Journal of Health and Social Behavior*, 24: 385–396.

Cohen, S. & Rodriguez, M. (2001) Stress, viral respiratory infections, and asthma, in D.P. Skoner (ed.), *Asthma and Respiratory Infections (Volume 154 of series Lung Biology in Health and Disease)*. New York: Marcel Dekker. pp. 193–208.

Cohn, L.D., Macfralane, S., Yanez, C. & Imai, W.K. (1995) Risk-perception: Differences between adolescents and adults, *Health Psychology*, 14: 217–222.

Colloca, L., Sigaudo, M. & Benedetti, F. (2008) The role of learning in nocebo and placebo effects, *Pain*, 136: 211–218.

Conner, M., Povey, R., Sparks, P., James, R. & Shepherd, R. (2003) Moderating role of attitudinal ambivalence within the theory of planned behaviour, *British Journal of Social Psychology*, 42: 75–94.

Conroy, T., Marchal, F. & Blazeby, J.M. (2006) Quality of life in patients with oesophageal and gastric cancer: An overview, *Oncology*, 70: 391–402.

Contrada, R.J. & Goyal, T.M. (2005) Individual differences, health and illness: The role of emotional traits and generalized expectancies, in S. Sutton et al. (eds), *SAGE Handbook of Health Psychology*. London: SAGE. pp. 143–168.

Cooke, D., Newman, S., Sacker, A., DeVellis, B., Bebbington, P. & Meltzer, H. (2007) The impact of physical illnesses on non-psychotic psychiatric morbidity, *British Journal of Health Psychology*, 12: 463–471.

Coplan, J.D. & Lydiard, R.B. (1998) Brain circuits in panic disorder, *Biological Psychiatry*, 44: 1264–1276.

Cordoni, A. & Cordoni, L.E. (2001) Eutectic mixture of local anaesthetics reduces pain during intravenous catheter insertion in the paediatric patient, *Clinical Journal of Pain*, 17: 115–118.

Coresh, J. et al. (2007) Prevalence of chronic kidney disease in the United States, *Journal of the American Medical Association*, 298: 2038–2047.

Cornman, D.H. et al. (2008) Clinic-based intervention reduces unprotected sexual behaviour among HIV-infected patients in KwaZulu Natal, South Africa: Results of a pilot study, *Journal of Aquired Immune Deficiency Syndromes*, 48: 553–560.

Coulibaly, R., Séguin, L., Zunzunegui, M.V. & Gauvin, L. (2006) Links between maternal breast-feeding duration and Québec infants' health: A population-based study. Are the effects different for poor children?, *Maternal & Child Health Journal*, 10: 537–543.

Courneya, K.S. & Friedenreich, C.M. (1999) Physical exercise and quality of life following cancer diagnosis: A literature review, *Annals of Behavioral Medicine, 21*: 171–179.

Cox, D.J. et al. (1991) Intensive versus standard glucose awareness training (BGAT) with insulin-dependent diabetes: Mechanisms and ancillary effects, *Psychosomatic Medicine, 53*: 453–462.

Critchley, J. & Capewell, S. (2004) Smoking cessation for the secondary prevention of coronary heart disease, *Cochrane Database of Systematic Reviews, 1*: Art. CD003041.

Croyle, R.T. & Sande, G.N. (1988) Denial and confirmatory search: Paradoxical consequences of medical diagnosis, *Journal of Applied Social Psychology, 18*: 473–490.

Cummings, J.H. & Bingham, S.A. (1998) Diet and the prevention of cancer, *British Medical Journal, 317*: 1636–1640.

Cunningham, A.J. & Watson, K. (2004) How psychological therapy may prolong survival in cancer patients: New evidence and a simple theory, *Integrative Cancer Therapies, 3*: 214–229.

Cushing, H.W. (1932) The basophil adenomas of the pituitary body and their clinical manifestations, *Bulletin of Johns Hopkins Hospital, 50*: 137–195.

Czarnocka, J. & Slade, P. (2000) Prevalence and predictors of post-traumatic stress symptoms following childbirth, *British Journal of Clinical Psychology, 39*: 35–51.

Daniels, H. (ed.) (1996) *An Introduction to Vygotsky*. London: Routledge.

Dannemiller, J.L. & Stephens, B.R. (1988) A critical test of infant pattern preference models, *Child Development, 59*: 210–216.

Davies, J., Hey, E., Reid, W. & Young, G. (1996) Prospective regional study of planned home births, *British Medical Journal, 313*: 1302–1306.

Davis, C. (1939) Results of the self-selection of diets by young children, *Canadian Medical Association Journal, 41*: 257–261.

Davis, C., Kleinman, J.T., Newhart, M., Gingis, L., Pawlak, M. & Hillis, A.E. (2008) Speech and language functions that require a functioning Broca's area, *Brain & Language, 105*: 50–58.

de Groot, M., Anderson, R.J., Freedland, K.E., Clouse, R.E. & Lustman, P.J. (2001) Association of depression and diabetes complications: A meta-analysis, *Psychosomatic Medicine, 63*: 619–630.

de Moor, C. et al. (2002) A pilot study of the side effects of expressive writing on psychological and behavioural adjustment in patients in a phase II trial of vaccine therapy for metastatic renal cell carcinoma, *Health Psychology, 21*: 615–619.

de Sanjosé, S. et al. (2007) Worldwide prevalence and genotype distribution of cervical human papillomavirus DNA in women with normal cytology: A meta-analysis, *Lancet Infectious Diseases, 7*: 453–459.

de Visser, R., Rissel, C., Richters, J. & Smith, A. (2007) The impact of sexual coercion on psychological, physical, and sexual well-being, *Archives of Sexual Behavior, 36*: 676–686.

de Visser, R., Rissel, C., Smith, A. & Richters, J. (2006) Sociodemographic correlates of smoking, drinking, injecting drug use, and sexual risk behaviour, *International Journal of Behavioral Medicine, 13*: 153–162.

de Visser, R. & Smith, A. (2001) Relationship between sexual partners influences rates and correlates of condom use, *AIDS Education and Prevention, 13*: 413–427.

de Visser, R. & Smith, J. (2007) Alcohol consumption and masculine identity among young men, *Psychology & Health, 22*: 595–614.

de Visser, R., Smith, A., Rissel, C., Richters, J. & Grulich, A. (2003) Sex in Australia: Safer sex and condom use, *Australian and New Zealand Journal of Public Health, 27*: 223–29.

Deecher, D., Andree, T.H., Sloan, D. & Schechter, L.E. (2008) From menarche to menopause: Exploring the underlying biology of depression in women experiencing hormonal changes, *Psychoneuroendocrinology, 33*: 3–17.

Delvaux, N., Razavi, D., Marchal, S., Bredart, A., Farvacques, C. & Slachmuylder, J.L. (2004) Effects of a 105 hour psychological training program on attitudes, communication skills and occupational stress in oncology: A randomised study, *British Journal of Cancer, 90*: 106–114.

Demyttenaere, K. (2001) Compliance and acceptance in antidepressant treatment, *International Journal of Psychiatry in Clinical Practice, 5 (Suppl.1)*: s29–s35.

Dennerstein, L., Guthrie, J.R., Clark, M., Lehert, P. & Henderson, V.W. (2004) A population-based study of negative mood in middle-aged, Australian-born women, *Menopause, 11*: 563–568.

Department of Health (2001) *Treatment Choice in Psychological Therapies and Counselling: Evidence Based Clinical Practice Guidelines.* London: Department of Health.

Department of Health & Human Services (1990) *The Health Benefits of Smoking Cessation: A Report of the Surgeon General.* Washington, DC: DHSS.

Descartes, R. (1637). Discours de la Méthode. Leiden, NL: Elsevier.

Dickens, C., McGowan, L., Clark-Carter, D. & Creed, F. (2002) Depression in rheumatoid arthritis: A systematic review of the literature with meta-analysis, *Psychosomatic Medicine, 64*: 52–60.

DiMatteo, M.R. (2004a) Variations in patients' adherence to medical recommendations: A quantitative review of 50 years of research, *Medical Care, 42*: 200–209.

DiMatteo, M.R. (2004b) Social support and patient adherence to medical treatment: A meta analysis, *Health Psychology, 23*: 207–218.

DiMatteo, M.R., Giordani, P.J., Lepper, H.S. & Croghan, T.W. (2002) Patient adherence and medical treatment outcomes: A meta-analysis, *Medical Care, 40*: 794–811.

DiMatteo, M.R., Haskard, K.B. & Williams, S.L. (2007) Health beliefs, disease severity, and patient adherence: A meta-analysis, *Medical Care, 45*: 521–528.

DiMatteo, M.R., Lepper, H.S. & Croghan, T.W. (2000) Depression is a risk factor for noncompliance with medical treatment: Meta-analysis of the effects of anxiety and depression on patient adherence, *Archives of Internal Medicine, 160*: 2101–2107.

Dinges, D.F. et al. (1997) Cumulative sleepiness, mood disturbance, and psychomotor vigilance performance decrements during a week of sleep restricted to 4–5 hours per night, *Sleep, 20*: 267–277.

Dixon, R.P., Roberts, L.M., Lawrie, S., Jones, L.A. & Humphreys, M.S. (2008) Medical students' attitudes to psychiatric illness in primary care, *Medical Education, 42*: 1080–1087.

Djernes, J.K. (2006) Prevalence and predictors of depression in populations of elderly: A review, *Acta Psychiatrica Scandinavica, 113*: 372–387.

Dolin, D.J. & Booth-Butterfield, S. (1995) Foot-in-the-door and cancer prevention, *Health Communication, 7*: 55–66.

Douglas, R.M., Hemilä, H., Chalker, E. & Treacy, B. (2007) Vitamin C for preventing and treating the common cold, *Cochrane Database of Systematic Reviews, 3* (Art. sCD000980).

Dray-Spira, R., Lert, F., Marimoutou, C., Bouhnik, A.-D. & Obadia, Y. (2003) Socio-economic conditions, health status and employment among persons living with HIV/AIDS in France in 2001, *AIDS Care, 15*: 739–748.

Driver, H.S. & Taylor, S.R. (2000) Exercise and sleep, *Sleep Medicine Reviews*, 4: 387–402.

Drossman, D.A., Camilleri, M., Mayer, E.A. & Whitehead, W.E. (2002) AGA technical review on irritable bowel syndrome, *Gastroenterology*, 123: 2108–2131.

Eagley, A. & Chaiken, S. (1993) *The Psychology of Attitudes*. Fort Worth, TX: Harcourt Brace.

Eaker, E.D., Sullivan, L.M., Kelly-Hayes, M., D'Agostino, R.B. & Benjamin, E.J. (2007) Marital status, marital strain, and risk of coronary heart disease or total mortality: The Framingham offspring study, *Psychosomatic Medicine*, 69: 509–513.

Eastridge, B.J. et al. (2003) Effect of sleep deprivation on the performance of simulated laparoscopic surgical skill, *American Journal of Surgery*, 186: 169–174.

Edwards, A., Elwyn, G. & Mulley, A. (2002) Explaining risks: Turning numerical data into meaningful pictures, *British Medical Journal*, 324: 827–830.

Egede, L.E. (2007) Major depression in individuals with chronic medical disorders: Prevalence, correlates and association with health resource utilization, lost productivity and functional disability, *General Hospital Psychiatry*, 29: 409–416.

Ehlers, A. & Clark, D.M. (2000) A cognitive model of posttraumatic stress disorder, *Behaviour Research and Therapy*, 38: 319–345.

Ehlers, A., Stangier, U. & Geiler, U. (1995) Treatment of atopic dermatitis: A comparison of psychological and dermatological approaches to relapse prevention, *Journal of Consulting and Clinical Psychology*, 63: 624–635.

Ekman, P. (1992) An argument for basic emotions, *Cognition and Emotion*, 6: 169–200.

Ekman, P. (1999) 'Basic emotions' in T. Dalgleish & T. Power (eds), *Handbook of Cognition and Emotion*. Chichester, UK: Wiley. pp. 45–60.

Elkind, D. (1967) Egocentrism in adolescence, *Child Development*, 38: 1025–1034.

Elsenbruch, S. et al. (2005) Effects of mind-body therapy on quality of life and neuroendocrine and cellular immune functions in patients with ulcerative colitis, *Psychotherapy and Psychosomatics*, 74: 277–287.

Emery, C.F., Kiecolt-Glaser, J.K., Glaser, R., Malarkey, W.B. & Frid, D.J. (2005) Exercise accelerates wound healing among healthy older adults: A preliminary investigation, *Journals of Gerontology, Series A*, 60: 1432–1436.

Engel, G. (1977) The need for a new medical model: The challenge for biomedicine, *Science*, 196: 129–136.

Engelhard, I.M., van den Hout, M.A. & Arntz, A. (2001) Posttraumatic stress disorder after pregnancy loss, *General Hospital Psychiatry*, 23: 62–66.

Erikson, E.H. (1950) *Childhood and Society*. New York: Norton.

Erikson, E.H. (1968) *Identity: Youth and Crisis*. New York: Norton.

Ernst, E. (2009) Massage therapy for cancer palliation and supportive care: A systematic review of randomised clinical trials, *Support Care Cancer*, 17: 333–337.

Esgate, A. & Groome, D. (2005) *An Introduction to Applied Cognitive Psychology*. Hove: Psychology Press.

Essex, H. & Pickett, K. (2008) Mothers without companionship during childbirth: Analysis within Millennium cohort study, *Birth*, 35: 266–276.

European Centre for Disease Prevention and Control (CPDC)/WHO Regional Office for Europe (2009) *HIV/AIDS Surveillance in Europe 2008*. Stockholm: European CDPC.

Evans, G.W., Wener, R.E., Phillips, D. (2002) The morning rush hour: Predictability and commuter stress, *Environment and Behavior, 34*: 521–530.

Eysenck, M.W. (2000) *Psychology: A Student's Handbook*. Hove: Psychology Press.

Ezzy, D. (2000) Illness narratives: Time, hope, and HIV, *Social Science & Medicine, 50*: 605–617.

Ezzy, D., de Visser, R. & Bartos, M. (1999) Poverty, disease progression and employment among people living with HIV/AIDS in Australia, *AIDS Care, 11*: 405–414.

Fagan, J., Galea, S., Ahern, J., Bonner, S. & Vlahov, D. (2003) Relationship of self-reported asthma severity and urgent health care utilization to psychological sequelae of the September 11, 2001 terrorist attacks on the World Trade Center among New York City area residents, *Psychosomatic Medicine, 65*: 993–996.

Farsides, T. (2009) What counseling is, in B. Alder, C. Abraham, E. van Teijlingen & M. Porter (eds), *Psychology and Sociology Applied to Medicine* (3rd edition). Edinburgh: Elsevier Science. pp. 132–133.

Faunce, G.J. (2002) Eating disorders and attentional bias: A review, *Eating Disorders, 10*: 125–239.

Feinstein, R.E., Blumenfield, M., Orlowski, B., Frishman, W.H. & Ovanessian, S. (2006) A national survey of cardiovascular physicians' beliefs and clinical care practices when diagnosing and treating depression in patients with cardiovascular disease, *Cardiology in Review, 14*: 164–169.

Fennel, M.J.V. (1998) Low self-esteem, in N. Tarrier, A. Wells & G. Haddock (eds), *Treating Complex Cases: The Cognitive Therapy Approach*. Chichester, UK: Wiley. pp. 217–240.

Fenton, K. et al. (2001) Sexual behaviour in Britain: Reported sexually transmitted infections, *Lancet, 358*: 1851–1854.

Fenton, K. et al. (2004) Recent trends in the epidemiology of sexually transmitted infections in the European Union, *Sexually Transmitted Infections, 80*: 255–263.

Ferner, R.E. & McDowell, S. E. (2006) Doctors charged with manslaughter in the course of medical practice, 1795–2005: A literature review, *Journal of the Royal Society of Medicine, 99*: 309–314.

Ferri, C.P. et al. (2005) Global prevalence of dementia, *Lancet, 366*: 2112–2117.

Festinger, L. (1957) *A Theory of Cognitive Dissonance*. Evanston, IL: Row, Peterson.

Field, T., Diego, M. & Hernandez-Reif, M. (2007) Massage therapy research, *Developmental Review, 27*: 75–89.

Finch, S.J. (2003) Pregnancy during residency: A literature review, *Academic Medicine, 78*: 418–428.

Finlay, I.G. et al. (2002) Palliative care in hospital, hospice, at home: Results from a systematic review, *Annals of Oncology, 13(Suppl. 4)*: 257–264.

Firth-Cozens, J. (2001) Medical student stress, *Medical Education, 35*: 6–7.

Fitts, S.S., Guthrie, M.R. & Blagg, C.R. (1999) Exercise coaching and rehabilitation counseling improve quality of life for predialysis and dialysis patients, *Nephron, 82*: 115–121.

Flaherty, R.J. (2007) *Medical Myths: Evidence-based Medicine for Student Health Services*. Available at http://www.montana.edu/wwwebm/myths.htm (last accessed 31/08/07).

Flocke, S.A., Miller, W.L. & Crabtree, B.F. (2002) Relationships between physician practice style, patient satisfaction, and attributes of primary care, *Journal of Family Practice, 51*: 835–840.

Floyd, D.L., Prentice-Dunn, S. & Rogers, R.W. (2000) A meta-analysis of research on protection motivation theory, *Journal of Applied Social Psychology, 30*: 407–429.

Folstein, M.F., Folstein, S.E. & McHugh, P.R. (1975) "Mini-mental state": A practical method for grading the cognitive state of patients for the clinician, *Journal of Psychiatric Research, 12*: 189–198.

Forcier, K. et al. (2006) Links between physical fitness and cardiovascular reactivity and recovery to psychological stressors: A meta-analysis, *Health Psychology, 25*: 723–739.

Ford, A.C., Talley, N.J., Schoenfeld, P.S., Quigley, E.M.M. & Moayyedi, P. (2009) Efficacy of antidepressants and psychological therapies in irritable bowel syndrome: Systematic review and meta-analysis, *Gut, 58*: 367–378.

Fortner, B.V. & Neimeyer, R.A. (1999) Death anxiety in older adults: A quantitative review, *Death Studies, 23*: 387–411.

Foster, M.C. et al. (2008) Overweight, obesity, and the development of stage 3 CKD: The Framingham Heart Study, *American Journal of Kidney Disease, 52*: 39–48.

Frank, M.G. & Benington, J.H. (2006) The role of sleep in memory consolidation and brain plasticity: Dream or reality?, *Neuroscientist, 12*: 477–488.

Franks, H.M. & Roesch, S.C. (2006) Appraisals and coping in people living with cancer: A meta-analysis, *Psycho-Oncology, 15*: 1027–1037.

Frasure-Smith, N. et al. (2000) Depression and health-care costs during the first year following myocardial infarction, *Journal of Pychosomatic Research, 36*: 471–478.

Frattaroli, J. (2006) Experimental disclosure and its moderators: A meta-analysis, *Psychological Bulletin, 132*: 823–865.

Freeman, E. W. & Sherif, K. (2007) Prevalence of hot flushes and night sweats around the world: A systematic review, *Climacteric, 10*: 197–214.

French, S.A., Leffert, N., Story, M., Neumark-Sztainer, D., Hannan, P. & Benson, P.L. (2001) Adolescent binge/purge and weight loss behaviors: Associations with developmental assets, *Journal of Adolescent Health, 28*: 211–221.

Freud, S. (1999 [1900]) *The Interpretation of Dreams* (translator: J. Crick). Oxford: Oxford University Press.

Friedman, H.S. & Booth-Kewley, S. (1987) The "disease-prone" personality: A meta-analytic view of the construct, *American Psychologist, 42*: 539–555.

Friedman, M. et al. (1986) Alteration of Type A behaviour and its effect on cardiac recurrences in post myocardial infarction patients, *American Heart Journal, 112*: 653–665.

Friedman, T. & Gath, D. (1989) The psychiatric consequences of spontaneous abortion, *British Journal of Psychiatry, 155*: 810–813.

Fries, J.F., Green, L.W. & Levine, S. (1989) Health promotion and the compression of morbidity, *Lancet, 333*: 481–483.

Frijda, N.H. (1986) *The Emotions: Studies in Emotion and Social Interaction*. New York: Cambridge University Press.

Furnham, A., Petrides, K.V., Sisterson, G. & Baluch, B. (2003) Repressive coping style and positive self-presentation, *British Journal of Health Psychology, 8*: 223–249.

Gale, C.R., Batty, G.D. & Deary, I.J. (2008) Locus of control at age 10 years and health outcomes and behaviors at age 30 years, *Psychosomatic Medicine*, 70: 397–403.

Gamble, J. & Creedy, D. (2001) Women's preference for a caesarean section: Incidence and associated factors, *Birth*, 28: 101–110.

Gangestad, S.W. & Cousins, A.J. (2001) Adaptive design, female mate preferences, and shifts across the menstrual cycle, *Annual Review of Sex Research*, 12: 145–185.

Garakani, A. et al. (2003) Comorbidity of irritable bowel syndrome in psychiatric patients: A review, *American Journal of Therapeutics*, 10: 61–67.

Garrett, V.D., Brantley, P.J., Jones, G.H. & McKnight, G.T. (1991) The relation between daily stress and Crohns disease, *Journal of Behavioral Medicine*, 14: 87–96.

Garssen, B. (2004) Psychological factors and cancer development: Evidence after 30 years of research, *Clinical Psychology Review*, 24: 315–338.

Gavin, L. et al. (2009) Sexual and reproductive health of persons aged 10–24 years – United States, 2002–2007, *Morbidity & Mortality Weekly Report Surveillance Summary*, 58(6): 1–58.

Gdalevich, M., Mimouni, D. & Mimouni, M. (2001a) Breast-feeding and the risk of bronchial asthma in childhood: A systematic review with meta-analysis of prospective studies, *Journal of Pediatrics*, 139: 261–266.

Gdalevich, M., Mimouni, D., David, M. & Mimouni, M. (2001b) Breast-feeding and the onset of atopic dermatitis in childhood: A systematic review and meta-analysis of prospective studies, *Journal of the American Academy of Dermatology*, 45: 520–527.

Geen, R.G. & O'Neal, E.C. (1969) Activation of cue-elicited aggression by general arousal, *Journal of Personality and Social Psychology*, 11: 289–292.

Geenen, R., van Middendorp, H. & Bijlsma, J.W.J. (2006) The impact of stressors on health status and hypothalamic-pituitary-adrenal axis and autonomic nervous system responsiveness in rheumatoid arthritis, *Annals of the New York Academy of Sciences*, 1069: 77–978.

Geeraerts, B. et al. (2005) Influence of experimentally induced anxiety on gastric sensorimotor function in humans, *Gastroenterology*, 129: 1437–1444.

Gehlert, S., Song, I.H., Chang, C.-H. & Hartlage, S.A. (2008) The prevalence of premenstrual dysphoric disorder in a randomly selected group of urban and rural women, *Psychological Medicine*, 39: 129–136.

Gelb, P. (1982) The experience of nonerotic contact in traditional psychotherapy: A critical investigation of the taboo against touch, *Dissertation Abstracts*, 43: 1–13.

Gelder, M., Mayou, R. & Geddes, J. (2005) *Psychiatry* (3rd edition). Oxford: Oxford University Press.

General Medical Council (2009) *Tomorrow's Doctors*. London: General Medical Council.

Gerhardt, S. (2004) *Why Love Matters: How Affection Shapes a Baby's Brain*. New York: Brunner-Routledge.

Ghosh, S. & Mitchell, R. (2007) Impact of inflammatory bowel disease on quality of life, *Journal of Crohn's and Colitis*, 1: 10–20.

Gielissen, M., Verhagen, C. & Bleijenberg, G. (2007) Cognitive behaviour therapy for fatigued cancer survivors: Long-term follow-up, *British Journal of Cancer*, 97: 612–618.

Gigerenzer, G., Gaissmaier, W., Kurz-Milcke, E., Schwartz, L.M. & Woloshin, S. (2008) Helping doctors and patients to make sense of health statistics, *Psychological Science in the Public Interest*, 8: 53–96.

Gil, K.M., Somerville, A.M., Cichowski, S. & Savitski, J.L. (2009) Distress and quality of life characteristics associated with seeking surgical treatment for stress urinary incontinence, *Health and Quality of Life Outcomes*, 7, 8 (doi:10.1186/1477-7525-7-8).

Gilbert, P. (2000) *Overcoming Depression: A Self-Help Guide Using Cognitive Behavioural Techniques*. London: Robinson.

GINA: Global Initiative for Asthma (2001) *Global Strategy for Asthma Management and Prevention*. Bethesda, MD: NIH NHLBI.

Girón, M., Manjón-Arce, P., Puerto-Barber, J., Sánchez-García, E. & Gómez-Beneyto, M. (1998) Clinical interview skills and identification of emotional disorders in primary care, *American Journal of Psychiatry*, 155: 530–535.

Glaser, B. & Strauss, A. (1966) *Awareness of Dying*. Chicago, IL: Aldine.

Glaser, R. & Kiecolt-Glaser, J.K. (2005) Stress-induced immune dysfunction: Implications for health, *Nature Reviews: Immunology*, 5: 243–251.

Glaser, R. et al. (1987) Stress-related immune suppression: Health implications, *Brain, Behavior & Immunity*, 1: 7–20.

Goebel, M.U., Neykadeh, N., Kou, W., Schedlowski, M. & Hengge, U.R. (2008) Behavioral conditioning of antihistamine effects in patients with allergic rhinitis, *Psychotherapy & Psychosomatics*, 77: 227–234.

Goffman, E. (1959) *The Presentation of Self in Everyday Life*. New York: Doubleday.

Goldstein, L.H. & Leigh, P.N. (1999) Motor neurone disease: A review of its emotional and cognitive consequences for patients and its impact on carers, *British Journal of Health Psychology*, 4: 193–208.

Goodwin, R.D., Cox, B.J. & Clara, I. (2006) Neuroticism and physical disorders among adults in the community: Results from the national comorbidity survey, *Journal of Behavioural Medicine*, 29: 229–238.

Gorman, J.M., Kent, J.M., Sullivan, G.M. & Coplan, J.D. (2000) Neuroanatomical hypothesis of panic disorder, revised, *American Journal of Psychiatry*, 157: 493–505.

Gott, M. (2006) Sexual health and the new ageing, *Age & Ageing*, 35: 106–107.

Gottlieb, B. (2007) Social support interventions, in S. Ayers et al. (eds), *Cambridge Handbook of Psychology, Health and Medicine* (2nd edition). Cambridge: Cambridge University Press. pp. 397–402.

Gottlieb, B. & Wachala, E. (2007) Cancer support groups: A critical review of empirical studies, *Psycho-Oncology*, 16: 379–400.

Gouin, J.P., Kiecolt-Glaser, J.K., Malarky, W.B. & Glaser, R. (2008) The influence of anger expression on wound healing, *Brain, Behaviour and Immunity*, 22: 699–708.

Gould, N. & Kendall, T. (2007) Developing the NICE/SCIE guidelines for dementia care: The challenges of enhancing the evidence base for social and health care, *British Journal of Social Work*, 37: 475–490.

Government Office for Science (2007) *Tackling Obesities: Future Choices – Project Report* (2nd edition). London: Government Office for Science.

Goyal, R.K. & Hirano, I. (1996) The enteric nervous system, *New England Journal of Medicine*, 334: 1106–1115.

Gracely, R.H. et al. (2004) Pain catastrophizing and neural responses to pain among persons with fibromyalgia, *Brain*, 127: 835–843.

Grant, B.F. et al. (2006) The epidemiology of DSM-IV panic disorder and agoraphobia in the United States, *Journal of Clinical Psychiatry, 67*: 363–374.

Gravely-Witte, S., Stewart, D.E., Suskin, N., Higginson, L., Alter, D.A. & Grace, S.L. (2008) Cardiologists' charting varied by risk factor, and was often discordant with patient report, *Journal of Clinical Epidemiology, 61*: 1073–1079.

Greenhalgh, T. (2006) *How to Read a Paper: The Basics of Evidence-Based Medicine* (3rd edition). Oxford: Blackwell.

Greenhalgh, T. & Hurwitz, B. (eds) (1998) *Narrative Based Medicine: Dialogue and Discourse in Clinical Practice*. London: British Medical Journal Books.

Greer, S., Morris, T. & Pettingale, K.W. (1979) Psychological responses to breast cancer: Effect on outcome, *Lancet, 393*: 785–787.

Griffin, J.E. & Ojeda, S.R. (2004) *Textbook of Endocrine Physiology* (5th edition). Oxford: Oxford University Press.

Grilo, C.M., Masheb, R.M. & Wilson, G.T. (2005) Efficacy of cognitive behavioral therapy and fluoxetine for the treatment of binge eating disorder: A randomized double-blind placebo controlled comparison, *Biological Psychology, 57*: 301–309.

Groeger, J.A., Zijlstra, FR.H. & Dijk, D.-J. (2004) Sleep quantity, sleep difficulties and their perceived consequences in a representative sample of some 2000 British adults, *Journal of Sleep Research, 13*: 359–371.

Gross, J.J. & Thompson, R.A. (2007) Emotion regulation; conceptual foundations, in J.J. Gross (ed.), *Handbook of Emotion Regulation*. London: Guilford. pp. 3–24.

Grover, S.A. et al. (2006) The prevalence of erectile dysfunction in the primary care setting: Importance of risk factors for diabetes and vascular disease, *Archives of Internal Medicine, 166*: 213–219.

Gruber, A.J. & Pope, H.G. (2000) Psychiatric and medical effects of anabolic-androgenic steroid use in women, *Psychotherapy & Psychosomatics, 69*: 19–26.

Grulich, A. et al. (2003) Sex in Australia: Sexually transmissible infection, *Australian and New Zealand Journal of Public Health, 27*: 234–241.

Guinjoan, S.M. et al. (2004) Cardiac parasympathetic dysfunction related to depression in older adults with acute coronary symptoms, *Journal of Psychosomatic Research, 56*: 83–88.

Gullette, E.C.D. et al. (1997) Effects of mental stress on myocardial ischaemia in daily life, *Journal of the American Medical Association, 277*: 1521–1526.

Gurevich, M., Bishop, S., Bower, J., Malka, M. & Nyhof-Young, J. (2004) (Dis)embodying gender and sexuality in testicular cancer, *Social Science & Medicine, 58*: 1597–1607.

Gustafson, J. & Welling, D. (2009) "No acid, no ulcer" – 100 years later: A review of the history of peptic ulcer disease, *Journal of American College of Surgeons, 210*: 110–116.

Gustafsson, P.A., Duchén, K., Birberg, U. & Karlsson, T. (2004) Breastfeeding, very long polyunsaturated fatty acids and IQ at 6½ years of age, *Acta Paediatrica, 93*: 1280–1287.

Gutman, D.A. & Nemeroff, C.B. (2003) Persistent central nervous system effects of an adverse early environment: Clinical and preclinical studies, *Physiology & Behaviour, 79*: 471–478.

Haas, J.S. et al. (2004) Changes in the health status of women during and after pregnancy, *Journal of General Internal Medicine, 20*: 45–51.

Hagedoorn, M., Kuijer, E.F., Buunk, V.P., DeJong, G., Wobbes, T. & Sanderman, R. (2000) Marital satisfaction in patients with cancer: Does support from intimate partners benefit those who need it the most?, *Health Psychology*, 19: 274–282.

Hahn, S. et al. (2008) Patient and visitor violence in general hospitals: A systematic review of the literature, *Aggression & Violent Behavior*, 13: 431–441.

Hall, E.T. (1966) *The Hidden Dimension*. Garden City, NY: Doubleday.

Hall, J.A. & Roter, D.L. (2002) Do patients talk differently to male and female physicians? A meta-analytic review, *Patient Education & Counseling*, 48: 217–224.

Halvorsen, L., Nerum, H., Øian, P. & Sørlie, T. (2008) Is there an association between psychological stress and request for caesarean section?, *Tidsskrift for den Norske Laegeforening*, 12: 1388–1391.

Hamer, M., Chida, Y. & Molloy, G.J. (2009) Psychological distress and cancer mortality, *Journal of Psychosomatic Research*, 66: 255–258.

Hanauer, S.B. (2008) Review article: Evolving concepts in treatment and disease modification in ulcerative colitis, *Alimentary Pharmacology & Therapeutics*, 27: 15–21.

Hancock, L., Windsor, A.C. & Mortensen, N.J. (2006) Inflammatory bowel disease: The view of the surgeon, *Colorectal Disease*, 8: 10–14.

Hardeman, W. et al. (2002) Application of the Theory of Planned Behaviour in behaviour change interventions: A systematic review, *Psychology of Health*, 17: 123–158.

Harlow, H.F. (1958) The nature of love, *American Psychologist*, 13: 673–685.

Harrigan, J.A., Oxman, T.E. & Rosenthal, R. (1985) Rapport expressed through nonverbal behaviour, *Journal of Nonverbal Behaviour*, 9: 95–110.

Harrington, P. & Ayers, S. (2008) *Systematic Review of Depression in People with Neurological Disease*. Falmer: Brighton & Sussex Medical School (unpublished).

Harrison, J.A., Mullen, P.D. & Green, L.W. (1992) A meta-analysis of studies of the Health Belief Model with adults, *Health Education Research*, 7: 107–116.

Hart, A. & Kamm, M.A. (2002) Review article: Mechanisms of initiation and perpetuation of gut inflammation by stress, *Alimentary Pharmacology & Therapeutics*, 16: 2017–2028.

Hashash, J. et al. (2008) Clinical trial: A randomized controlled cross-over study of flupenthixol & melitracen in functional dyspepsia, *Alimentary Pharmacology & Therapeutics*, 27: 1148–1155.

Hawks, S.R., Madanat, H.N. & Christley, H.S. (2008) Psychosocial associations of dietary restraint: Implications for healthy weight promotion, *Ecology of Food and Nutrition*, 47: 450–483.

Hayes, S.C. (2004) Acceptance and commitment therapy and the new behaviour therapies: Mindfulness, acceptance, and relationship, in S.C. Hayes, V.M. Follette & M.M. Linehan (eds), *Mindfulness and Acceptance: Expanding the Cognitive Behavioural Tradition*. New York: Guilford pp. 1–29.

Hayes, S.C., Strosahl, K.D. & Wilson, N.G. (1999) *Acceptance and Commitment Therapy: An Experimental Approach to Behaviour Change*. New York: Guilford.

Hay-Smith, J. & Dumoulin, C. (2006) Pelvic floor muscle training versus no treatment, or inactive control treatments, for urinary incontinence in women, *Cochrane Database of Systematic Reviews*, 1 (Art. CD005654).

Healthcare Commission (2007) *Caring for Dignity*. London: Healthcare Commission.

Heinrichs, N., Hoffman, E.C. & Hofmann, S.G. (2001) Cognitive-Behavioral Treatment for social phobia in Parkinson's disease: A single-case study, *Cognitive & Behavioral Practice, 8*: 328–335.

Hemilä, H., Chalker, E., Treacy, B. & Douglas, B. (2007) Vitamin C for preventing and treating the common cold, *Cochrane Database of Systematic Reviews, Issue 3* (Art. CD000980).

Herbert, T.B. & Cohen, S. (1993) Depression and immunity: A meta-analytic review, *Psychological Bulletin, 113*: 472–486.

Heron, M.P. (2007) *Deaths: Leading Causes for 2004*. Hyattsville, MD: National Center for Health Data and Methods.

Herzog, D.B. et al. (2000) Mortality in eating disorders: A descriptive study, *International Journal of Eating Disorders, 28*: 20–26.

Hettama, J., Steele, J. & Miller, W.R. (2005) Motivational interviewing, *Annual Review of Clinical Psychology, 1*: 91–111.

Hettema, J., Neale, M.C. & Kendler, K.S. (2001) A review and meta-analysis of the genetic epidemiology of anxiety disorders, *American Journal of Psychiatry, 158*: 1568–1578.

Hewitt, J.K. & Turner, J.R. (1995) Behavior genetic studies of cardiovascular responses to stress, in J.R. Turner, L.R. Cardon & J.K. Hewitt (eds), *Behavior Genetic Approaches in Behavioral Medicine*. New York: Plenum. pp. 87–103.

Heyn, P., Abreu, B.C. & Ottenbacher, K.J. (2004) The effects of exercise training on elderly persons with cognitive impairment and dementia: A meta-analysis, *Archives of Physical Medicine and Rehabilitation, 85*: 1694–1704.

Higgins, E.T. (1987) Self-discrepancy: A theory relating self and affect, *Psychological Review, 94*: 319–340.

Hill, C., Abraham, C. & Wright, D.B. (2007) Can theory-based messages in combination with cognitive prompts promote exercise in classroom settings?, *Social Science & Medicine, 65*: 1049–1058.

Hobson, J.A. & McCarley, R.W. (1977) The brain as a dream state generator: an activation-synthesis hypothesis of the dream process, *American Journal of Psychiatry, 134*: 1335–1348.

Hodnett, E., Gates, S., Hofmeyr, G.J. & Sakala, C. (2007) Continuous support for women during childbirth, *Cochrane Database of Systematic Reviews, 3* (Art. CD003766).

Hoey, L.M., Ieropoli, S.C., White, V.M. & Jefford, M. (2008) Systematic review of peer-support programs for people with cancer, *Patient Education and Counselling, 70*: 315–337.

Hofling, C.K., Brotzman, E., Dalrymple, S., Graves, N. & Pierce, C.M. (1966) An experimental study of nurse-physician relationships, *Journal of Nervous and Mental Disease, 143*: 171–180.

Hogg, M.A. & Vaughan, G.M. (2008) *Social Psychology* (5th edition). Harlow: Pearson Prentice-Hall.

Holman, E.A., Silver, R.C., Poulin, M., Andersen, J., Gil-Rivas, V. & McIntosh, D.N. (2008) Terrorism, acute stress, and cardiovascular health: A 3-year national study following the September 11th attacks, *Archives of General Psychiatry, 65*: 73–80.

Hong, C.C.H. et al. (1996) Language in dreaming and regional EEG alpha power, *Sleep, 19*: 232–235.

Horowitz, M.J., Duff, D.F. & Stratton, L.O. (1969) Body-buffer zones, *Archives of General Psychiatry, 11*: 651–656.

Houts, P.S., Doak, C.C., Doak, L.G. & Loscalzo, M.J. (2006) The role of pictures in improving health communication: A review of research on attention, comprehension, recall, and adherence, *Patient Education and Counseling, 61*: 173–190.

Howard, F.M. (2003) Chronic pelvic pain, *Obstetrics & Gynecology, 101*: 594–611.

Huddart, R.A. et al. (2005) Fertility, gonadal and sexual function in survivors of testicular cancer, *British Journal of Cancer, 93*: 200–207.

Hudson, J.I., Hiripi, E., Pope, H.G. & Kessler, R.C. (2007) The prevalence and correlates of eating disorders in the National Comorbidity Survey Replication, *Biological Psychiatry, 61*: 348–358.

Hui, W.M., Shiu, L.P. & Lam, S.K. (1999) The perception of life events and daily stress in nonulcer dyspepsia, *American Journal of Gastroenterology, 86*: 292–296.

Hull, K.L. & Harvey, S. (2003) Growth hormone therapy and quality of life: Possibilities, pitfalls and mechanisms, *Journal of Endocrinology, 179*: 311–333.

Hunter, M., Ussher, J., Cariss, M., Browne, S. & Jelly, R. (2002) A randomised comparison of psychological (cognitive behaviour therapy, CBT), medical (fluoxetine) and combined treatment for women with Premenstrual Dysphoric Disorder, *Journal of Psychosomatic Obstetrics and Gynaecology, 23*: 193–199.

Huntley, A., White, A. & Ernst, E. (2002) Relaxation therapies for asthma: A systematic review, *Thorax, 57*: 127–131.

Hydén, L.C. (1997) Illness and narrative, *Sociology of Health and Illness, 19*: 48–69.

Ingersoll, K.S. & Jessye Cohen, J. (2008) The impact of medication regimen factors on adherence to chronic treatment: a review of literature, *Journal of Behavioural Medicine, 31*: 213–224.

Institute of Medicine (2005) *Estimating the Contributions of Lifestyle-Related Factors to Preventable Death: A Workshop Summary*. Washington: National Academies Press.

Ishigami, T. (1919) The influence of psychic acts on the progress of pulmonary tuberculosis, *American Review of Tuberculosis, 2*: 470–484.

Izard, C.E. (1991) *The Psychology of Emotions*. New York: Plenum.

Jackson, L.A. & Ervin, K.S. (1992) Height stereotypes of women and men: The liabilities of shortness for both sexes, *Journal of Social Psychology, 132*: 433–445.

Jacobsen, P.B., Bovbjerg, D.J. & Redd, W.H. (1993) Anticipatory anxiety in patients receiving cancer chemotherapy, *Health Psychology, 12*: 469–475.

Jané-Llopis, E. & Matytsina, I. (2006) Mental health and alcohol, drugs and tobacco: A review of the comorbidity between mental disorders and the use of alcohol, tobacco and illicit drugs, *Drug and Alcohol Review, 25*: 515–536.

Janis, I.L. & Mann, L. (1977) *Decision Making: A Psychological Analysis of Conflict, Choice, and Commitment*. New York: Free.

Janz, N.K. & Becker, M.H. (1984) The Health Belief Model: A decade later, *Health Education Quarterly, 11*: 1–47.

Jeffery, R.W., Adlis, S.A. & Forster, J.L. (1991) Prevalence of dieting among working men and women: The healthy worker project, *Health Psychology, 10*: 274–281.

Jin, J., Sklar, G.E., Oh, V.M.S. & Li, S.C. (2008) Factors affecting therapeutic compliance: A review from the patient's perspective, *Therapeutics & Clinical Risk Management, 4*: 269–286.

Joekes, K. (2007) Breaking bad news, in S. Ayers et al. (eds), *Cambridge Handbook of Psychology, Health and Medicine* (2nd edition). Cambridge: Cambridge University Press. pp. 423–426.

Johnson, W.D. et al. (2009) Behavioral interventions to reduce risk for sexual transmission of HIV among men who have sex with men, *Cochrane Database of Systematic Reviews, 3* (Art. CD001230).

Johnston, M. & Vogele, C. (1993) Benefits of psychological preparation for surgery: A meta-analysis, *Annals of Behavioral Medicine, 15*: 245–256.

Jonker-Pool, G. et al. (2001) Sexual functioning after treatment for testicular cancer: Review and meta-analysis of 36 empirical studies between 1975–2000, *Archives of Sexual Behavior, 30*: 55–74.

Jopson, N. & Moss-Morris, R. (2003) The role of illness severity and illness representations in adjusting to multiple sclerosis, *Journal of Psychosomatic Research, 54*: 503–511.

Jordan, J. & Neimeyer, R. (2003) Does grief counselling work?, *Death Studies, 27*: 765–786.

Kanayama, G., Hudson, J.I. & Pope, H.G. (2008) Long-term psychiatric and medical consequences of anabolic-androgenic steroid abuse: A looming public health concern?, *Drug & Alcohol Dependence, 98*: 1–12.

Kangas, M., Henry, J.L. & Bryant, R.A. (2002) Posttraumatic stress disorder following cancer: A conceptual and empirical review, *Clinical Psychology Review, 22*: 499–524.

Kaplan, G.A. & Reynolds, P. (1988) Depression and cancer mortality and morbidity: Prospective evidence from the Alameda County Study, *Journal of Behavioral Medicine, 11*: 1–13.

Kaplan, G.A., Seeman, T.E., Cohen, R.D., Knudsen, L.P. & Garulnik, J. (1987) Mortality among the elderly in the Alameda County Study: Behavioral and demographic risk factors, *American Journal of Public Health, 77*: 307–312.

Kaplan, K.A. & Harvey, A.G. (2009) Hypersomnia across mood disorders: A review and synthesis, *Sleep Medicine Reviews, 13*: 275–285.

Kaplan, R. (1990) Behavior as the central outcome in health care, *American Psychologist, 70*: 1211–1220.

Kapur, S. & Remington, G. (1996) Serotonin-dopamine interaction and its relevance to schizophrenia, *American Journal of Psychiatry, 153*: 466–476.

Kato, P.M. & Mann, T. (1999) A synthesis of psychological interventions for the bereaved, *Clinical Psychology Review, 19*: 275–296.

Katon, W.J. & Walker, E.A. (1998) Medically unexplained symptoms in primary care, *Journal of Clinical Psychiatry, 59 (suppl. 20)*: s15–s21.

Kaye, J.A. & Jick, H. (2003) Incidence of erectile dysfunction and characteristics of patients before and after the introduction of sildenafil in the United Kingdom: Cross sectional study with comparison patients, *British Medical Journal, 326*: 424–425.

Keegan, T.H.M., Gomez, S.L., Clarke, C.A., Chan, J.K. & Glaser, S.L. (2007) Recent trends in breast cancer incidence among 6 Asian groups in the Greater Bay Area of Northern California, *International Journal of Cancer, 120*: 1324–1329.

Kellett, S. & Gilbert, P. (2001) Acne: A biopsychosocial and evolutionary perspective with a focus on shame, *British Journal of Health Psychology*, 6: 1–24.

Kendrick, A.H., Higgs, C.M.B., Whitfield, M.J. & Laszlo, G. (1993) Accuracy of perception of severity of asthma: Patients treated in general practice, *British Medical Journal,* 307: 422–424.

Kennedy, R.M., Luhmann, J. & Zempsky, W.T. (2008) Clinical implications of unmanaged needle-insertion pain and distress in children, *Pediatrics*, 122: 130–133.

Kennedy, T.M. et al. (2006) Cognitive behavioural therapy in addition to antispasmodic therapy for irritable bowel syndrome in primary care: Randomised controlled trial, *British Medical Journal, 331*: 435–440.

Kenny, D.T. (2007) Stress management, in S. Ayers et al. (eds), *Cambridge Handbook of Psychology, Health and Medicine* (2nd edition). Cambridge: Cambridge University Press. pp. 403–407.

Kessels, R.P.C. (2003) Patients' memory for medical information, *Journal of the Royal Society of Medicine, 96*: 219–222.

Khaw, K.T., Wareham, N., Bingham, S., Welch, A., Luben, R. & Day, N. (2008) Combined impact of health behaviours and mortality in men and women: The EPIC-Norfolk prospective population study. *PLOS Medicine, 5*: e12.

Kiecolt-Glaser, J.K. & Glaser, R. (2002) Depression and immune function: Central pathways to morbidity and mortality, *Journal of Psychosomatic Research, 53*: 873–876.

Kiecolt-Glaser, J.K., McGuire, L., Robles, T.F. & Glaser, R. (2002a) Psychoneuroimmunology: Psychological influences on immune function and health, *Journal of Consulting and Clinical Psychology, 70*: 537–547.

Kiecolt-Glaser, J.K., McGuire, L., Robles, T.F. & Glaser, R. (2002b) Emotions, morbidity, and mortality: New perspectives from psychoneuroimmunology, *Annual Review of Psychology, 53*: 83–107.

Kiernan, J. (2002) The experience of therapeutic touch in the lives of five postpartum women, *The American Journal of Maternal Child Nursing*, 27: 47–53.

Kim, S. et al. (2008) Self-reported experience and outcomes of care among stomach cancer patients at a median follow-up time of 27 months from diagnosis, *Supportive Care in Cancer, 16*: 831–839.

Kinsman, R.A., Dirks, J.F. & Jones, N.F. (1982) Psychomaintenance of chronic physical illness, in T. Millon, C. Green & R. Meagher (eds), *Handbook of Clinical Health Psychology*. New York: Plenum. pp. 435–466.

Kirsch, I. (2007) Placebos, in S. Ayers et al. (eds), *Cambridge Handbook of Psychology, Health and Medicine* (2nd edition). Cambridge: Cambridge University Press. pp. 161–167.

Kirsch, I., Deacon, B.J., Huedo-Medina, T.B., Scoboria, A., Moore, T.J. & Johnson, B.T. (2008) Initial severity and antidepressant benefits: A meta-analysis of data submitted to the Food and Drug Administration, *PloS Medicine, 5*: 260–268.

Kirschner-Hermanns, R. & Jakse, G. (2002) Quality of life following radical prostatectomy, *Critical Reviews in Oncology and Hematology, 43*: 141–151.

Kisely, S., Goldberg, D. & Simon, G. (1997) A comparison between somatic symptoms with and without clear organic cause: Results of an international study, *Psychological Medicine, 27*: 1011–1019.

Klein, C.T.F. & Helweg-Larsen, M. (2002) Perceived control and the optimistic bias: A meta-analytic review, *Psychology and Health*, 17: 437–446.

Ko, W.F. & Sawatzky, J.A. (2008) Understanding urinary incontinence after radical prostatectomy, *Clinical Journal of Oncology Nursing*, 12: 647–654.

Kok, G. (2007) Health promotion, in S. Ayers et al. (eds), *Cambridge Handbook of Psychology, Health and Medicine* (2nd edition). Cambridge: Cambridge University Press. pp. 355–359.

Koob, G.F. (2006) The neurobiology of addiction: A neuroadaptational view relevant for diagnosis, *Addiction, 101 (suppl.1)*: s23–s30.

Kraaij, V., Arensman, E. & Spinhoven, P. (2002) Negative life events and depression in elderly persons: A meta-analysis, *Journals of Gerontology: Series B: Psychological Sciences & Social Sciences*, 57B: 87–94.

Kramer, M.S. et al. (2008) Breastfeeding and child cognitive development: New evidence from a large randomized trial, *Archives of General Psychiatry*, 65: 578–584.

Krantz, D.S. & McCeney, M.K. (2002) Effects of psychological and social factors on organic disease: A critical assessment of research on coronary heart disease, *Annual Review of Psychology, 53*: 341–369.

Krantz, D.S., Helmers, K.F., Bairey, N., Nebel, L.E., Hedges, S.M. & Rozanski, A. (1991) Cardiovascular reactivity and mental stress-induced myocardial ischaemia in patients with coronary artery disease, *Psychosomatic Medicine*, 53: 1–12.

Kroenke, K. (2003a) Patients presenting with somatic complaints: Epidemiology, psychiatric comorbidity and management, *International Journal of Methods in Psychiatric Research*, 12: 34–43.

Kroenke, K. (2003b) The interface between physical and psychological symptoms, *Journal of Clinical Psychiatry, 5 (suppl.7)*: s11–s18.

Kübler-Ross, E. (1969) *On Death and Dying*. New York: Macmillan.

Kunkel, E.J., Bakker, J.R., Myers, R.E., Oyesanmi, O. & Gomella, L.G. (2000) Biopsychosocial aspects of prostate cancer, *Psychosomatics*, 41: 85–94.

Kurtz, S.M. & Silverman, J.D. (1996) The Calgary-Cambridge observation guides: An aid to defining the curriculum and organizing the teaching in communication training programmes, *Medical Education, 30*: 83–89.

Kwekkeboom, K.L. & Gretarsdottir, E. (2006) Systematic review of relaxation interventions for pain, *Journal of Nursing Scholarship*, 38: 269–277.

Lackner, J.M. et al. (2004) Psychological treatments for irritable bowel syndrome: A systematic review and meta-analysis, *Journal of Consulting and Clinical Psychology*, 72: 1100–1113.

Ladomenou, F., Kafatos, A. & Galanakis, E. (2007) Risk factors related to intention to breastfeed, early weaning and suboptimal duration of breastfeeding, *Acta Paediatrica*, 96: 1441–1444.

Laessle, R.G. & Schulz, S. (2009) Stress-induced laboratory eating behavior in obese women with binge eating disorder, *International Journal of Eating Disorders, 42*: 505–510.

LaFrance, M. & Ickes, W. (1981) Posture mirroring and interactional involvement: Sex and sex typing effects, *Journal of Nonverbal Behaviour*, 5: 139–154.

Lahtinen, V., Lonka, K. & Lindblom-Ylänne, S. (1997) Spontaneous study strategies and the quality of knowledge construction, *British Journal of Educational Psychology, 67*: 13–24.

Lai, H., Lai, S., Krongrad, A., Trapido, E., Page, J.B. & McCoy, C.B. (1999) The effect of marital status on survival in late-stage cancer patients, *International Journal of Behavioral Medicine*, 6: 150–176.

Lang, P.J. & Davis, M. (2006) Emotion, motivation, and the brain: Reflex foundations in animal and human research, *Progress in Brain Research*, 156: 3–29.

Larkin, M., Clifton, E. & de Visser, R. (2009) Making sense of "consent" in a constrained environment, *International Journal of Law & Psychiatry*, 32: 176–183.

Larson, R.W., Richards, M.H., Moneta, G. & Holmbeck, G.C. (1996) Changes in adolescents' daily interactions with their families from ages 10 to 18: Disengagement and transformation, *Developmental Psychology*, 32: 744–754.

Larsson, S.C. & Wolk, A. (2006) Meat consumption and risk of colorectal cancer: A meta-analysis of prospective studies, *International Journal of Cancer*, 119: 2657–2664.

Larsson, S.C. & Wolk, A. (2007) Obesity and colon and rectal cancer risk: A meta-analysis of prospective studies, *American Journal of Clinical Nutrition*, 86: 556–565.

Latané, B. & Darley, J.M. (1970) *The Unresponsive Bystander*. New York: Appleton Century Crofts.

Laumann, E.O., Gagnon, J.H., Michael, R.T. & Michaels, S. (1994) *The Social Organization of Sexuality: Sexual Practices in the United States*. Chicago: University of Chicago Press.

Laumann, E.O., Paik, A. & Rosen, R.C. (1999) Sexual dysfunction in the United States: Prevalence and predictors, *Journal of the American Medical Association*, 281: 537–544.

Lavie, P. (2001) Sleep-wake as a biological rhythm, *Annual Review of Psychology*, 52: 277–303.

Lawler, M. & Nixon, E. (2010) Body dissatisfaction among adolescent boys and girls: The effects of body mass, peer appearance culture and internalization of appearance ideals, *Journal of Youth & Adolescence* [Epub ahead of print].

Lawrie, S.M. et al. (1998) General practitioners' attitudes to psychiatric and medical illness, *Psychological Medicine*, 28: 1463–1467.

Layard, R. (2006) *The Depression Report: A New Deal for Depression and Anxiety Disorders*. London: London School of Economics.

Lazarus, R.S. & Folkman, S. (1984) *Stress, Appraisal and Coping*. New York: Springer.

Lazarus, R.S., Opton, E.M., Nomikos, S.M. & Rankin, N.O. (1965) The principle of short-circuiting of threat: Further evidence, *Journal of Personality*, 33: 622–635.

Le Doux, J.E. (1996) *The Emotional Brain*. New York: Simon & Schuster.

Leichsenring, F. (2005) Are psychodynamic and psychoanalytic psychotherapies effective? A review of empirical data, *International Journal of Psychoanalysis*, 86: 841–868.

Leiter, M.P. & Maslach, C. (2000) Burnout and health, in A. Baum, T. Revenson & J. Singer (eds), *Handbook of Health Psychology*. Hillsdale, NJ: Lawrence Erlbaum. pp. 415–426.

Lepore, S.J., Helgeson, V.S., Eton, D.T. & Schulz, R. (2003) Improving quality of life in men with prostate cancer: A randomized controlled trial of group education interventions, *Health Psychology*, 22: 443–452.

Leserman, J. (2008) Role of depression, stress, and trauma in HIV disease progression, *Psychosomatic Medicine*, 70: 539–545.

Leserman, J. et al. (1999) Progression to AIDS: The effects of stress, depressive symptoms, and social support, *Psychosomatic Medicine*, 61: 397–406.

Lett, H.S. et al. (2004) Depression as a risk factor for coronary artery disease: Evidence, mechanisms, and treatment, *Psychosomatic Medicine, 66*: 305–315.

Levav, I. et al. (2000) Cancer incidence and survival following bereavement, *American Journal of Public Health, 90*: 1601–1607.

Levenstein, S. (2000) The very model of a modern etiology: A biopsychosocial view of peptic ulcer, *Psychosomatic Medicine, 62*: 176–185.

Leventhal, H., Brissette, I. & Leventhal, E.A. (2003) The common-sense model of self-regulation of health and illness, in L.D. Cameron & H. Leventhal (eds), *The Self-Regulation of Health and Illness Behaviour*. London: Routledge. pp. 42–65.

Leventhal., H., Nerenz, D.R. & Steele, D.J. (1984) Illness representations and coping with health threats, in A. Baum et al. (eds), *Handbook of Psychology and Health*. Hillsdale, NJ: Lawrence Erlbaum. pp. 219–252.

Lewin, B. (2007) Coronary heart disease: Rehabilitation, in S. Ayers et al. (eds), *Cambridge Handbook of Psychology, Health and Medicine* (2nd edition). Cambridge: Cambridge University Press. pp. 656–659.

Lewin, B. et al. (1992) Effects of self-help post myocardial infarction rehabilitation on psychological adjustment and use of health services, *Lancet, 339*: 1036–1040.

Lewis, E. & Casement, P. (1986) The inhibition of mourning by pregnancy: A case study, *Psychoanalytic Psychotherapy, 2*: 45–52.

Lewis, G. & Wesseley, S. (1992) The epidemiology of fatigue: More questions than answers, *Journal of Epidemiology and Community Health, 46*: 92–97.

Lexchin, J. (2006) Bigger and better: How Pfizer redefined erectile dysfunction, *PLoS Medicine, 3*(4): e132.

Ley, P. (1997) Recall by patients, in A. Baum et al. (eds), *Cambridge Handbook of Psychology Health & Medicine*. Cambridge: Cambridge University Press. pp. 315–317.

Leza, J.C. & Menchen, L. (2008) Editorial [Hot topic: Stress-induced deleterious consequences in the gastrointestinal tract], *Current Molecular Medicine, 8*: 244–246.

Lichtman, J.H. et al. (2008) Depression and coronary heart disease: Recommendations for screening, referral, and treatment, *Circulation, 118*: 1768–1775.

Lightener, J.M. (1980) Competition of external and internal information in an exercise setting, *Journal of Personality and Social Psychology, 39*: 165–174.

Lill, M.M. & Wilkinson, T.J. (2005) Judging a book by its cover: Descriptive survey of patients' preferences for doctors' appearance and mode of address, *British Medical Journal, 331*: 524–1527.

Lin, H.R. & Bauer-Wu, S.M. (2003) Psycho-spiritual well-being in patients with advanced cancer: An integrative review of the literature, *Journal of Advanced Nursing, 44*: 69–80.

Linkins, R.W. & Comstock, G.W. (1990) Depressed mood and development of cancer, *American Journal of Epidemiology, 132*: 962–972.

Lintz, K. et al. (2003) Prostate cancer patients' support and psychological care needs: Survey from a non-surgical oncology clinic, *Psychooncology, 12*: 769–783.

Lipp, M.R. (1986) *Respectful Treatment: A Practical Handbook of Patient-Care*. New York: Elsevier.

Little, A.C., Jones, B.C. & Burriss, R.P. (2007) Preferences for masculinity in male bodies changes across the menstrual cycle, *Hormones and Behavior, 51*: 633–639.

Lloyd, M. & Bor, R. (2004) *Communication Skills for Medicine* (2nd edition). Edinburgh: Churchill Livingstone.

Lok, I.H. & Neugebauer, R. (2007) Psychological morbidity following miscarriage, *Best Practice & Research in Clinical Obstetrics & Gynaecology*, 21: 229–247.

Lorber, W., Mazzoni, G. & Kirsch, I. (2007) Illness by suggestion: Expectancy, modeling, and gender in the production of psychosomatic symptoms, *Annals of Behavioral Medicine*, 33: 112–116.

Lorig, K.R., Ritter, P., Stewart, A.L. et al. (2001) Chronic disease self-management program: 2-year health status and health care utilization outcomes, *Medical Care*, 39: 1217–1223.

Lovallo, W.R. (2004) *Stress & Health: Biological and Psychological Interactions*. Thousand Oaks, CA: SAGE.

Lowe, C.F., Dowey, A. & Horne, P. (1998) Changing what children eat, in A. Murcott (ed.), *The Nation's Diet: The Social Science of Food Choice*. Harlow: Addison Wesley Longman. pp. 57–80.

Luebbert, K., Dahme, B. & Hasenbring, M. (2001) The effectiveness of relaxation training in reducing treatment-related symptoms and improving emotional adjustment in acute non-surgical cancer treatment: A meta-analytical review, *Psycho-Oncology*, 10: 490–502.

Luria, A.R. (1963 [1948]) *Restoration of Function after Brain Injury*. New York: Macmillan.

Lustman, P.J., Anderson, R.J., Freedland, K.E., de Groot, M., Carney, R.M. & Clouse, R.E. (2000) Depression and poor glycemic control: A meta-analytic review of the literature, *Diabetes Care*, 23: 934–942.

Lynch, J.W., Kaplan, G.A., Cohen, R.D., Tuomilehto, J. & Solonen, J.T. (1996) Do cardiovascular risk factors explain the relation between socioeconomic status, risk of all-cause mortality, cardiovascular mortality, and acute myocardial infarction?, *American Journal of Epidemiology*, 144: 934–942.

Lyons, A.C. & Willott, S.A. (2008) Alcohol consumption, gender identities and women's changing social positions, *Sex Roles*, 59: 694–712.

MacDonald, G.M., Higgins, J.P.T. & Ramchandani, P. (2006) Cognitive-behavioural interventions for children who have been sexually abused, *Cochrane Database of Systematic Reviews*, 4 (Art. CD001930).

Madey, S.F. & Gomez, R. (2003) Reduced optimism for perceived age-related medical conditions, *Basic and Applied Social Psychology*, 25: 213–219.

Magos, A.L. & Studd, J.W.W. (1988) A simple method for the diagnosis of the premenstrual syndrome by use of a self-assessment disk, *American Journal of Obstetrics and Gynecology*, 158: 1024–1028.

Mahajan, N.N. et al. (2009) Adjustment to infertility: The role of interpersonal and intrapersonal resources/vulnerabilities, *Human Reproduction*, 24: 906–912.

Mahoney, L., Ayers, S. & Seddon, P. (2010) The influence of parents and healthcare professionals on children's coping and distress during venepuncture, *Journal of Pediatric Psychology*, doi: 10.1093/jpepsy/jsq009.

Mainio, A., Hakko, H. Niemelä, A., Koivukangas, J. & Räsänen, P. (2005) Depression and functional outcome in patients with brain tumors: A population-based 1-year follow-up study, *Journal of Neurosurgery*, 103: 841–847.

Mancia, M. (ed.) (2006) *Psychoanalysis and Neuroscience*. New York: Springer.

Manne, S. (2007) Cancers of the digestive tract, in S. Ayers et al. (eds) *Cambridge Handbook of Psychology, Health and Medicine* (2nd edition). Cambridge: Cambridge University Press. pp. 581–584.

Manuck, S.B., Harvey, A., Lecheiter, S. & Neil, K. (1978) Effects of coping on blood pressure responses to threat of aversive stimulation, *Psychophysiology, 15*: 544–549.

Mapes, D.L. et al. (2004) Health-related quality of life in the Dialysis Outcomes and Practice Patterns Study (DOPPS), *American Journal of Kidney Disease, 44 (Suppl 2)*: 54–60.

Marsh, A.A. & Blair, R.J. (2008) Deficits in facial affect recognition among antisocial populations: A meta-analysis, *Neuroscience and Biobehavioral Reviews, 32*: 454–465.

Marsland, A.L., Cohen, S. & Bachen, E. (2007) Cold, common, in S. Ayers et al. (eds), *Cambridge Handbook of Psychology, Health and Medicine* (2nd edition). Cambridge: Cambridge University Press. pp. 637–638.

Marteau, T.M. & Weinman, J. (2004) Communicating about health threats and treatments, in S. Sutton et al. (eds), *The SAGE Handbook of Health Psychology*. London: SAGE. pp. 270–298.

Martinez Devesa, P., Waddell, A., Perera, R. & Theodoulou, M. (2007) Cognitive behavioural therapy for tinnitus, *Cochrane Database of Systematic Reviews, 1* (Art. CD005233).

Marucha, P.T., Kiecolt-Glaser, J.K. & Favagehi, M. (1998) Mucosal wound healing is impaired by examination stress, *Psychosomatic Medicine, 60*: 362–365.

Maslach, C. (2007) Burnout in health professionals, in S. Ayers et al. (eds) *Cambridge Handbook of Psychology, Health and Medicine* (2nd edition). Cambridge: Cambridge University Press. pp. 427–430.

Matarazzo, J. (1980) Behavioral health and behavioural medicine: Frontiers of a new health psychology, *American Psychologist, 35*: 807–817.

Mazzeo, S.E., Mitchell, K.S., Bulik, C.M., Reichborn-Kjennerud, T., Kendler, K.S. & Neale, M.C. (2009) Assessing the heritability of anorexia nervosa symptoms using a marginal maximal likelihood approach, *Psychological Medicine, 39*: 463–473.

McCaffery, J.M. et al.. (2006) Common genetic vulnerability to depressive symptoms and coronary artery disease: A review and development of candidate genes related to inflammation and serotonin, *Psychosomatic Medicine, 68*: 187–200.

McClenahan, C., Shevlin, M., Adamson, G., Bennett, C. & O'Neill, B. (2007) Testicular self-examination: A test of the health belief model and the theory of planned behaviour, *Health Education Research, 22*: 272–284.

McCrae, R.R. & Costa, P.T. (2003) *Personality in Adulthood: A Five-Factor Theory Perspective* (2nd edition). New York: Guilford.

McDonald, H.P., Garg, A.X. & Haynes, R.B. (2002) Interventions to enhance patient adherence to medication prescriptions: Scientific review, *Journal of the American Medical Association, 288*: 2868–2879.

McEwen, B.S. (1998) Protective and damaging effects of stress mediators, *New England Journal of Medicine, 338*: 171–179.

McGregor, B.A. & Antoni, M.H. (2009) Psychological intervention and health outcomes among women treated for breast cancer: A review of stress pathways and biological mediators, *Brain, Behaviour & Immunity, 23*: 159–166.

McKinstry, B. (2000) Do patients wish to be involved in decision-making in the consultation? A cross sectional survey with video vignettes, *British Medical Journal, 321*: 867–871.

McManus, F., Sacadura, C. & Clark, D.M. (2008) Why social anxiety persists: An experimental investigation of the role of safety behaviours as a maintaining factor, *Journal of Behavior Therapy & Experimental Psychiatry, 39*: 147–161.

McManus, I.C., Keeling. A. & Paice, E. (2004) Stress, burnout and doctors' attitudes to work are determined by personality and learning style: A twelve year longitudinal study of UK medical graduates, *BMC Medicine, 2*: 1–12.

McWhinney, I. (1989) The need for a transformed clinical method, in M.Stewart & D. Roter (eds), *Communicating with Medical Patients*. Newbury Park, CA: SAGE. pp.25–40.

Meechan, G., Collins, J. & Petrie, K.J. (2003) The relationship of symptoms and psychological factors to delay in seeking medical care for breast symptoms, *Preventive Medicine, 36*: 374–378.

Meissner, C.A. & Brigham, J.C. (2001) Thirty years of investigating the own-race bias in memory for faces: A meta-analytic review, *Psychology, Public Policy & Law, 7*: 3–35.

Melby, M.K., Lock, M. & Kaufert, P. (2005) Culture and symptom reporting at menopause, *Human Reproduction Update, 11*: 495–512.

Meltzoff, A.N. & Moore, M.K. (1977) Imitation of facial and manual gestures by human neonates, *Science, 198*: 75–78.

Melzack, R. (1999) From the gate to the neuromatrix, *Pain, 82 (suppl.1)*: s121–s126.

Melzack, R. & Wall, P. (1965) Pain mechanisms: A new theory, *Science, 150*: 971–979.

Mendle, J., Turkheimer, E. & Emery, R.E. (2007) Detrimental psychological outcomes associated with early pubertal timing in adolescent girls, *Developmental Review, 27*: 151–171.

Menz, R. & Al-Roubaie, A. (2008) Interruptions, status, and gender in medical interviews: The harder you brake the longer it takes, *Discourse Society, 19*: 645–666.

Mercer, C. et al. (2005) Who reports sexual function problems?, *Sexually Transmitted Infections, 81*: 394–399.

Mesmer-Magnus, J. & DeChurch, L. (2009) Information sharing and team performance: A meta-analysis, *Journal of Applied Psychology, 94*: 535–546.

Meyer, D., Levental, H. & Guttman, M. (1985) Common-sense models of illness: The example of hypertension, *Health Psychology, 4*: 115–135.

Milgram, S. (1974) *Obedience to Authority*. New York: Harper & Row.

Millar, K., Purushotham, A.D., McLatchie, E., George, W.D. & Murray, G.D. (2005) A 1-year prospective study of individual variation in distress and illness perceptions, after treatment for breast cancer, *Journal of Psychosomatic Research, 58*: 335–342.

Miller, G.A. (1956) The magic number seven, plus or minus two: Some limits on our capacity for processing information, *Psychological Review, 63*: 81–93.

Miller, G.E. & Cohen. S. (2000) Psychological interventions and the immune system: A meta-analytic review and critique, *Health Psychology, 20*: 47–63.

Miller, M., Mangano, C., Park, Y., Goel, R., Plotnick, G.D. & Vogel, R.A. (2006) Impact of cinematic viewing on endothelial function, *Heart, 92*: 261–262.

Miller, T.Q., Smith, T.W., Turner, C.W., Guijarro, M.L. & Hallet, A.J. (1996) A meta-analytic review of research on hostility and physical health, *Psychological Bulletin, 119*: 322–348.

Miller, W.C. & Zenilman, J.M. (2005) Epidemiology of chlamydial infection, gonorrhea, and trichomoniasis in the United States – 2005, *Infectious Disease Clinics of North America*, 19: 281–296.

Miller, W.R. (1995) *Motivational Enhancement Therapy with Drug Abusers*. Albuquerque, NM: University of New Mexico.

Mioshi, E., Dawson, K., Mitchell, J., Arnold, R. & Hodges, J.R. (2006) Addenbrooke's Cognitive Examination Revised (ACE-R), *International Journal of Geriatric Psychiatry*, 21: 1078–1085.

Miskovic, D. et al. (2008) Randomized controlled trial investigating the effect of music on the virtual reality laparoscopic learning performance of novice surgeons, *Surgical Endoscopy*, 22: 2416–2420.

Mitte, K. (2005) Meta-analysis of cognitive-behavioral treatments for generalized anxiety disorder: A comparison with pharmacotherapy, *Psychological Bulletin*, 131: 785–795.

Mohr, D.C. & Cox, D. (2001) Multiple sclerosis: Empirical literature for the clinical health psychologist, *Journal of Clinical Psychology*, 57: 479–499.

Molloy, G.J., Stamatakis, E., Randall, G. & Hamer, M. (2009) Marital status, gender and cardiovascular mortality: Behavioural, psychological distress and metabolic explanations, *Social Science & Medicine*, 69: 223–228.

Monahan, J.L., Murphy, S.T. & Zajonc, R.B. (2000) Subliminal mere exposure: Specific, general and diffuse effects, *Psychological Science*, 11: 462–467.

Montgomery, P. & Dennis, J. (2002) Cognitive behavioural interventions for sleep problems in adults aged 60+, *Cochrane Database of Systematic Reviews*, 2 (Art. CD003161).

Monz, B. et al. (2005) Patient-reported impact of urinary incontinence – results from treatment seeking women in 14 European countries, *Maturitas*, 52 (suppl.2): s24–s34.

Moore, P.J., Sickel, A.E., Malat, J., Williams, D., Jackson, J. & Adler, N.E. (2004) Psychosocial factors in medical and psychological treatment avoidance: The role of the doctor-patient relationship, *Journal of Health Psychology*, 9: 421–433.

Moos, R.H. & Schaefer, J.A. (1984) The crisis of physical illness: An overview and conceptual approach, in R.H. Moos (ed.), *Coping with Physical Illness: Vol 2: New Perspectives*. New York: Plenum. pp. 3–25.

Morey, M.C., Pieper, C.F., Crowley, G.M., Sullivan, R.J. & Puglisi, C.M. (2002) Exercise adherence and 10-year mortality in chronically ill older adults, *Journal of the American Geriatric Society*, 50: 2089–2091.

Morley, S. (2007) Pain management, in S. Ayers et al. (eds), *Cambridge Handbook of Psychology, Health and Medicine* (2nd edition). Cambridge: Cambridge University Press. pp. 370–374.

Morley, S., Eccleston, C. & Williams, A. (1999) Systematic review and meta-analysis of randomized controlled trials of cognitive behaviour therapy and behaviour therapy for chronic pain in adults, excluding headache, *Pain*, 80: 1–13.

Mortensen, E.L., Michaelsen, K.F., Sanders, S.A. & Reinisch, J.M. (2002) The association between duration of breastfeeding and adult intelligence, *Journal of the American Medical Association*, 287: 2365–2371.

Moseley, J.B. et al. (2002) A controlled trial of arthroscopic surgery for osteoarthritis of the knee, *New England Journal of Medicine*, 347: 81–88.

Moser, G. et al. (1993) Inflamatory bowel disease: Patients' beliefs about the etiology of their disease, *Psychosomatic Medicine, 55*: 131.

Mozurkewich, E.L., Luke, B., Avni, M. & Wolf, F.M. (2000) Working conditions and adverse pregnancy outcome: A meta-analysis, *Obstetrics and Gynecology, 95*: 623–635.

Mulligan, K. & Newman, S. (2007) Self-management interventions, in S. Ayers et al. (eds), *Cambridge Handbook of Psychology, Health and Medicine* (2nd edition). Cambridge: Cambridge University Press. pp. 393–397.

Mullington, J.M., Haack, M., Toth, M., Serrador, J.M. & Meier-Ewert, H.K. (2009) Cardiovascular, inflammatory, and metabolic consequences of sleep deprivation, *Progress in Cardiovascular Diseases, 51*: 294–302.

Murphy, C.C., Schei, B., Myhr, T.L. & Du Mont, J. (2001) Abuse: A risk factor for low birth weight? A systematic review and meta-analysis, *Canadian Medical Association Journal, 164*: 1567–1572.

Murray, E., Charles, C. & Gafni, A. (2006) Shared decision-making in primary care: Tailoring the Charles et al. model to fit the context of general practice, *Patient Education & Counseling, 62*: 205–211.

Murray, M.A., Fiset, V., Young, S. & Kryworuchko, J. (2009) Where the dying live: A systematic review of determinants of place of end-of-life cancer care, *Oncology Nursing Forum, 36*: 69–77.

Myers, L.B. & Midence, K. (1998) Concepts and issues in adherence, in L.B. Myers & K. Midence (eds), *Adherence to Treatment in Medical Conditions*. Amsterdam: Harwood. pp. 1–24.

Myunclestu (2005) *Biopsychosocialism*. Available at http://www.amazon.com/gp/product/1580461026/ref=olp_product_details/002-7908524-1290461?ie=UTF8&seller= (last accessed 6 January 2010).

Naliboff, B.D. et al. (1997) Evidence for two distinct perceptual alterations in irritable bowel syndrome, *Gut, 41*: 505–512.

National Center for Health Statistics (NCHS) (2007) *Health, United States, 2007*. Hyattsville, MD: NCHS.

National Institute for Clinical Excellence (2005) *Post-Traumatic Stress Disorder (PTSD). The Management of PTSD in Adults and Children in Primary and Secondary Care. Clinical Guideline 26*. London: NICE.

National Institute for Health and Clinical Excellence (NICE) (2006) *Urinary Incontinence: The Management of Urinary Incontinence in Women*. London: RCOG Press. Available at www.nice.org.uk/CG040.

National Institute of Allergy and Infectious Diseases (NIAID) (2006) *The Common Cold*. Avilable at http://www3.niaid.nih.gov/healthscience/healthtopics/colds/ (last accessed 18 September 2009).

Nausheen, B., Gidron, Y., Peveler, R. & Moss-Morris, R. (2009) Social support and cancer progression: A systematic review, *Journal of Psychosomatic Research, 67*: 403–415.

Navarro, X., Vivó, M. & Valero-Cabré, A. (2007) Neural plasticity after peripheral nerve injury and regeneration, *Progress in Neurobiology, 82*: 163–201.

Nelson, C.J., Lee, J.S., Gamboa, M.C. & Roth, A.J. (2008) Cognitive effects of hormone therapy in men with prostate cancer: A review, *Cancer, 115*: 1097–1106.

Nelson, J.E. (1999) Saving lives and saving deaths, *Annals of Internal Medicine, 130*: 776–777.

Nelson, L.D. & Morrison, E.L. (2005) The symptoms of resource scarcity: Judgements of food and finances influence preferences for potential partners, *Psychological Science, 16*: 167–173.

Nelson, M.D., Saykin, A.J., Flashman, L.A. & Riordan, H.J. (1998) Hippocampal volume reduction in schizophrenia as assessed by Magnetic Resonance Imaging: A meta-analytic study, *Archives of General Psychiatry, 55*: 433–440.

Newton, T.L. (2009) Cardiovascular functioning, personality, and the social world: The domain of hierarchical power, *Neuroscience and Biobehavioral Reviews, 33*: 145–159.

Nishino, S., Ripley, B., Overeem, S., Lammers, G.J. & Mignot, E. (2000) Hypocretin (orexin) deficiency in human narcolepsy, *Lancet, 355*: 39–40.

Nitti, V.W. (2001) The prevalence of urinary incontinence, *Reviews in Urology, 3(Suppl.1)*: s2–s6.

Nitzan, U. & Lichtenberg, P. (2004) Questionnaire survey on use of placebo, *British Medical Journal, 329*: 944–946.

Noble, L.M. (1998) Doctor-patient communication and adherence to treatment, in L.B. Myers & K. Midence (eds), *Adherence to Treatment in Medical Conditions*. Amsterdam: Harwood. pp. 51–82.

Nolan, K., Shope, C.B., Citrome, L. & Volavka, J. (2009) Staff and patient views of the reasons for aggressive incidents, *Psychiatric Quarterly, 80*: 167–172.

Nykamp, K., Rosenthal, L., Folkerts, M., Roehrs, T., Guido, P. & Roth, T. (1998) The effects of REM sleep deprivation on the level of sleepiness/alertness, *Sleep, 21*: 609–614.

O'Connor, T.G. et al. (2000) The effects of global severe privation on cognitive competence, *Child Development, 71*: 376–390.

O'Connor, T.G., Heron, J., Golding, J., Beveridge, M. & Glover, V. (2002) Maternal antenatal anxiety and children's behavioural/emotional problems at 4 years, *British Journal of Psychiatry, 180*: 502–508.

O'Donovan, D. (2008) *The Atlas of Health: Mapping the Challenges and Causes of Disease*. London: Earthscan.

O'Hara, M.W. & Swain, A.M. (1996) Rates and risks of postpartum depression: A meta-analysis, *International Review of Psychiatry, 8*: 37–54.

O'Leary, C.J. (2007) Psoriasis, in S. Ayers et al. (eds), *Cambridge Handbook of Psychology, Health and Medicine* (2nd edition). Cambridge: Cambridge University Press. pp. 833–835.

Oddens, B.J., den Tonkelaar, I. & Nieuwenhuyse, H. (1999) Psychosocial experiences in women facing fertility problems – a comparative survey, *Human Reproduction, 14*, 255–261.

Odegård, S., Finset, A., Mowinckel, P., Kvien, T.K. & Uhlig, T. (2007) Pain and psychological health status over a 10-year period in patients with recent onset rheumatoid arthritis, *Annals of Rheumatic Disease, 66*: 1195–1201.

Oerlemans, M.E.J., van den Akker, M., Schuurman, A.G., Kellen, E. & Buntinx, R. (2007) A meta-analysis on depression and subsequent cancer risk, *Clinical Practice and Epidemiology in Mental Health, 3*: 1–11.

Office for National Statistics (2000) *Key Health Statistics from General Practice 1998: Series MB6, no.2.* London: ONS.

Office for National Statistics (2002a) *Tobacco, Alcohol and Drug Use and Mental Health.* London: ONS.

Office for National Statistics (2002b) *Households in Receipt of Benefit: By Type of Benefit, 2001/02: Regional Trends 38.* Available at www.statistics.gov.uk/STATBASE/ssdataset. asp?vlnk=7755 (last accessed 1 August 2009).

Office for National Statistics (2008) *Birth Statistics.* Newport: ONS.

Office of the Surgeon General (2004) *The Health Consequences of Smoking.* Available at http:// www.surgeongeneral.gov/library/smokingconsequences (last accessed 29 September 2009).

Ogden, J., Reynolds, R. & Smith, A. (2006) Expanding the concept of parental control: A role for overt and covert control in children's snacking behaviour, *Appetite, 47*: 100–106.

Ogutmen, B. et al. (2006) Health-related quality of life after kidney transplantation in comparison to intermittent hemodialysis, peritoneal dialysis, and normal controls, *Transplantation Proceedings, 38*: 419–421.

Okano, H. & Sawamoto, K. (2008) Neural stem cells: Involvement in adult neurogenesis and CNS repair, *Philosophical Transactions of the Royal Society B, 363*: 2111–2122.

Ong, L.M.L., de Haes, J.C.J.M., Hoos, A.M. & Lammes, F.B. (1995) Doctor-patient communication: A review of the literature, *Social Science & Medicine, 40*: 903–918.

Osterberg, L. & Blaschke, T. (2005) Adherence to medication, *New England Journal of Medicine, 353*: 487–497.

Ott, M. et al. (2002) The trade-off between hormonal contraceptives and condoms, *Perspectives on Sexual & Reproductive Health, 34*: 6–14.

Ott, M.J., Norris, R.L. & Bauer-Wu, S.M. (2009) Mindfulness meditation for oncology patients: A discussion and critical review, *Integrative Cancer Therapies, 5*: 98–108.

Ouimet, A.J., Gawronski, B. & Dozois, D.J.A. (2009) Cognitive vulnerability to anxiety: A review and an integrative model, *Clinical Psychology Review, 29*: 459–470.

Owen, N., Spathonis, K. & Leslie, E. (2007) Physical activity and health, in S. Ayers et al. (eds), *Cambridge Handbook of Psychology, Health and Medicine* (2nd edition). Cambridge: Cambridge University Press. pp. 155–160.

Pae, C.U., Masand, P.S., Ajwani, N., Lee, C. & Patkar, A.A. (2007) Irritable bowel syndrome in psychiatric perspectives: A comprehensive review, *International Journal of Clinical Practice, 61*: 1708–1718.

Paniagua, F.A. (1999) Commentary on the possibility that Viagra may contribute to transmission of HIV and other sexual diseases among older adults, *Psychological Reports, 85*: 942–944.

Pantanetti, P., Sonino, N., Arnaldi, G. & Boscaro, M. (2002) Self image and quality of life in acromegaly, *Pituitary, 5*: 17–19.

Park, N.W. & Ingles, J.L. (2000) Effectiveness of attention training after an acquired brain injury: A meta-analysis of rehabilitation studies, *Brain and Cognition (Special Issue), 44*: 5–9.

Parry, C.H. (1825) *Collections From the Unpublished Writings of the Late C.H. Parry. Vol 2.* London: Underwoods.

Parsons, T. (1975) The sick role and the role of the physician reconsidered, *Millbank Memorial Fund Quarterly, 53*: 257–278.

Paulsen, J.S. et al. (2005) Depression and stages of Huntington's disease, *Journal of Neuropsychiatry & Clinical Neuroscience, 17*: 496–502.

Payne, S., Horn, S. & Relf, M. (1999) *Loss and Bereavement*. Buckingham: Open University Press.

Pearson, R. M., Cooper, R.M., Penton-Voak, I.S., Lightman, S.L. & Evans, J. (2009) Depressive symptoms in early pregnancy disrupt attentional processing of infant emotion, *Psychological Medicine 40*: 621–631.

Pennebaker, J. W. & Lightner, J.M. (1980) Hara, M.W. & Swain, A.M. (1996) Rates and risks of postpartum depression: A meta-analysis, *International Review Psychiatry, 8*: 37–54.

Perlman, R.L. et al. (2005) Quality of life in chronic kidney disease (CKD), *American Journal of Kidney Disease, 45*: 658–666.

Petrie, K.J. & Pennebaker, J.W. (2004) Health-related cognitions, in S.Sutton et al. (eds), *The SAGE Handbook of Health Psychology*. London: SAGE. pp. 127–142.

Petrie, K.J., Broadbent, E. & Meechan, G. (2003) Self-regulatory interventions for improving the self management of chronic illness, in L.D. Cameron & H. Leventhal (eds), *The Self-Regulation of Health and Illness Behaviour*. London: Routledge. pp. 257–277.

Petrie, K.J., Buick, D.L., Weinman, J. & Booth, R.J. (1999) Positive effects of illness reported by myocardial infarction and breast cancer patients, *Journal of Psychosomatic Research, 47*: 537–543.

Petrie, K.J., Cameron, L.D., Ellis, C.J., Buick, D. & Weinman, J. (2002) Changing illness perceptions after myocardial infarction: an early intervention randomized controlled trial, *Psychosomatic Medicine, 64*: 580–586.

Petrie, K.J., Moss-Morris, R., Grey, C. & Shaw, M. (2004) The relationship of negative affect and perceived sensitivity to symptom reporting following vaccination, *British Journal of Health Psychology, 9*: 101–111.

Petrie, K.J., Weinman, J., Sharpe, N. & Buckley, J. (1996) Role of patients' view of their illness in predicting return to work and functioning after myocardial infarction: Longitudinal study, *British Medical Journal, 312*: 1191–1194.

Petscher, E.S., Rey, C. & Bailey, J.S. (2009) A review of empirical support for differential reinforcement of alternative behaviour, *Research in Developmental Disabilities, 30*: 409–425.

Petticrew, M., Bell, R. & Hunter, D. (2002) Influence of psychological coping on survival and recurrence in people with cancer: Systematic review, *British Medical Journal, 325*: 1–10.

Phillips, A.C., Gallagher, S. & Carroll, D. (2009) Social support, social intimacy, and cardiovascular reactions to acute psychological stress, *Annals of Behavioral Medicine, 37*: 38–45.

Piaget, J. (1954) *The Construction of Reality in the Child*. New York: Basic.

Picardi, A. & Abeni, D. (2001) Stressful life events and skin diseases: Disentangling evidence from myth, *Psychotherapy and Psychosomatics, 70*: 118–136.

Picardi, A., Abeni, D., Melchi, C.F., Puddu, P. & Paquini, P. (2000) Psychiatric morbidity in dermatological outpatients: An issue to be recognized, *British Journal of Dermatology, 143*: 920–921.

Pierce, T.W., Grim, R.D. & King, J.S. (2005) Cardiovascular reactivity and family history, *Psychophysiology, 42*: 125–131.

Piliavin, I.M., Rodin, J. & Piliavin, J.A. (1969) Good Samaritanism: An underground phenomenon?, *Journal of Personality and Social Psychology, 1*: 289–299.

Pincus, T., Griffith, J., Pearce, S. & Isenberg, D. (1996) Prevalence of self-reported depression in patients with rheumatoid arthritis, *British Journal of Rheumatology, 35*: 879–883.

Pinel, J.P.J. (2007) *Biopsychology* (7th edition). Boston, MA: Pearson.

Plotsky, P.M., Owens, M.J. & Nemeroff, C.B. (1998) Psychoneuroendocrinology of depression: hypothalamic-pituitary-adrenal axis, *Psychiatric Clinics of North America, 21*: 293–307.

Ponsford, J. (2004) Rehabilitation following traumatic brain injury and cerebrovascular accident, in J. Ponsford (ed.), *Cognitive and Behavioral Rehabilitation*. New York: Guildford. pp. 299–342.

Pope, H.G. et al. (2006) Binge eating disorder: A stable syndrome, *American Journal of Psychology, 163*: 2181–2183.

Popham, F. & Mitchell, R. (2006) Leisure time exercise and personal circumstances in the working age population, *Journal of Epidemiology and Community Health, 60*: 270–274.

Porcelli, P., Leoci, C., Guerra, V., Taylor, G.J. & Bagby, R.M. (1996) A longitudinal study of alexithymia and psychological distress in inflammatory bowel disease, *Journal of Psychosomatic Research, 41*: 569–573.

Posner, M.I. & Petersen, S.E. (1990) The attention system of the human brain, *Annual Review of Neuroscience, 13*: 25–42.

Powers, M.B., Vedel, E. & Emmelkamp, P.M.G. (2008) Behavioural couples therapy (BCT) for alcohol and drug use disorders: A meta-analysis, *Clincial Psychology Review, 28*: 952–962.

Pressman, S. D. & Cohen, S. (2005) Does positive affect influence health?, *Psychological Bulletin, 131*: 925–971.

Presson, P.K. & Benassi, V.A. (1996) Locus of control orientation and depressive symptomatology: A meta-analysis, *Journal of Social Behavior & Personality, 11*: 201–212.

Price, D.D. et al. (2007) Placebo analgesia is accompanied by large reductions in pain-related brain activity in irritable bowel syndrome patients, *Pain, 127*: 63–72.

Price, J. et al. (2006) Attitudes of women with chronic pelvic pain to the gynaecological consultation, *British Journal of Obsetrics & Gynaecology, 113*: 446–452.

Price, J.R. & Couper, J. (2000) Cognitive behaviour therapy for chronic fatigue syndrome in adults, *Cochrane Database of Systematic Reviews*, Issue 1. (Art. CD001027).

Priest, R.G., Vize, C., Roberts, A., Roberts, M. & Tylee, A. (1996) Lay people's attitudes to treatment of depression: Results of opinion poll for Defeat Depression Campaign just before its launch, *British Medical Journal, 313*: 858–859.

Prigatano, G.P. (1999) *Principles of Neuropsychological Rehabilitation*. Oxford: Oxford University Press.

Prochaska, J.O. & DiClemente, C.C. (1983) Stages and processes of self-change of smoking: toward an integrative model of change, *Journal of Consulting and Clinical Psychology, 51*: 390–395.

Prochaska, J.O., Velicer, W.F., Fava, J.L., Rossi, J.S. & Tsoh, J.Y. (2001) Evaluating a population-based recruitment approach and a stage-based expert system intervention for smoking cessation, *Addictive Behaviors, 26*: 583–602.

Proudfoot, J. et al. (2004) Clinical efficacy of computerised cognitive-behavioural therapy for anxiety and depression in primary care: randomised controlled trial, *British Journal of Psychiatry, 185*: 46–54.

Proudfoot, J., Goldberg, D. P., Mann, A. et al. (2003) Computerised, interactive, multimedia cognitive behaviour therapy for anxiety and depression in general practice, *Psychological Medicine, 33*: 217–227.

Pyett, P. et al. (2005) Using hormone treatment to reduce the adult height of tall girls: Are women satisfied with the decision in later years?, *Social Science & Medicine, 61*: 1629–1639.

Rajaratnam, S.M.W. et al. (2009) Melatonin agonist tasimelteon (VEC-162) for transient insomnia after sleep-time shift: Two randomised controlled multicentre trials, *Lancet, 373*: 482–491.

Ramchand, R., Marshall, G.N., Schell, T.L. & Jaycox, L.H. (2008) Posttraumatic distress and physical functioning: A longitudinal study of injured survivors of community violence, *Journal of Consulting and Clinical Psychology, 76*: 668–676.

Ramirez, A.J. et al. (1996) Mental health of hospital consultants: The effects of stress and satisfaction at work, *Lancet, 347*: 724–728.

Ranson, K.E. & Urichuk, L.J. (2008) The effect of parent-child attachment relationships on child biopsychosocial outcomes: A review, *Early Child Development and Care, 178*: 129–152.

Rao, J.K., Anderson, L.A., Inui, T.S. & Frankel, R.M. (2007) Communication interventions make a difference in conversations between physicians and patients: a systematic review of the evidence, *Medical Care, 45*: 340–349.

Rapkin, A. (2003) A review of treatment of premenstrual syndrome & premenstrual dysphoric disorder, *Psychoneuroendocrinology, 28*: 39–53.

Raven, B.H. (1965) Social influence and power, in I.D.Steiner & M.Fishbein (eds), *Current Studies in Social Psychology*. New York: Holt, Reinhart & Winston. pp. 399–444.

Read, J., van Os, J., Morrison, A.P. & Ross, C.A. (2005) Childhood trauma, psychosis and schizophrenia: A literature review with theoretical and clinical implications, *Acta Psychiatrica Scandinavica, 112*: 330–350.

Rees, K., Bennett, P., West, R., Davey, S.G. & Ebrahim, S. (2004) Psychological interventions for coronary heart disease, *Cochrane Database of Systematic Reviews, 2* (CD002902).

Rehman, S.U., Neater, P.J., Cope, D.W. & Kilpatrick, A.O. (2005) What to wear today? Effect of doctor's attire on the trust and confidence of patients, *American Journal of Medicine, 118*: 1279–1286.

Reiche, E.M.V., Nunes, S.O.V. & Morimoto, H.K. (2004) Stress, depression, the immune system, and cancer, *Lancet Oncology, 5*: 617–625.

Reiss, S., Peterson, R.A., Gursky, D.M. & McNally, R.J. (1986) Anxiety sensitivity, anxiety frequency and the prediction of fearfulness, *Behaviour Research & Therapy, 24*: 1–8.

Rey, E. & Talley, N.J. (2009) Irritable bowel syndrome: Novel views on the epidemiology and potential risk factors, *Digestive and Liver Disease, 41*: 772–780.

Reynolds, C.F., Kupfer, D.J., Hoch, C.C., Stack, J.A., Houck, P.R. & Berman, S.R. (1986) Sleep deprivation in healthy elderly men and women: Effects on mood and on sleep during recovery, *Sleep, 9*: 492–501.

Rhudy, J.L. & Meagher, M.W. (2000) Fear and anxiety: Divergent effects on human pain thresholds, *Pain, 84*: 65–75.

Rice, F., Jones, I. & Thapar, A. (2007) The impact of gestational stress and prenatal growth on emotional problems in offspring: A review, *Acta Psychiatrica Scandinavica*, 115: 171–183.

Richardson, P. (2006) National Clinical Practice Guidelines (NICE Guidelines on Depression) – Core interventions in the management of depression in primary & secondary care, *APP Newsletter*, 34: 2–5.

Richters, J. et al. (2003a) Sexual difficulties, *Australian and New Zealand Journal of Public Health*, 27: 164–170.

Richters, J. et al. (2003b) Sexual and emotional satisfaction in regular relationships, *Australian and New Zealand Journal of Public Health*, 27: 171–179.

Ridsdale, L. et al. (2001) Chronic fatigue in general practice: Is counselling as good as cognitive behaviour therapy? A UK randomised trial, *British Journal of General Practice*, 51: 19–24.

Rissel, C.E., Richters, J., Grulich, A.E., de Visser, R.O. & Smith A.M.A. (2003) Attitudes towards sex in a representative sample of adults, *Australian & New Zealand Journal of Public Health*, 27: 118–123.

Ritz, T. & Roth, W.T. (2003) Behavioral interventions in asthma, *Behavior Modification*, 27: 710–730.

Roberts, A.R. (2005) *Crisis Intervention Handbook: Assessment, Treatment, and Research* (3rd edition). Oxford: Oxford University Press.

Robertson, I.M., Jordan, J.M. & Whitlock, F.A. (1975) Emotions and skin (II): The conditioning of scratch responses in cases of lichen simplex, *British Journal of Dermatology*, 92: 407–412.

Robine, J.M. et al. (2007) Who will care for the oldest people in our ageing society?, *British Medical Journal*, 334: 570–571.

Rogers, C. (1951) *Client-centered Therapy: Its Current Practice, Implications and Theory*. London: Constable.

Roig, E., Castaner, A., Simmons, B., Patel, R., Ford, E. & Cooper, R. (1987) In-hospital mortality rates from acute myocardial infarction by race in US hospitals: Findings from the National Hospital Discharge Survey, *Circulation*, 76: 280–288.

Ropacki, S.A. & Jeste, D.V. (2005) Epidemiology of and risk factors for psychosis of Alzheimer's Disease, *American Journal of Psychiatry*, 162: 2022–2030.

Rosen, M.I., Ryan, C. & Rigsby, M. (2002) Motivational enhancement and MEMS review to improve medication adherence, *Behaviour Change*, 19: 183–190.

Rosenblatt, A. & Leroi, I. (2000) Neuropsychiatry of Huntington's Disease and other basal ganglia disorders, *Psychosomatics*, 41: 24–30.

Rosenstock, I.M. (1974) Historical origins of the Health Belief Model, *Health Education Monographs*, 2: 1–8.

Ross, L. (1977) The intuitive psychologist and his shortcomings, in L. Berkowitz (ed.), *Advances in Experimental Social Psychology, Vol.10*, Orlando, FL: Academic. pp. 173–240.

Ross L.E. & McLean, L.M. (2006) Anxiety disorders during pregnancy and the postpartum period: A systematic review, *Journal of Clinical Psychiatry*, 67: 1285–98.

Roter, D.L. & Hall, J.A. (2004) Physician gender and patient-centered communication: A critical review of empirical research, *Annual Review of Public Health*, 25: 497–519.

Roter, D.L., Hall, J.A. & Katz, N.R. (1988) Patient-physician communication: A descriptive summary of the literature, *Patient Education & Counseling*, 12: 99–119.

Roth, A. & Fonagy, P. (2004) *What Works for Whom? A Critical Review of Psychotherapy Research* (2nd edition). New York: Guilford.

Rothman, A.J. & Salovey, P. (1997) Shaping perceptions to motivate healthy behavior: The role of message framing, *Psychological Bulletin, 121*: 3–19.

Rowles, S.V., Prieto, L., Badia, X., Shalet, S.M., Webb, S.M. & Trainer, P.J. (2005) Quality of Life (QOL) in patients with acromegaly is severely impaired, *Journal of Clinical Endocrinology & Metabolism, 90*: 3337–3341.

Rozin, P., Haidt, J. & McCauley, C.R. (2000) Disgust, in M. Lewis & J.M. Haviland Jones (eds), *Handbook of Emotions* (2nd edtion). New York: Guilford. pp. 637–652.

Rudberg, L., Nilsson, S., Wikblad, K. & Carlsson, M. (2005) Testicular cancer and testicular self-examination: Knowledge and attitudes of adolescent Swedish men, *Cancer Nursing, 28*: 256–262.

Rusted, J. (2007) Dementias, in S. Ayers et al. (eds), *Cambridge Handbook of Psychology, Health and Medicine* (2nd edition). Cambridge: Cambridge University Press. pp. 667–670.

Rutishauser, C., Esslinger, A., Bond, L. & Sennhauser, F.H. (2003) Consultations with adolescents: The gap between their expectations and their experiences, *Acta Pædiatrica, 92*: 1322–1326.

Ryback, R.S. & Lewis, O.F. (1971) Effects of prolonged bed rest on EEG sleep patterns in young, healthy volunteers, *Electroencephalography & Clinical Neurophysiology, 31*: 395–399.

Sabini, J. & Silver, M. (2005) Ekman's basic emotions: Why not love and jealousy?, *Cognition & Emotion, 19*: 693–712.

Sackett, D.L., Rosenberg, W.M.C., Gray, J.A.M., Haynes, R.B. & Richardson, W.S. (1996) Evidence based medicine: What it is and what it isn't, *British Medical Journal, 312*: 71–72.

Salkovskis, P. M., Hackmann, A., Wells, A., Gelder, M.G. & Clark, D.M. (2006) Belief disconfirmation versus habituation processes to situational exposure in panic disorder with agoraphobia: A pilot study, *Behaviour Research and Therapy, 45*: 877–885.

Sandberg, S. et al. (2000) The role of acute and chronic stress in asthma attacks in children, *Lancet, 356*: 982–987.

Sanders, S. & Reinisch, J. (1999) Would you say you 'had sex' if ... ?, *Journal of the American Medical Association, 281*: 275–277.

Santos, J., Alonso, C., Vicario, M., Ramos, L., Lobo, B. & Malagelada, J.R. (2008) Neuropharmacology of stress-induced mucosal inflammation: Implications for inflammatory bowel disease and irritable bowel syndrome, *Current Molecular Medicine, 8*: 258–273.

Saracci, R. (1997) The World Health Organisation needs to reconsider its definition of health, *British Medical Journal, 314*: 1409.

Sarafino, E.P. (2002) *Health Psychology: Biopsychosocial Interactions* (5th edition). New Jersey: Wiley.

Saunders, K.A. & Hawton, K. (2001) Suicidal behaviour and the menstrual cycle, *Psychological Medicine, 36*: 901–912.

Savage, L.J. (1954) *The Foundations of Statistics*. New York: Wiley.

Sawyer, A., Ayers, S. & Field, A. (2010) Posttraumatic growth and adjustment among individuals with cancer or HIV/AIDS: A meta-analysis, *Clinical Psychology Review, 30* (4): 436–447.

Sayette, M.A. (2007) Alcohol abuse, in S. Ayers et al. (eds) *Cambridge Handbook of Psychology, Health and Medicine* (2nd edition). Cambridge: Cambridge University Press. pp. 534–537.

Sayin, A., Mutluay. R. & Sindel, S. (2007) Quality of life in hemodialysis, peritoneal dialysis, and transplantation patients, *Transplantation Proceedings*, 39: 3047–3053.

Scharloo, M., Kaptein, A.A., Weinman, J., Hazes, J.M., Breedveld, F.C. & Rooijmans, H.G.M. (1999) Predicting functional status in patients with rheumatoid arthritis, *Journal of Rheumatology*, 26: 1686–1693.

Schedlowski, M. & Tewes, U. (1992) Physiological arousal and perception of bodily state during parachute jumping, *Psychophysiology*, 29: 95–103.

Scheier, M.F., Carver, C.S. & Bridges, M.W. (1994) Distinguishing optimism from neuroticism (and trait anxiety, self-mastery, and self-esteem): A re-evaluation of the Life Orientation Test, *Journal of Personality and Social Psychology*, 67: 1063–1078.

Schneider, M.L., Moore, C.F., Roberts, A.D. & Dejesus, O. (2001) Prenatal stress alters early neurobehavior, stress reactivity and learning in non-human primates: A brief review, *Stress*, 4: 183–193.

Schout, B.M.A., Hendrikx, A.J.M., Scheele, F., Bemelmans, B.M.H. & Scherpbier, A.J.J.A. (2010) Validation and implementation of surgical simulators: A critical review of present, past, and future, *Surgery & Endoscopy*, 24: 536–546.

Schouten, B.C. & Meeuwesen, L. (2006) Cultural differences in medical communication: A review of the literature, *Patient Education and Counselling*, 64: 21–34.

Schwartz, G. (1982) Testing the biopsychosocial model: The ultimate challenge facing behavioural medicine?, *Journal of Consulting and Clinical Psychology*, 50: 1040–1053.

Schwarz, J.K. (2004) Responding to persistent requests for assistance in dying: a phenomenological inquiry, *International Journal of Palliative Nursing*, 10: 225–235.

Seale, C. (1998) *Constructing Death: The Sociology of Dying and Bereavement*. Cambridge: Cambridge University Press.

Sechrest, L. & Wallace, J. (1964) Figure drawings and naturally occurring events: Elimination of the expansive euphoria hypothesis, *Journal of Educational Psychology*, 55: 42–44.

Segal, Z.V., Williams, J.M.G. & Teasdale, J.D. (2002) *Mindfulness-Based Cognitive Therapy for Depression: A New Approach for Preventing Relapse*. New York: Guilford.

Segerstrom, S.C., Taylor, S.E., Kemeny, M.E. & Fahey, J.L. (1998) Optimism is associated with mood, coping, and immune change in response to stress, *Journal of Personality and Social Psychology*, 74: 1646–1655.

Segerstrom, S.C. (2005) Optimism and immunity: Do positive thoughts always lead to positive effects?, *Brain, Behavior, and Immunity*, 19: 195–200.

Segerstrom, S.C. & Miller, G.E. (2004) Psychological stress and the human immune system: A meta-analytic study of 30 years of inquiry, *Psychological Bulletin*, 130: 601–630.

Seibt, B., Häfner, M. & Deutsch, R. (2007) Prepared to eat: How immediate affective and motivational responses to food cues are influenced by food deprivation, *European Journal of Social Psychology*, 37: 359–379.

Seligman, M.E.P. (1975) *Helplessness: On Depression, Development, and Death*. San Francisco, CA: W.H. Freeman.

Selye, H. (1956) *The Stress of Life*. New York: McGraw-Hill.

Shack, L. et al. (2008) Variation in incidence of breast, lung and cervical cancer and malignant melanoma of the skin by socioeconomic group in England, *BMC Cancer*, 8: 1–10.

Shapiro, D.E., Boggs, S.R, Melamed, B.G. & Graham-Pole, J. (1992) The effect of varied physician affect on recall, anxiety, and perceptions in women at risk for breast cancer: An analogue study, *Health Psychology, 11*, 61–66.

Sharpley, C.F., Halat, J., Rabinowicz, T., Weiland, B. & Stafford, J. (2001) Standard posture, postural mirroring, and client-perceived rapport, *Counselling Psychology Quarterly, 14*: 267–280.

Sheeran, P. et al. (1999) Psychosocial correlates of condom use, *Psychological Bulletin, 125*: 90–132.

Sheps, D.S. et al. (2002) Mental stress-induced ischemia and all-cause mortality in patients with coronary artery disease: Results from the psychophysiological investigations of myocardial ischemia study, *Circulation, 105*: 1780–1784.

Shields, C.G. et al. (2009) Patient-centered communication and prognosis discussions with cancer patients, *Patient Education and Counseling, 77*: 437–442.

Silverman, D.H.S., Munakata, J.A., Ennes, H., Mandelkern, M.A., Hoh, C.K. & Mayer, E.A. (1997) Regional cerebral activity in normal and pathological perception of visceral pain, *Gastroenterology, 112*: 64–72.

Simoni, J.M., Pearson, C.R., Pantalone, D.W., Marks, G. & Crepaz, N. (2006) Efficacy of interventions in improving highly active antiretroviral therapy adherence and HIV-1 RNA viral load: A meta-analytic review of randomized controlled trials, *Journal of Acquired Immune Deficiency Syndromes, 43*: s23–s35.

Singh, S., Graff, L.A. & Bernstein, C.N. (2009) Do NSAIDs, antibiotics, infections, or stress trigger flares in IBD?, *American Journal of Gastroenterology, 104*: 1298–1313.

Sirois, F. (1992) Denial in coronary heart disease, *Canadian Medical Association Journal, 147*: 315–321.

Skinner, B.F. (1957) *Verbal Behaviour*. Acton, MA: Copley.

Slachter, R.B. & Pennebaker, J.W. (2007) Emotional expression and health, in S. Ayers et al. (eds), *Cambridge Handbook of Psychology, Health and Medicine* (2nd edition). Cambridge: Cambridge University Press. pp. 84–87.

Sloboda, J.A., Davidson, J.W. & Howe, M.J.A. (1994) Is everyone musical?, *The Psychologist, 7*: 349–354.

Smedslund, G., Dalsb, T.K., Steiro, A.K., Winsvold, A. & Clench-Aas, J. (2007) Cognitive behavioural therapy for men who physically abuse their female partner, *Cochrane Database of Systematic Reviews, 3* (Art. CD006048).

Smith, J. (2007) From base evidence through to evidence base: A consideration of the NICE guidelines, *Psychoanalytic Psychotherapy, 21*: 40–60.

Smith, T.P., Kennedy, S.L. & Fleshner, M. (2004) Influence of age and physical activity on the primary in vivo antibody and T cell–mediated responses in men, *Journal of Applied Physiology, 97*: 491–498.

Smith, T.W. & MacKenzie, J. (2006) Personality and risk of physical illness, *Annual Review of Clinical Psychology, 2*: 435–467.

Soo, C. & Tate, R. (2007) Psychological treatment for anxiety in people with traumatic brain injury, *Cochrane Database of Systematic Reviews, 3* (Art. CD005239).

Speigel, D. & Giese-Davis, J. (2003) Depression and cancer: mechanisms and disease progression, *Biological Psychiatry, 54*: 269–282.

Spiegel, B., Schoenfeld, P. & Naliboff, B. (2007) Systematic review: The prevalence of suicidal behaviour in patients with chronic abdominal pain and irritable bowel syndrome, *Alimentary Pharmacology & Therapeutics, 26*: 183–193.

Spiegel, D., Bloom, J.R., Kraemer, H.C. & Gottheil, E. (1989) Effect of psychosocial treatment on survival of patients with metastatic breast cancer, *Lancet, 334*: 888–891.

Squier, R.W. (1990) A model of empathic understanding and adherence to treatment regimens in practitioner-patient relationships, *Social Science & Medicine, 30*: 325–339.

Stabler, B. et al. (1996) Links between growth hormone deficiency, adaptation and social phobia, *Hormone Research, 45*: 30–33.

Stahl, S.M. (2000) *Essential Psychopharmacology of Depression and Bipolar Disorder.* Cambridge: Cambridge University Press.

Stangier, U. (2007) Skin disorders, in S. Ayers et al. (eds) *Cambridge Handbook of Psychology, Health and Medicine* (2nd edition). Cambridge: Cambridge University Press. pp. 880–883.

Stangier, U. & Ehlers, A. (2000) Stress and anxiety in dermatological disorders, in D.I. Mostofsky & D.H. Barlow (eds), *The Management of Stress and Anxiety in Medical Disorders.* Needham Heights, MA: Allyn & Bacon. pp. 304–333.

Stapleton, A.B., Lating, J., Kirkhart, M. & Everly, G.S. (2006) Effects of medical crisis intervention on anxiety, depression, and posttraumatic stress symptoms: A meta-analysis, *Psychiatric Quarterly, 77*: 231–238.

Stead, L.F., Bergson, G. & Lancaster, T. (2008) Physician advice for smoking cessation (review), *Cochrane Library*, issue 1. (Art. CD000165).

Steadman, L. & Quine, L. (2004) Encouraging young males to perform testicular self-examination: A simple, but effective, implementation intentions intervention, *British Journal of Health Psychology, 9*: 479–487.

Steinberg, L. & Silverberg, S. (1986) The vicissitudes of autonomy in early adolescence, *Child Development, 57*: 841–851.

Steptoe, A. (2006) *Depression and Physical Illness.* Oxford: Oxford University Press.

Steptoe, A. & Ayers, S. (2005) Stress, health and illness, in S.Sutton et al. (eds), *SAGE Handbook of Health Psychology.* London: SAGE. pp. 169–196.

Steptoe, A. & Brydon, L. (2009) Emotional triggering of cardiac events, *Neuroscience and Biobehavioral Reviews, 33*: 63–70.

Steptoe, A. & Vogele, C. (1986) Are stress responses influenced by cognitive appraisal? An experimental comparison of coping strategies, *British Journal of Psychology, 77*: 243–255.

Stevens, L. & Rodin, I. (2001) *Psychiatry.* Edinburgh: Churchill Livingstone.

Stevenson, F.A., Barry, C.A., Britten, N., Barber, N. & Bradley, C.P. (2000) Doctor-patient communication about drugs: The evidence for shared decision making, *Social Science & Medicine, 50*: 829–840.

Stewart, M.A. et al. (1997) *The Impact of Patient-Centred Care on Patient Outcomes in Family Practice.* London, ON: University of Western Ontario.

Stice, E. & Shaw, H. (2007) Eating disorders, in S. Ayers et al. (eds), *Cambridge Handbook of Psychology, Health and Medicine* (2nd edition). Cambridge: Cambridge University Press. pp. 690–693.

Stice, E., Shaw, H. & Marti, C.N. (2008) A meta-analytic review of eating disorder prevention programs, *Annual Review of Clinical Psychology, 3*: 207–231.

Stickgold, R., Hobson, J.A., Fosse, R. & Fosse, M. (2001) Sleep, learning, and dreams: Off-line memory reprocessing, *Science, 294*: 1052–1057.

Stiles, W.B., Barkam, M., Twigg, E., Mellor-Clark, J. & Cooper, M. (2006) Effectiveness of cognitive-behavioural, person-centred and psychodynamic therapies as practised in the UK National Health Service settings, *Psychological Medicine, 36*: 555–566.

Stockhorst, U. et al. (1998) Effects of overshadowing on conditioned nausea in cancer patients: An experimental study, *Physiology & Behaviour, 64*: 743–753.

Stockhorst, U., Steingrueber, H.J., Enck, P. & Klosterhalfen, S. (2006) Pavlovian conditioning of nausea and vomiting, *Autonomic Neuroscience: Basic & Clinical, 129*: 50–57.

Stone, A.A., Neale, J.M., Cox, D.S., Napoli, A., Valdimarsdottir, H. & Kennedy-Moore, E. (1994) Daily events are associated with a secretory immune response to an oral antigen in men, *Health Psychology, 13*: 440–446.

Stone, N. & Ingham, R. (2003) When and why do young people in the United Kingdom first use sexual health services?, *Perspectives on Sexual & Reproductive Health, 35*: 114–120.

Stone, S.V. & McCrae, R.R. (2007) Personality and health, in S. Ayers et al. (eds), *Cambridge Handbook of Psychology, Health and Medicine* (2nd edition). Cambridge: Cambridge University Press. pp. 151–155.

Stones, W., Cheong, Y.C. & Howard, F.M. (2005) Interventions for treating chronic pelvic pain in women, *Cochrane Database of Systematic Reviews, 2* (Art. CD000387).

Straus, S.E., Richardson, W.S., Glasziou, P. & Haynes, R.B. (2005) *Evidence-Based Medicine: How to Practice and Teach EBM*. London: Elsevier.

Strecher, V.J., Chapion, V.L. & Rosenstock, I.M. (1997) The Health Belief Model and health behaviour, in D.S. Gochman (ed.), *Handbook of Health Behavior Research I: Personal and Social Determinants*. New York, NY: Plenum Press. pp.71–91.

Street, R.L., Makoul, G., Arora, N.K. & Epstein, R.M. (2009) How does communication heal? Pathways linking clinician–patient communication to health outcomes, *Patient Education & Counseling, 74*: 295–301.

Striegel-Moore, R.H. & Franko, D.L. (2008) Should binge eating disorder be included in the DSM-V? A critical review of the state of the evidence, *Annual Review of Clinical Psychology, 4*: 305–324.

Stroebe, M., Schut, H. & Stroebe, W. (2007) Coping with bereavement, in S. Ayers et al. (eds), *Cambridge Handbook of Psychology, Health and Medicine* (2nd edition). Cambridge: Cambridge University Press. pp. 41–46.

Sturm, L.A., Mays, R.M. & Zimet, G.D. (2005) Parental beliefs and decision making about child and adolescent immunization: from polio to sexually transmitted infections, *Journal of Developmental & Behavioral Pediatrics, 26*: 441–452.

Subramanian, S.W., Elwert, F. & Christakis, N. (2008) Widowhood and mortality among the elderly: The modifying role of neighborhood concentration of widowed individuals, *Social Science & Medicine, 66*: 873–884.

Sullivan, P.F., Neale, M.C. & Kendler, K.S. (2000) Genetic epidemiology of major depression: Review and meta-analysis, *American Journal of Psychiatry, 157*: 1552–1562.

Sullivan, P.F., Kendler, K. & Neale, M. (2003) Schizophrenia as a complex trait: Evidence from a meta-analysis of twin studies, *Archives of General Psychiatry, 60*: 1187–1192.

Suls, J., Martin, R. & Wheeler, L. (2002) Social comparison: Why, with whom and with what effect?, *Current Directions in Psychological Science, 11*: 159–163.

Surtees, P.G., Wainwright, N.W.J., Luben, R.N., Wareham, N.J., Bingham, S.A. & Khaw, K.T. (2008) Depression and ischemic heart disease mortality: Evidence from the EPIC-Norfolk United Kingdom prospective cohort study, *American Journal of Psychiatry, 165*: 515–523.

Sutton, S. (2007) Transtheoretical model of behaviour change, in S. Ayers et al. (eds), *Cambridge Handbook of Psychology, Health and Medicine* (2nd edition). Cambridge: Cambridge University Press. pp. 228–232.

Swami, V. & Tovee, M.J. (2006) Does hunger influence judgements of female physical attractiveness?, *British Journal of Psychology, 97*: 353–363.

Tajfel, H. & Turner, J. (1986) An integrative theory of intergroup conflict, in S. Worchel & W. Austin (eds), *Psychology of Intergroup Relations*. Chicago: Nelson-Hall. pp. 2–24.

Talge, N.M., Neal, C. & Glover, V. (2007) Antenatal maternal stress and long-term effects on child neurodevelopment: How and why?, *Journal of Child Psychology and Psychiatry, 48*: 245–261.

Tallis, R.C. (1996) Burying Freud, *The Lancet, 347*: 669–671.

Taylor, C.B., Miller, N.H., Smith, P.M. & DeBusk, R.F. (1997) The effect of a home-based, case-managed, multifactorial risk-reduction program on reducing psychological distress in patients with cardiovascular disease, *Journal of Cardiopulmonary Rehabilitation, 17*: 157–162.

Taylor, R.S. et al. (2004) Exercise-based rehabilitation for patients with coronary heart disease: Systematic review and meta-analysis of randomized controlled trials, *American Journal of Medicine, 116*: 682–692.

Taylor, S.E. (2007) Social support, in H.S. Friedman and R.C. Silver (eds), *Foundations of Health Psychology*. New York: Oxford University Press. pp. 145–171.

Taylor, S.E., Cousino Klein, L., Lewis, B.P., Gruenewald, T.L., Gurung, R.A.R. & Updegraff, J.A. (2000) Biobehavioral responses to stress in females: Tend-and-befriend, not fight-or-flight, *Psychological Review, 107*: 411–429.

Taylor, S.E., Welch, W.T., Kim, H.S. & Sherman, D.K. (2007) Cultural differences in the impact of social support on psychological and biological stress responses, *Psychological Science, 18*: 831–837.

Tedstone, J.E. & Tarrier, N. (2003) Posttraumatic stress disorder following medical illness and treatment, *Clinical Psychology Review, 23*: 409–448.

Teri, L. et al. (1999) Anxiety of Alzheimer's disease: Prevalence, and comorbidity, *Journals of Gerontology Series A, 54*: 348–352.

Teutsch, C. (2003) Patient-doctor communication, *Medical Clinics of North America, 87*: 1115–1145.

The, A.M., Hak, T., Koeter, G. & van der Wal, G. (2000) Collusion in doctor-patient communication about imminent death: An ethnographic study, *British Medical Journal, 321*: 1376–1381.

Thiblin, I. & Petersson, A. (2004) Pharmacoepidemiology of anabolic androgenic steroids: A review, *Fundamental & Clinical Pharmacology, 19*: 27–44.

Thomas, J.J. & Brownell, J.D. (2007) Obesity, in S.Ayers et al. (eds), *Cambridge Handbook of Psychology, Health and Medicine* (2nd edition). Cambridge: Cambridge University Press. pp. 797–800.

Thomas, P.W., Thomas, S., Hillier, C., Galvin, K. & Baker, R. (2006) Psychological interventions for multiple sclerosis, *Cochrane Database of Systematic Reviews*, Issue 1 (Art.: CD004431).

Thorburn, A.W. (2005) Prevalence of obesity in Australia, *Obesity Review*, 6: 187–189.

Tian, J., Chen, Z.C. & Hang, L.F. (2009) Effects of nutritional and psychological status of the patients with advanced stomach cancer on physical performance status, *Support Care Cancer*, 17: 1263–1268.

Timmons, B.H. & Ley, R. (1994) *Behavioral and Psychological Approaches to Breathing Disorders*. New York: Plenum.

Tomlinson, J. (ed.) (2004) *ABC of Sexual Health* (2nd edition). London: Wiley.

Towle, A., Godolphin, W. & van Staalduinen, S. (2006) Enhancing the relationship and improving communication between adolescents and their health care providers: A school based intervention by medical students, *Patient Education & Counseling*, 62: 189–192.

Treasure, J. & Maissi, E. (2007) Motivational interviewing, in S. Ayers et al. (eds), *Cambridge Handbook of Psychology, Health and Medicine* (2nd edition). Cambridge: Cambridge University Press. pp. 363–366.

Treiber, F.A., Kamarck, T., Schneiderman, N., Sheffield, D., Kapuku, G. & Taylor, T. (2003) Cardiovascular reactivity and development of preclinical and clinical disease states, *Psychosomatic Medicine*, 65: 46–62.

Trenholm, C. et al. (2008) Impacts of abstinence education on teen sexual activity, risk of pregnancy, and risk of sexually transmitted diseases, *Journal of Policy Analysis and Management*, 27: 255–276.

Trojian, T.H., Mody, K. & Chain, P. (2007) Exercise and colon cancer: Primary and secondary prevention, *Current Sports Medicine Reports*, 6: 120–124.

Trufelli, D.C. et al. (2008) Burnout in cancer professionals: A systematic review and meta-analysis, *European Journal of Cancer Care*, 17: 524–531.

Trzepacz, P.T. & Baker, R.W. (1993) *The Psychiatric Mental Status Examination*. Oxford: Oxford University Press.

Tsai, Y.-C. et al. (in press) Quality of life predicts risks of end-stage renal disease and mortality in patients with chronic kidney disease, *Nephrology Dialysis Transplantation*.

Tsakanikos, E. (2006) Perceptual biases and positive schizotypy: The role of perceptual load, *Personality and Individual Differences*, 41: 951–958.

Tsugane, S. (2005) Salt, salted food intake, and risk of gastric cancer: Epidemiological evidence, *Cancer Science*, 96: 1–6.

Tucker, L.A. & Bates, L. (2009) Restrained eating and risk of gaining weight and body fat in middle-aged women: A 3-year prospective study, *American Journal of Health Promotion*, 23: 187–194.

Turk Charles, S., Gatz, M., Kato, K. & Pedersen, N.L. (2008) Physical health 25 years later: The predictive ability of neuroticism, *Health Psychology*, 27: 369–378.

Turton, P., Hughes, P., Evans, C.D.H. & Fainman, D. (2001) Incidence, correlates, and predictors of post-traumatic stress disorder in the pregnancy after stillbirth, *British Journal of Psychiatry*, 178: 556–560.

Tversky, A. & Kahneman, D. (1974) Judgment under uncertainty: Heuristics and biases, *Science*, 185: 1124–1130.

UK ECT Review Group (2003) Efficacy and safety of electroconvulsive therapy in depressive disorders: a systemic review and meta-analysis, *Lancet*, 361: 799–808.

UNAIDS/WHO (2009) *AIDS Epidemic Update*. Geneva: UNAIDS.

Ünal, B., Critchley, J.A., Fidan, D. & Capewell, S. (2005) Life-years gained from modern cardiological treatments and population risk factor changes in England and Wales, 1981–2000, *American Journal of Public Health*, 95: 103–108.

UNICEF Innocenti Research Centre (2001) *A League Table of Teenage Births in Rich Nations*. Florence: UNICEF.

Ussher, J.M., Hunter, M. & Cariss, M. (2002) A woman-centred psychological intervention for premenstrual symptoms, drawing on cognitive-behavioural and narrative therapy, *Clinical Psychology and Psychotherapy*, 9: 319–331.

Ussher, M. (2007) Physical activity interventions, in S. Ayers et al. (eds), *Cambridge Handbook of Psychology, Health and Medicine* (2nd edition). Cambridge: Cambridge University Press. pp. 375–379.

Valentiner, D.P., Holahan, C.J. & Moos, R.H. (1994) Social support, appraisals of event controllability, and coping: An integrative model, *Journal of Personality and Social Psychology*, 66: 1094–1102.

van der Bruggen, C.O., Stams, G.J., Bogels, S.M. (2008) Research review: The relation between child and parent anxiety and parental control, *Journal of Child Psychology and Psychiatry, and Allied Disciplines*, 49: 1257–1269.

van der Klink, J.J.L., Blonk, R.W.B., Schene, A.H. & van Dijk, F.J.H. (2001) The benefits of interventions for work-related stress, *American Journal of Public Health*, 91: 270–276.

van Dixhoorn, J. & White, A. (2005) Relaxation therapy for rehabilitation and prevention in ischaemic heart disease: A systematic review and meta-analysis, *European Journal of Cardiovascular Prevention and Rehabilitation*, 12: 193–202.

van Ijzendoorn, M.H. & Kroonenberg, P.M. (1988) Cross-cultural patterns of attachment: A meta-analysis of the Strange Situation, *Child Development*, 59: 147–156.

van Londen, W.M., Juffer, F. & van Izendoorn, M.H. (2007) Attachment, cognitive and motor development in adopted children: Short-term outcomes after international adoption, *Journal of Pediatric Psychology*, 32: 1259–1263.

Van Oudenhove, L. & Aziz, Q. (2009) Recent insights on central processing and psychological processes in functional gastrointestinal disorders, *Digestive and Liver Disease*, 41: 781–787.

Venn, A. et al. (2004) The use of oestrogen to reduce the adult height of tall girls: Long term effects on fertility, *Lancet*, 364: 1513–1518.

Vertes, R.P. & Eastman, K.E. (2000) The case against memory consolidation in REM sleep, *Behavioral and Brain Sciences*, 23: 867–876.

Villanacci, V. et al. (2008) Enteric nervous system abnormalities in inflammatory bowel diseases, *Neurogastroenterol Motility*, 20: 1009–1016.

Vogel, T., Brechat, P.H., Leprêtre, P.M., Kaltenbach, G., Berthel, M. & Lonsdorfer, J. (2009) Health benefits of physical activity in older patients: A review, *International Journal of Clinical Practice*, 63: 203–320.

Vos, M.S. & de Haes, J.C.J.M. (2007) Denial in cancer patients: An explorative review, *Psycho-Oncology*, 16: 12–25.

Voth, J. & Sirois, F.M. (2009) The role of self-blame and responsibility in adjustment to inflammatory bowel disease, *Rehabilitation Psychology*, 54: 99–108.

Vuilleumier, P. (2005) How brains beware: Neural mechanisms of emotional attention, *Trends in Cognitive Sciences, 9*: 585–594.

Vuilleumier, P. & Huang, Y.M. (2009) Emotional attention: Uncovering the mechanisms of affective biases in perception, *Current Directions in Psychological Science, 18*: 148–152.

Walker, J. (2001) *Control and the Psychology of Health*. Buckingham: Open University Press.

Wallston, K.A. (2007) Perceived control, in S. Ayers et al. (eds), *Cambridge Handbook of Psychology, Health and Medicine* (2nd edition). Cambridge: Cambridge University Press. pp.148–150.

Wallston, K.A., Wallson, B.S. & DeVellis, R. (1978) Development of the multidimensional health locus of control (MHLC) scales, *Health Education Monographs, 6*: 160–170.

Walsh, J.C., Lynch, M., Murphy, A.W. & Daly, K. (2004) Factors influencing the decision to seek treatment for symptoms of acute myocardial infarction: An evaluation of the Self-Regulatory Model of illness behaviour, *Journal of Psychosomatic Research, 56*: 67–73.

Wampold, B.E., Minami, T., Tierney, S.C., Baskin, T.W. & Bhati, D.S. (2005) The placebo is powerful: Estimating placebo effects in medicine and psychotherapy from randomised clinical trials, *Journal of Clinical Psychology, 61*: 835–854.

Wardle, J., Griffith, J., Johnson, F. & Rapoport, L. (2000) Intentional weight control and food choice habits in a national representative sample of adults in the UK, *International Journal of Obesity, 24*: 534–540.

Wardle, J., Steptoe, A., Burckhardt, R., Vögele, C., Vila, J. & Zarczynski, Z. (1994) Testicular self-examination: Attitudes and practices among young men in Europe, *Preventive Medicicne, 23*: 206–210.

Wardle, J., Steptoe, A., Oliver, G. & Lipsey, Z. (2000) Stress, dietary restraint and food intake, *Journal of Psychosomatic Research, 48*: 195–202.

Watson, D. & Tellegen, A. (1985) Toward a consensual structure of mood, *Psychological Bulletin, 98*: 219–223.

Watson, P.W.B. & McKinstry, B. (2009) A systematic review of interventions to improve recall of medical advice in healthcare consultations, *Journal of the Royal Society of Medicine, 102*: 235–243.

Webb, E., Ashton, C.H., Kelly, P. & Kamali, F. (1996) Alcohol and drug use in university students, *Lancet, 348*: 922–925.

Wegner, D.M. (2003) The mind's best trick: How we experience conscious will, *TRENDS in Cognitive Science, 7*: 65–69.

Weinman, J., Ebrecht, M., Scott, S., Walburn, J. & Dyson, M. (2008) Enhanced wound healing after emotional disclosure intervention, *British Journal of Health Psychology, 13*: 95–102.

Weinstein, N.D. (1987) Unrealistic optimism about susceptibility to health problems: Conclusions from a community-wide sample, *Journal of Behavioral Medicine, 10*: 481–500.

Weiser, E.B. (2007) The prevalence of anxiety disorders among adults with asthma: A meta-analytic review, *Journal of Clinical Psychology in Medical Settings, 14*: 297–307.

Weisz, G. & Knaapen, L. (2009) Diagnosing and treating premenstrual syndrome in five western nations, *Social Science & Medicine, 68*: 1498–1505.

Weiten, W. (2004) *Psychology Themes and Variations* (6th edition). Belmont, CA: Wadsworth/ Thomson Learning.

Welch, J.L. & Thomas-Hawkins, C. (2005) Psycho-educational strategies to promote fluid adherence in adult hemodialysis patients: A review of intervention studies, *International Journal of Nursing Studies*, 42: 597–608.

Wells, A. (1997) *Cognitive Therapy of Anxiety Disorders: A Practice Manual and Conceptual Guide.* New York: Wiley.

West, R. (2006) *Theory of Addiction.* Oxford: Blackwell.

West, R. & Hardy, A. (2007) Tobacco use, in S. Ayers et al. (eds), *Cambridge Handbook of Health Psychology* (2nd edition). Cambridge: Cambridge University Press. pp. 908–912.

Wettergren, L., Kettis-Lindblad, A., Sprangers, M. & Ring, L. (2009) The use, feasibility and psychometric properties of an individualised quality-of-life instrument: A systematic review of the SEIQoL-DW, *Quality of Life Research*, 18: 737–746.

White, J., Levinson, W. & Roter, D. (1994) "Oh by the way" – the closing moments of the medical interview, *Journal of General Internal Medicine*, 9: 24–28.

Whitten, C.E., Donovan, M. & Cristobal, K. (2005) Treating chronic pain: New knowledge, more choices, *The Permanente Journal*, 9: 9–18.

Wiklund, I., Edman, G. & Andolf, E. (2007) Cesarean section on maternal request: Reasons for the request, self-estimated health, expectations, experience of birth and signs of depression among first-time mothers, *Acta Obstetricia et Gynecologica Scandinavica*, 86: 451–456.

Wilbert-Lampen, U. et al. (2008) Cardiovascular events during World Cup soccer, *New England Journal of Medicine*, 358: 475–483.

Wilfley, D.E., Wilson, G.T. & Agras, W.S. (2003) The clinical significance of binge eating disorder, *International Journal of Eating Disorders*, 34 (suppl.1): s96–s106.

Wilhelmsen, I. (2000) Brain-gut axis as an example of the bio-psycho-social model, *Gut, 47 (Suppl.IV)*: iv5–iv7.

Williams, J.M. & Binnie, L.M. (2002) Children's concepts of illness: An intervention to improve knowledge, *British Journal of Health Psychology*, 7: 129–147.

Williams, S., Weinman, J. & Dale, J. (1998) Doctor-patient communication and patient satisfaction: A review, *Family Practice*, 15: 480–492.

Wills, T.A. & Ainette, M.G. (2007) Social support and health, in S. Ayers et al. (eds), *Cambridge Handbook of Psychology, Health and Medicine* (2nd edition). Cambridge: Cambridge University Press. pp. 202–207.

Wilson, B.A. (2007) Neuropsychological rehabilitation, in S. Ayers et al. (eds), *Cambridge Handbook of Psychology, Health and Medicine* (2nd edition). Cambridge: Cambridge University Press. pp. 367–369.

Winstanley, S. (2005) Cognitive model of patient aggression towards health care staff: The patient's perspective, *Work & Stress*, 19: 340–350.

Winterich, J.A. et al. (2009) Masculinity and the body: How African American and white men experience cancer screening exams involving the rectum, *American Journal of Men's Health*, 3: 300–309.

Witte, K. & Allen, M. (2000) A meta-analysis of fear appeals: Implications for effective public health campaigns, *Health Education & Behavior*, 27: 591–615.

Wolf, F.M., Guevera, J.P., Grum, C.M., Clark, N.M. & Cates, C.J. (2003) Educational interventions for asthma in children, *Cochrane Library,* issue 2 (Art. CD000326).

Wolitzky-Taylor, K.B., Horowitz, J.D., Powers, M.B. & Telch, M.J. (2008) Psychological approaches in the treatment of specific phobias: A meta-analysis, *Clinical Psychology Review,* 28: 1021–1037.

Women's Health Initiative (2009) *Postmenopausal Hormone Therapy Trials.* Available at http://www.nhlbi.nih.gov/whi/index.html. (last accessed 21 July 2009).

Wong, J.G., Clare, I.C.H., Gunn, M.J. & Holland, A.J. (1999) Capacity to make health care decisions: Its importance in clinical practice, *Psychological Medicine,* 29: 437–446.

Worden, J.W. (1991) *Grief Counselling and Grief Therapy: A Handbook for the Mental Health Practitioner* (2nd edtion). New York: Springer.

World Association for Sexual Health (2007) *Definitions Accepted by the WAS General Assembly, 17 April 2007, Sydney Australia.* Available at http://www.worldsexology.org/doc/definitions-of-specialties.pdf

World Health Organisation (1992) *Basic Documents* (39th edition). Geneva: WHO.

World Health Organisation (1996) *Diagnostic and Management Guidelines for Mental Disorders in Primary Care. ICD-10 Chapter V Primary Care Version.* Geneva: WHO.

World Health Organisation (2002) *Global Strategy on Infant and Young Child Feeding.* Geneva: WHO.

World Health Organisation (2004) *International Statistical Classification of Diseases and Health Related Problems (The) ICD-10* (2nd edition). Geneva: WHO.

World Health Organisation (2005) *Gender, Health & Alcohol Use.* Geneva: WHO.

World Health Organisation (2008) *The Top Ten Causes of Death: Fact Sheet Number 310.* Geneva: WHO.

World Health Organisation (2009) *Mortality Database.* Available at http://apps.who.int/whosis/database/mort/table1.cfm (last accessed 30 July 2009).

Wright, D.B. & Loftus, E.F. (2008) Eyewitness memory, in G. Cohen & M. Conway (eds), *Memory in the Real World* (3rd edtion). New York: Psychology. pp. 91–105.

Wright, R.J. et al. (2004) Community violence and asthma morbidity, *American Journal of Public Health,* 94: 625–632.

Wyatt, K., Dimmock, P., Jones, P., Obhrai, M. & O'Brien, S. (2001) Efficacy of progesterone and progestogens in management of premenstrual syndrome: Systematic review, *British Medical Journal,* 323: 776–780.

Xi, J. & Zhang, S.-C. (2008) Stem cells in development of therapeutics for Parkinson's disease: A perspective, *Journal of Cellular Biochemistry,* 105: 1153–1160.

Yabroff, K.R. & Mandelblatt, J.S. (1999) Interventions targeted towards patients to increase mammography use, *Cancer Epidemiology Biomarkers and Prevention,* 8: 749–775.

Yamamoto, T., Nakahigashi, M. & Saniabadi, A.R. (2009) Diet and inflammatory bowel disease – epidemiology and treatment, *Alimentary Pharmacology & Therapeutics,* 30: 99–112.

Yarzebski, J., Goldberg, R.J., Gore, J.M. & Alpert, J.S. (1994) Termporal trends and factors associated with extent of delay to hospital arrival in patients with acute myocardial infarction, *American Heart Journal,* 128: 255–263.

Yedidia, M.J. et al. (2003) Effect of communications training on medical student performance, *Journal of the American Medical Association, 290*: 1157–1165.

Yorke, J., Fleming, S.L. & Shuldham, C.M. (2004) Psychological interventions for adults with asthma, *Cochrane Database of Systematic Reviews, 1* (Art. CD002982).

Yoshida, F. & Hori, H. (1989) Personal space as a function of eye-contact and spatial arrangements of a group, *Japanese Journal of Psychology, 60*: 53–56.

Young, J.E., Klosko, J.S. & Weishaar, M.E. (2004) Cognitive therapy of borderline personality disorder, *Bipolar Disorders, 5*: 14–21.

Young, K.D. (2005) Pediatric procedural pain, *Annals of Emergency Medicine, 45*: 160–171.

Young, Q.R., et al. (2007) Brief screen to identify 5 of the most common forms of psychosocial distress in cardiac patients: Validation of the screening tool for psychological distress (STOP-D), *Journal of Cardiovascular Nursing, 22*: 525–534.

Zellner, D.A., Garriga-Trillo, A., Centeno, S. & Wadsworth, E. (2004) Chocolate craving and the menstrual cycle, *Appetite, 42*: 119–121.

Zhang, Q.-L. & Rothenbacher, D. (2008) Prevalence of chronic kidney disease in population-based studies: Systematic review, *BMC Public Health, 8*: 117.

Zillmer, E.A., Spiers, M.V. & Culbertson, W.C. (2008) *Principles of Neuropsychology* (2nd edition). Belmont, CA: Wadsworth.

Zondervan, K.T. et al. (2001) The community prevalence of chronic pelvic pain in women and associated illness behaviour, *British Journal of General Practice, 51*: 541–547.

Zorrilla, E.P. et al. (2001) The relationship of depression and stressors to immunological assays: A meta-analytic review, *Brain, Behavior, and Immunity, 15*: 199–226.

Zvolensky, M.J. & Eifert, G.H. (2001) A review of psychological factors/processes affecting anxious responding during voluntary hyperventilation and inhalations of carbon dioxide-enriched air, *Clinical Psychology Review, 21*: 375–400.

Zweifel, J.E. & O'Brien, W.H. (1997) A meta-analysis of the effect of hormone replacement therapy upon depressed mood, *Psychoneuroendocrinology, 22*: 189–212.

Zweyer, K., Velker, B. & Willibald, R. (2004) Do cheerfulness, exhilaration, and humor production moderate pain tolerance?, *Humor: International Journal of Humor Research, 17*: 85–119.

INDEX

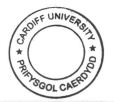